OXFORD MEDICAL PUBLICATIONS

Practising health for all

Practising health for all

Edited by

DAVID MORLEY

JON E. ROHDE

GLEN WILLIAMS

OXFORD NEW YORK TORONTO
OXFORD UNIVERSITY PRESS

Oxford University Press, Walton Street, Oxford OX2 6DP

Oxford New York Toronto
Delhi Bombay Calcutta Madras Karachi
Kuala Lumpur Singapore Hong Kong Tokyo
Nairobi Dar es Salaam Cape Town
Melbourne Auckland

and associated companies in
Beirut Berlin Ibadan Nicosia

Oxford is a trade mark of Oxford University Press

First published 1983
Reprinted 1984, 1986

British Library Cataloguing in Publication Data
Practising health for all. – (Oxford medical publications)
1. Medical care
I. Morley, David   II. Rohde, Jon E.
III. Williams, Glen
362.1   RA 393
ISBN 0-19-261445-2

Library of Congress Cataloging in Publication Data
Main entry under title:
Practising health for all.
(Oxford medical publications)
Includes bibliographies and index.
1. Underdeveloped areas – Community health services
– Case studies. 2. Community health services – Case
studies. I. Morley, David. II. Rohde, Jon E.
III. Williams, Glen. IV. Series
RA441.5.P73 1983   362.1'09172'4   83-12099
ISBN 0-19-261445-2 (pbk.)

Printed in Great Britain by
M & A Thomson Litho Ltd.
East Kilbride

This book is dedicated to the World Health Organization and the United Nations Children's Fund. These two international agencies, working together with national governments, voluntary agencies, and community organizations throughout the world, have shown that Health for All need not be an impossible dream.

Foreword

by **David Morley**

Over the past 30 years the international community has come to understand that hospitals, large and small, do not provide the sort of health care which most people need. As a result, governments and voluntary organizations have attempted to introduce new systems of 'primary health care', emphasizing disease prevention rather than cure and community participation rather than over-dependence on medical personnel for health services. The Alma Ata Declaration of 1978, proclaiming primary health care as the way to achieving 'Health for All by the Year 2000', gave fresh impetus to this new approach.

Yet primary health care programmes are not moving into a total void. On the contrary, they have to find a way through a maze of political, socioeconomic, organizational, and technical problems. *Practising Health for All* presents a wide range of case studies depicting typical problems that arise in the implementation of primary health care — and how these can be overcome. We are not offering a 'cook book' on how to run a primary health care programme. This would be an impossible task, given the widely varying situations of individual countries and regions throughout the world. But there are important lessons and principles to be drawn from the successful programmes analysed in this book, and perhaps even more important ones from the failures.

Any book involving 21 different contributors scattered around the world demands patience, sensitivity, and unique editorial skills. These have been provided by Glen Williams, who has worked on this book over the past three years. Thanks to his contacts through OXFAM, New Internationalist Publications, and his own travels and wide correspondence, he has identified many interesting health programmes about which little or nothing has so far been published. He has also shouldered much of the responsibility for obtaining illustrations linked to key points in the book.

Collecting the material, editing, and typing articles has involved considerable expense, and we are heavily indebted to Misereor for funding this work so generously. We are also very grateful to OXFAM and the Swedish International Development Authority for financial assistance in the later stages of production. This support has allowed us, in co-operation with the Oxford University Press, to offer *Practising Health for All* as a low-cost book.

Preface

The gap between the health of people in the affluent nations — the 'North' — and those in the so-called developing nations — the 'South' — is vast. In the South, death claims 6–25 of every 100 births within the first year of life, one in every four children suffers from malnutrition, and life expectancy is 30 per cent lower than in the North.

These discrepancies, and the reasons for their existence, are glaringly obvious. Most people in the North, and the elite of the South, enjoy all the determinants of good health: adequate income, nutrition, education, sanitation, safe drinking water, and comprehensive health care. Governments in the North can afford to spend large amounts on health services. Public expenditure on health in the North now averages US $320 per capita compared with US $11 in the South. Even the small amounts available for health in the South are maldistributed through health structures heavily biased in favour of curative services for the urban elite. In most developing countries only 10–20 per cent of the population enjoys ready access to health services of any kind; technologies and problems are mismatched; low coverage programmes and costly solutions are devised for health problems which are uncommon; and western models are followed in medical education, the allocation of financial and human resources, the design and construction of facilities, the choice of pharmaceuticals and the orientation of research. In short, throughout most of the South, the prevailing tendency has been to favour high cost, low coverage, low impact, elite-oriented health services.

Yet this is not the whole picture. During the past 30 years a number of effective health programmes reaching the poorest people in rural areas have been developed by governments and voluntary agencies in countries as diverse as Cuba, Indonesia, China, India, Nigeria, Bangladesh, and Guatemala. Ten years ago WHO and UNICEF carried out a joint study to identify the key factors in the success of these and some other successful health programmes. Two WHO publications present the most interesting of these experiences and the lessons that can be drawn from them — Djukanovic and Mach's *Alternative approaches to meeting health needs in developing countries* (1975) and Newell's *Health by the people* (1975).

In 1978, at the joint WHO-UNICEF Conference in Alma Ata, the governments of 134 countries and many voluntary agencies endorsed the concept of primary health care (PHC) as the way to 'Health for All by the Year 2000'. PHC was defined as 'essential health care made universally accessible to individuals and families in the community by means acceptable to them, through their full participation and at a cost that the community and country can afford'. The Declaration of Alma Ata declared that PHC should include:

1. Education about prevailing health problems and methods of preventing and controlling them.
2. Promotion of food supply and proper nutrition.
3. An adequate supply of safe water and basic sanitation.
4. Maternal and child health, including family planning.
5. Immunization against infectious diseases.
6. Prevention and control of endemic diseases.
7. Appropriate treatment of common diseases and injuries.
8. Provision of essential drugs.

We endorse the concept of PHC and contend that there is no valid technical reason to question 'Health for All by the Year 2000' as a feasible goal. But are there solid grounds for hoping that the world could be 'on the threshold of a new era', as Newell, almost a decade ago, suggested in *Health by the people*? In an attempt to shed some light on this question, *Practising Health for All* analyses PHC programmes in 17 developing countries.

Our contributors do not analyse in detail the technologies available for the control of specific health problems. We are convinced that effective and affordable health technologies do exist for dealing with the major health problems of. the South. The main obstacles to the implementation of these technologies, however, are not technical but political and organizational. The chapters of our book are. therefore interwoven by the themes of political commitment and community participation in the organization of PHC. We contend that future developments in these two fields will determine whether 'Health for All by the Year 2000' proves to be a realistic objective or a utopian dream.

Our book is divided into four parts:

Part I. Political commitment to PHC: accounts of success and failure revealing some of the tangled links between political structures and the people's health.

Part II. Community participation: programmes ranging from a city in Indonesia to a rural area of the Dominican Republic. These experiences demonstrate that community participation means not just the mobilization of resources, but a process by which people gain more control over the factors affecting their health.

Part III. The process of programme development: detailed accounts of the interaction between health planners, political decision-makers, and community organizations, resulting in innovative national programmes in three countries.

Part IV. Practising health for all: lessons from previous experience and principles of success and failure in planning, implementing, and evaluating primary health care.

The 19 chapters of our book include a number of 'success stories' and also several accounts of programmes that fell far short of their original goals. We are convinced that these experiences of PHC demonstrate that high levels of health are achievable even with modest levels of income — provided that strong political commitment to equitable development exists; and that people in low-income communities can take responsibility for improving their health — provided they are encouraged to make decisions and trained appropriately. When properly informed, involved, and supported, people working together in communities of various types and sizes can bring about healthier and happier lives for themselves and their children. That is what this book is about.

London, Port-au-Prince, Oxford   D.M.
                                                                              J.E.R.
February 1983   G.W.

Acknowledgements

Numerous illustrations emphasize key points throughout this book. The editors are greatly indebted to Kanchan Dasgupta, David Kyungu, Jan Martin, Derek Matthews, Clive Offley, Gillian Oliver, and David Werner for contributing their artistic and graphic skills to *Practising Health for All*.

Contents

Part I

Political commitment

INTRODUCTION

The example of the Chinese 'barefoot doctor' has attracted widespread acclaim and inspired many imitators throughout the world. Yet China's great achievements in public health are not due primarily to this well-publicised paramedical worker. The crucial element in China's health revolution is total political commitment at all levels of government and society to health as an integral part of social equity. Health is everyone's right and everyone's responsibility. The 'barefoot doctor' is simply the most visible symbol of this approach, not its sole instrument. Yet today, while China is regarded as a model for other developing countries' health systems, the Chinese themselves are stressing greater modernization and professionalization of health services. These trends, if continued, could undermine the very principles of China's successful public health system.

Cuba's political commitment to 'Health for All' is clear and unequivocal. Since the revolution in 1959 the Cuban state has established a highly disciplined social order based on equity and social justice. Levels of public health have risen dramatically and are now the highest in the Caribbean and Latin American region. Yet whether the Cuban health system could − or should − be adopted by other developing countries is questionable. David Werner argues that Cuba's heavy reliance on doctor-centred medicine is too costly and tends to make the health system into a form of social control rather than one of collective and individual liberation.

India, with a more pluralistic political system than China and Cuba, has a long-standing official commitment to social equity. Yet India has so far failed to establish a viable PHC system serving the needs of the poor majority of its vast population. A combination of non-health factors − including political turbulence, the vested interests of the medical profession and drug manufacturers, inequitable social structures, and uneven economic development − has bedeviled successive efforts to put PHC on a firm footing at national level.

The government of Tanzania is well known for its commitment to social justice and equitable development. Yet a close examination of Tanzania's health and development policies gives a rather different picture: heavy urban bias in government expenditure; inadequate administrative decentralization; and a strong emphasis on curative, hospital-centred care. In Tanzania, as in many other countries, the gap between the rhetoric of 'Health for All' and the reality of 'health for some' is glaringly obvious.

The Indian State of Kerala has demonstrated that, in a democratic system with a strong political commitment to equitable socioeconomic development, high levels of health can be achieved even on modest levels of income. Widespread people's participation in political processes in Kerala has resulted in more equitable distribution of land, income, and public services − including health and education − than elsewhere in India. Although Kerala is one of the poorest States in the country, its people are better educated, healthier, live longer, enjoy higher average incomes, are more secure in their jobs and have fewer children

than the population of any other Indian State. The Kerala experience demonstrates that the basic causes of ill-health and malnutrition are socioeconomic and
political. If 'Health for All' is to be more than a mere slogan, structural changes
based on equity considerations are essential in many countries.

1 Health for all in China: principles and relevance for other countries

Jon Rohde identifies and analyses the elements widely held responsible for the success of primary health care in China, and assesses the possible relevance of the Chinese health system to other countries.

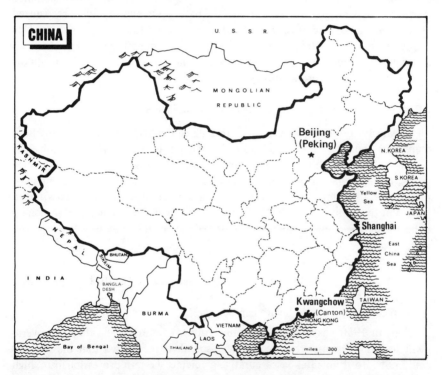

Jon Rohde, M.D., is currently Head of the Management Sciences for Health team working with the Department of Health in Haiti. He is also a consultant to WHO, UNICEF, and the World Bank in national programming in nutrition, primary health care, mass communications, training, and logistics.

The opening of China to international visitors over the past decade has produced a vast literature documenting the impressive improvements in health and well-being of the Chinese population. Accounts cover a wide field, including in-depth studies of particular topics such as schistosomiasis and nutrition, as well as descriptions of medical education, health economics, public health, acupuncture, and the use of traditional Chinese medicines. Whilst most reports are anecdotal, they are unanimous in their finding that 'health for all' — at least in a very basic sense — is being provided to the citizens of China today. Widespread acclaim for the Chinese health system also played a large part in motivating the World Health Organization to promote primary health care with the slogan 'Health for All by the Year 2000'.

Yet health services in China continue to evolve rapidly, and do not necessarily represent a consistent strategy or approach. As in other sectors of Chinese national development, there has been an ebb and flow of policies supporting alternative and sometimes contrasting activities affecting health. The current emphasis on modernization characterizing the Chinese social and political milieu is seen by many observers as a reversal of the basic principles so widely recognized as accounting for the success of health services for the Chinese masses. One highly relevant but still unanswered question is whether village level workers can be professionalized and yet retain their accountability to — and close rapport with — their fellow peasant workers.

HEALTH CAMPAIGNS AND BAREFOOT DOCTORS

The greatest attention has been given to date to the 'barefoot doctor', of whom there were about two million in 1980. Yet, while it is important to recognize the responsibilities, capabilities, and characteristics of this health worker, it also should be remembered that the barefoot doctor did not arrive on the scene until the mid-1960s, after almost two decades of important preparatory activities in the realm of public health. In 1950, just after Liberation, the national principles of health care were enunciated, with four main areas of emphasis:

- service to the people;
- disease-prevention;
- integration of traditional and modern systems of health, both preventive and curative;
- mass movements, or health campaigns.

China in 1950 was an extremely unhealthy environment, and the new government had few material resources at its disposal. It recognized that the country could not afford hospital-based curative medicine, western professionalism, high technology, or a health programme delivered to society by a centrally paid cadre of professionals and para-professional workers. The decision to approach the major health problems through mass movements was thus an early beginning to the demystification of health by a series of massive, continuous, saturation health campaigns. Public awareness of health issues was increased through extensive participation — often forced, at least in the early stages — in disease-preventive programmes. Eventually, widespread acceptance of the responsibility of the individual for critical elements of his own and the community's health led to the control of major public health problems.

The success of the mass campaigns of the 1950s and 1960s accounts for the major improvements in health in China since Liberation. These campaigns emanated from the very highest political levels but were considered an integral part of a person's participation in the sociopolitical life of the community. Conceived and supported by Mao Zedong, the campaigns owed much of their success to Zhou Enlai's skill in managing the Communist Party apparatus. Significantly, medical doctors were neither extensively involved in nor critical to the success of the campaigns. Auxiliary workers were recruited and trained for specific vertical programmes in vaccination against smallpox, elimination of venereal disease, control of schistosomiasis and malaria, and broad vaccination campaigns. Environmental improvement began with the elimination of pests: flies, mosquitoes, rats, and bed bugs, and with the installation and maintenance of sanitary facilities. The control and productive use of human wastes was also an integral part of health improvement. Specific programmes with clearly defined targets, well articulated and widely promoted by slogans, radio, public announcements, bill boards, and the particular brand of Chinese patriotic play brought total involvement of the population and major improvements in health care.

By the late 1960s the mass public health campaigns had largely reached fruition. The work of professional medical personnel, however, remained focused mainly on urban areas, where only 20 per cent of the population lived. At this point Mao, as part of the Cultural Revolution, launched a massive onslaught on the privileged position of the medical establishment, demanding a radical reallocation of health resources to the rural population. At least one-third of China's health professionals were ordered to the rural areas. For ten or more years, through permanent or periodic service, they remained in the villages, working in mobile medical teams providing health services to the rural population. Several top academic and public health officials have described to the author their own experiences in these early years of rural health. The mobile teams recognized that they could not handle the vast burden of ill-health in the rural areas, nor could they hope to return to urban institutions unless an alternative rural health service could be developed. It was at this point that the decision to recruit and train village-level health workers – barefoot doctors – was taken. Thus, to some extent, the commitment of health professionals to training barefoot doctors was aimed at freeing themselves from direct involvement in providing health care in rural areas. They thus were able to return to urban institutions and assume what they felt to be a more important long-term development and advisory role as teachers, supervisors, and specialists managing referred cases of illness.

A subtle but important shift in the nature of rural health services in China occurred simultaneously with this massive exodus of urban-trained, curative-oriented workers to the rural areas. Barefoot doctors were multipurpose health workers, in contrast to the previously trained auxiliaries and medical assistants, who generally were specialists in a narrow or particular field of health care.

Continued responsibility and attention were given to preventive activities such as environmental improvement, vaccination, and family planning. But the training and responsibilities of barefoot doctors shifted their emphasis to the diagnosis and treatment of illness. Indeed, most observers have identified an increasing tendency over the past decade for these health workers to confine their attention and activities to curative work. This may be appropriate, in view of the wide success of preventive programmes which no longer demand as complete attention from health personnel as previously. Owing to the genuine integration of these activities into the life-styles in modern China, vaccination coverage remains high, family planning is widely accepted and effective, and environmental cleanliness is generally good. Yet the high rate of cigarette smoking, increasing prevalence of obesity, crowded housing conditions, difficulty in managing the disposal of human waste in the cities, and public habits of expectoration are all examples of public-health problems yet to be tackled.

BAREFOOT DOCTORS TODAY

Selection and training

Barefoot doctors are chosen by their communities and are paid — as are other peasants and workers — on the basis of work points entitling them to a share in the production of their commune. Their responsibility is entirely to the community which selects and maintains them. Thus there is not the divided responsibility which so often characterizes health systems where workers are government employees and often more interested in satisfying the political demands of their superiors than the needs of the community. Initial training of barefoot doctors has been almost entirely pragmatic, short, and carried out close to the workplace (usually in the commune health centre). On the other hand, there has also been a noticeable lack of standardization of training or of norms, guidelines, and standards of treatment. Although the English-speaking world has been impressed by the *Barefoot Doctor Manual*, there is little evidence that it is in wide use in China. A critical revision of this encyclopedic work would be both timely and useful.

Recent trends indicate a tendency towards more specialized, institutional training, stressing curative medical care with the greatest accent on theory provided through a series of lectures. In addition, objective tests of theoretical knowledge are now being enforced much more rigorously. Previously the failure of trainees to pass tests was taken either as an indication that teachers needed to improve their teaching methods or as a justification for trainees to repeat part of their course. Now, however, failure in tests can result in trainees being excluded completely from their course.

Continuing education

By far the greatest emphasis on training amongst the barefoot doctors is the role of continuing education. This is done both through weekly visits to work in the local health centre and supervisory visits by health-centre staff to the brigade posts at which the barefoot doctors work. These supervisory activities, though undoubtedly providing continuing motivation and improving particular skills, do not follow any standard criteria or procedures. The lack of a unified reporting system, of supervision by measurable criteria and of specific, detailed information feedback systems makes technical supervision difficult. Refresher courses lasting from one to six months, however, are increasingly frequent. In addition, advanced training from six months to two years leading to a medical assistant degree is provided to many barefoot doctors. Preference for entry into medical school for qualified barefoot doctors is attracting many into this professional advancement. While career opportunities of this type are attractive, it is not clear what effect this trend will have on the general status of either the barefoot doctor *vis-à-vis* the community or the commitment of the individual health worker to the basic principle of 'serving the people'.

Communication services

Observation of the materials dispensed by the average barefoot doctor, his training and work shows that in the vast majority of cases, he is presented with symptomatic minor ailments which he can treat competently. In the face of serious disease, however, he functions as a 'connector', bringing the individual rapidly into contact with the appropriate levels of a well-developed health care delivery system capable of handling the problem. There are excellent communications by telephone and usually by vehicle from the health post to the commune health centre and from there to the county hospital and provincial tertiary facilities. Without this extensive, well-staffed and equipped support system of health services, it seems highly unlikely that the barefoot doctor could alleviate many serious or life-threatening diseases. This comes as no surprise, but should be emphasized to avoid the apparently frequent assumption that significant improvements in life expectancy and reduction in mortalities in China are due mainly to interventions by the barefoot doctor. The entire health-care system is essential. The barefoot doctor is indeed a critical *link* in a system which provides total health care to the whole population starting at the commune or neighbourhood hospital or health centre, which typically may contain 20 beds and 15-20 personnel, laboratory, X-ray equipment, operating room, pharmacy, and other basic facilities. The county hospital, of 100-300 beds, contains specialists of all basic medical services and an array of modern curative medical equipment. The barefoot doctor thus is no short-cut to providing technically adequate, well-supported health services. He rather functions more as a communicator and connector, facilitating early and appropriate use of this health system.

Accountability

Self-accountability — the extensive use of criticism and public dialogue aimed at improving performance and acceptability of services — ensures the continued evolution of the health service system. The people thus have a voice in decisions about what health services are most appropriate for their needs.

The organization of this vast nation into cooperative units also allows communities to allocate labour to health work, paying for it from the general pool of community revenues. This is not a form of insurance, but rather a form of shared work in which an entire population accepts a division of labour and the diversification of tasks with a centralization of payment and compensation.

THE PRIMARY HEALTH CARE SYSTEM

Decentralization

While policy is centrally directed and programme strategies often are planned and, to some extent, funded by the centre, the development of health services has been decentralized both in planning and administration. This has led to a high degree of flexibility, local control, and self-reliance on the part of the community being served. Participation in health services in China means financial autonomy and responsibility at the family, production team, brigade, and commune level.

The only exceptions appear to be the provision of free medical care for government officials and students and a form of medical insurance of industrial workers and their families. The vast majority of the population, particularly in rural areas, receives primary health care which is totally funded by the people

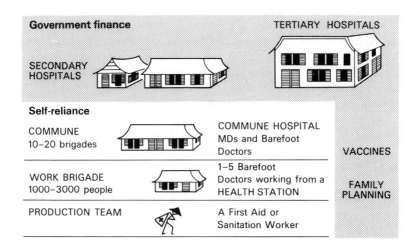

Fig. 1.1. Paying for health care in China.

themselves, with the exception of vaccines and family planning supplies. The effectiveness, credibility, and viability of such a system, however, would not have been possible without the prior implementation of a nationwide network of county hospitals, well-staffed, and funded by the government at that level (200 000–400 000 population). These were further backed up by tertiary institutions in the provinces and major cities, often associated with medical schools and training programmes for health workers, who in turn staff the commune health centres and train first-line health workers from the factories and the fields.

Traditional medicine

The pragmatic integration of traditional and modern medicine has provided China with numerous advantages. It enabled the immediate acceptance of the vast manpower resource of traditional practitioners (15–20 times as many as allopathic medical doctors) into the health services. This in turn substantially reduced the cost of medical care, even if attention to quality of care and outcome was neither documented nor perhaps even considered important. The extensive use of locally produced herbal medicines reduced demands for modern and expensive chemical drugs. In time, this integrated system effectively sorted out clinical conditions amenable to this low-cost therapy as well as responding to the sociological, psychological, and cultural demands of the population. There can be no question that in countries relying exclusively on modern allopathic medicine vast expenditures for manpower, medical procedures, and medications are made with little scientific justification or evidence of efficacy. The integration of traditional and modern medicine in China brought not only scientific benefits, but also – and perhaps more importantly – an affordable system to meet the felt needs of all. There is, however, a need for standardization of a national formulary along the lines of the World Health Organization's list of essential drugs, and the determination of the levels at which each can be used.

Monitoring and evaluation

The lack of standard information systems throughout China makes it difficult not only for valid international comparisons but also for a critical continuing monitoring of the health situation. While most communities are aware of vital events (births, deaths, etc.) and can articulate trends, little data on overall morbidity or cause-specific mortality is available. While nutritional status generally is regarded as good, such important basic health-promotive measures such as monitoring child growth through weighing are not being done. Thus it is difficult, even within the system, to carry out critical objective monitoring based on measurable health indicators. The monitoring of political attitudes such as service to the community and adherence to the goals of mass campaigns long has been deemed more important than the development of technical indicators of success.

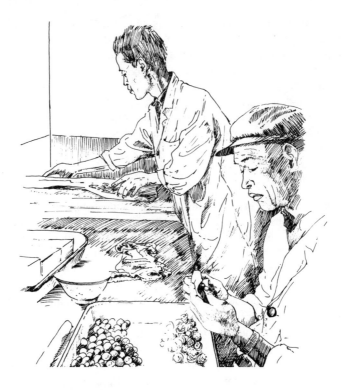

Fig. 1.2. Use of locally produced herbal medicines has reduced the demand for expensive chemical drugs in China.

Recent developments

Recent pronouncements by health authorities of plans to retrain health workers – including two million barefoot doctors – appear to reflect official concern to improve abilities in diagnosis and treatment of disease, including the use of a wider range of medications. In general, a process of greater professionalization and medicalization of the health system is under way. This process includes greater emphasis on improved 'quality' of doctor education, with a return to the seven-year medical curriculum. There are also plans to build research centres and massive modern hospitals in the cities, to train more specialists, and to develop more technologically sophisticated interventions. The increasingly wide availability of western drugs is also a cause for concern, as it seems certain to cause unrecognized iatrogenic illness. Ironically, while the rest of the developing world studies and attempts to emulate China's success in primary health care, China now appears to be trying to copy industrialized countries by placing greater emphasis on health advances of a purely technical nature.

WIDER RELEVANCE

In assessing the possible relevance of the Chinese health system for other countries, the following basic principles underlying the Chinese system should be considered:

- Politics and the health system are inextricably linked.
- Health is an integral part of national development.
- Self-reliance fostered by total participation of the community in the health system is essential.
- Health workers are selected, maintained, and controlled by their own community.
- Universal access to all levels of health care services is assured.
- The use of traditional medicine, including acupuncture and herbal drugs, has made the health system more affordable and acceptable to the Chinese people.

Considering each basic principle in turn:

Politics and the health system

From the highest political levels through to revolutionary committees and production brigades, China's health care system is deeply embedded in political institutions and processes which emphasize self-reliance and the equitable distribution of resources. Supervision of health care personnel at all levels is primarily political and assures that health services correspond to the needs of the people, rather than being controlled by an elite of health professionals.

Few other developing countries have shown a degree of political commitment to *equitable* socioeconomic development comparable to that of post-Liberation China. In many countries the medical profession, dominated mainly by male doctors, maintains its grip on health care oriented towards the needs of the middle-class, urban-dwelling minority. Despite rhetorical commitment to ideals of equity and social justice, many Third World governments have failed to build political institutions and administrative structures capable of ensuring a fair distribution of health services and other resources throughout their populations.

Health and other sectors of national development

China has succeeded in integrating health services with other sectors of national life such as education, housing, sanitation, food production and distribution, communications, employment, and industry. Health is viewed not only as a universal right, but, even more importantly, as a prerequisite to increased production and economic development. Control of births would not have been possible had it not been made part of the political, social, and economic milieu, leading to the achievement of overall national goals. The extent to which today's health standards in China can be attributed to health services alone is unclear. Improvements in food availability, work environments, education, and the status of women have proceeded rapidly and contributed greatly to improving the health of the Chinese people during the past two decades.

Although virtually all countries pay lip-service to the ideal of integrating health services with other sectors of national development, this ideal is usually honoured in the breach rather than the observance. Policies and priorities in certain sectors frequently clash with those in others; long-standing inter-departmental rivalries continue to block inter-sectoral cooperation; and the personal interests of politicians and public servants often assume greater importance than the real needs of the people they are supposed to serve. In these conditions many dedicated health workers may decide to insulate their work from that of other sectors, rather than getting bogged down in seemingly endless bureaucratic wrangles, obstructions, and power struggles.

Self-reliance and total community participation

A popular Chinese slogan is 'Do today what can be done today and improve on it in the future'. The Chinese practice — in contrast to many other countries — has been to compromise if necessary and get *something* done on long-term tasks. Tales of moving mountains one stone at a time are relevant to the story of the development of primary health care in China. Numerous examples can be cited of a community making a modest start rather than waiting until the ideal means to a distant goal were at their disposal. The vast participation in mass movements and careful social engineering through apt slogans and well-targeted campaigns made community participation and self-reliance the hallmarks of primary health care in China. Total health coverage was achieved through total involvement of the people.

Even in countries whose national governments have failed to demonstrate political commitment to primary health care, there have been many examples of small communities, voluntary agencies, and sections of the Health Service itself making a start to improve community health, nutrition, and living standards. Yet, inspiring as these initiatives may be, they will never achieve widespread coverage of the population without a radical restructuring of economic, social, and political institutions.

Health workers and the community

Rather than being accountable to an individual on a higher rung of the institutional hierarchy, China's barefoot doctors are accountable to the communities which originally selected them, continue to maintain them and of which they are equal members. This system of decentralized management and control serves to reinforce community commitment to provide better health services for all, while at the same time strengthening the motivation of barefoot doctors to serve the people. With a number of notable exceptions, most developing countries appear to lack the institutions needed to select, maintain and control village health workers. In many countries such a high degree of community participation in decision-making would be viewed with suspicion and alarm by governments unrepresentative of the people under their control.

Access to all levels of health services

Almost universal access to all levels of health services has been achieved in China through a cadre of para-professional health workers backed up by a network of reliable communications and well-staffed and equipped health facilities at secondary and tertiary levels. Barefoot doctors and other health workers at community level ensure that curative services are used early and that preventive and promotive programmes achieve total coverage of the population. The existence of the *total* system, rather than any single element, assures the comprehensiveness necessary to handle the health problems of the vast Chinese population. Many developing countries appear to place their faith in simply training a cadre of paraprofessionals — village health workers — but without making adequate provision for referrals, technical back-up, and administrative support. This approach reflects an inadequate understanding of the Chinese barefoot doctor 'model', which has always stressed the *whole* health system rather than any single element.

Traditional medicine

The use of traditional medicine, including acupuncture and herbal drugs, has helped to make primary health care more affordable and acceptable to the Chinese people. Peasants and workers in an extremely traditional culture have been brought into contact with modern curative and preventive services. While the efficacy of only a few of the vast array of therapeutic agents has been tested scientifically to date, important advances in studying this materia medica undoubtedly will lead to new therapeutic agents and a better understanding of existing ones. Herbal and other forms of traditional medicine continue to enjoy widespread popularity in developing countries. There is a need, however, to identify and promote the most efficacious traditional remedies and to establish norms for their usage. It is also urgent to halt the indiscriminate marketing of brand-name drugs by multinational companies — especially of drugs for conditions readily responsive to traditional medicine.

CONCLUSION

During the past three decades China has achieved good nutrition, life expectancy of 65 or more, and low rates of infant mortality and population growth — all this despite low per capita income. Yet it is open to question whether governments and voluntary agencies in other developing countries can take certain elements of the Chinese health system and implement them, even with modifications, in a totally different context. Without supportive political, socioeconomic, and administrative structures, efforts to 'transplant' parts of the Chinese health system — such as barefoot doctors — are bound to encounter serious difficulties. Finally it should be noted that recent trends towards the modernization of health services and the professionalization of health workers may well carry China *away* from the very principles which first brought success. While these recent trends may be the easiest for other developing countries to emulate, they are unlikely to contribute to making 'Health for All by the Year 2000' a reality.

2 Health care in Cuba: a model service or a means of social control – or both?

David Werner outlines the remarkable achievements of the Cuban health care system since the Revolution of 1959, but questions the system's heavy reliance on highly trained doctors and centralized control.

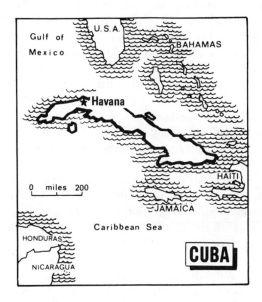

David Werner, a biologist by training, spent 14 years as a community health worker in an upland region of Mexico. Now based at Palo Alto in California, he is co-author of two widely used manuals for health workers — *Where There Is No Doctor* and *Helping Health Workers Learn.*

BACKGROUND

Before the Revolution of 1959, most of Cuba's people suffered from much the same social and physical hardships, poor health, and inadequate health care as does the poor majority of most of Latin America today. Life expectancy was low, infant and maternal mortality were high. Over half of the children were mal-nourished. More than 50 per cent of the doctors and 70 per cent of the hospital facilities were in the capital province of Havana where their costly services catered to the fortunate few. Most of the land and industry were in the hands of a small, wealthy minority, largely under foreign (US) control. For the working people, housing, water, and sanitation were inadequate; wages were low, agricultural work was seasonal only; workers' rights were minimal; unemployment was high. Government, representing primarily the interests of the rich, was corrupt, repressive, and, under Batista in the years preceding the Revolution, blatantly in violation of the constitution.

A new man

The Cuban Revolution changed things radically. It was spearheaded by a small group of strong-willed idealists with popular support. Their vision, in keeping with that of the Cuban poet and political philosopher Jose Marti, was to create a saner and fairer social order, free of corruption and exploitation, to work toward an idealistic yet pragmatic society in which meeting the basic needs of the many would be given top priority. As Fidel Castro declared in 1953, when the Revolution was still only a dream, 'The problem of land, the problem of industrialization, the problem of housing, the problem of unemployment, the problem of education and the problem of people's health; these are the six problems we would take immediate steps to solve along with the restoration of civil liberties and political democracy.'

According to the revolutionaries' vision, the new social order would be created by, and in turn help to create, the so-called *hombre nuevo* or 'new man' – a more truly human being whose first sense of responsibility would be to help better the lot of all people; for whom the joy and comraderie of working together for the common good would be its own greatest reward. Thus, the Cuban Revolution was founded on enormous personal reverence for ordinary working people, their innate capacity, and their idealized potential.

Today everyone in Cuba has adequate food. Everyone has access to comprehensive health care. Although sufficient housing is still a problem, a great effort is being made to provide adequate low-cost living quarters for everyone; the rapid progress toward this goal has been outstanding. Primary education is compulsory and almost universal; soon secondary education will be. Today there is virtually no unemployment. To a large extent, equal education and employment opportunities exist irrespective of race or sex. Differences in earnings between labourers and professionals, while still apparent, average in the order of 1:3 or 1:4 rather than 1:15 and 1:30, as in most of Latin America (and as in Cuba before the Revolution). Most remarkable of all, government corruption is relatively minimal. If it were not, Cuba could not have begun to accomplish what it has.

Impact on health

Cuba's vital statistics reflect the far-reaching sociopolitical changes that have taken place. Although per capita income remains that of a developing country,

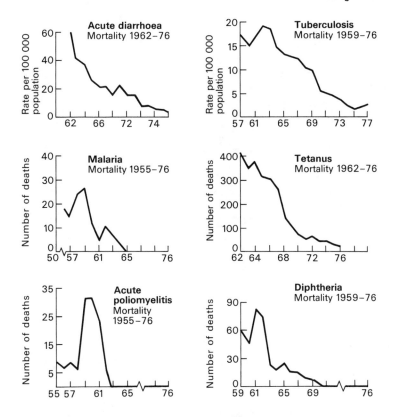

Fig. 2.1. Year by year mortality from infectious and contagious diseases in Cuba. (Adapted from *Cuba Review* **VIII**, No. 1, March 1978.)

infant and maternal mortality have fallen nearly to the levels of industrialized countries. Today Cuba's infant mortality is 25 per 1000, the lowest in Latin America and the Caribbean. Life expectancy is now 72 years — the highest in the region. Before 1959 the most common causes of death were typical of poor countries: malnutrition, diarrhoea, pneumonia, tuberculosis, malaria, and epidemic diseases. In recent years, the major causes of death have become more similar to those in industrialized countries: heart disease, stroke, cancer automotive accidents, and non-infectious pulmonary disease.

Figure 2.1 shows the impressive impact of the Cuban Public Health System since the Revolution on several common infectious and contagious diseases. It is noteworthy that although malaria and polio are still serious problems throughout much of Latin America, both have been entirely eliminated in Cuba. No other Latin American country can match Cuba's record in reducing infectious and contagious disease.

Table 2.1 provides a comparison of various indicators of the state of physical health and social well-being in Cuba and different Latin American countries. It

Table 2.1. Comparison of Latin American countries

Country	Population (millions)	GNP per capita (US$)	Infant mortality (deaths per 1000 live births)	Birth rate (per 1000 population)	Adult literacy rate (per cent)	Life expectancy	Type of government
Peru	17.1	930	86	38	80	58 years	Military-dominated
Guatemala	6.8	1020	N.A.	40	N.A.	59 years	Military junta
Cuba	9.8	1410	25	18	96	72 years	Communist
Mexico	65.5	1640	60	36	82	66 years	Authoritarian single party control
Chile	10.9	1690	55	23	N.A.	67 years	Military junta
Brazil	116.5	1780	92	29	76	63 years	Military-dominated
Argentina	27.3	2230	N.A.	21	94	70 years	Military junta
Venezuela	14.5	3120	40	35	82	67 years	Civilian democracy

Source: World Bank, *World Development Report, 1981*.

is evident that in terms of equalizing wealth, extending basic services, improving living standards, and radically reducing the physical and the most iniquitous social causes of poor health, Cuba is head and shoulders above the rest of Latin America, including even Venezuela, which has a per capita GNP (gross national product per person) nearly three times that of Cuba.

Birthrate and family planning

One of the most brow-raising statistics of modern Cuba is the birthrate, which has been declining steadily in recent years even though the Cuban government has never conducted a campaign to push family planning, as do nearly all Latin American governments today. The birthrate in Cuba is at present (with the possible exception of Barbados) the lowest in Latin America. From a reported 28.3 live births per 1000 inhabitants annually before the Revolution, the recorded number rose shortly after the Revolution to 35 per 1000.[1] From 1963 to the present, however, the birthrate has steadily declined. By 1979 the birthrate had dropped to 18.0 per 1000 (see Fig. 2.2), a figure that corresponds more closely with the birthrate in the United States (17 per 1000) than most of the Caribbean and tropical Latin America (Haiti, 41 per 1000; Honduras, 46 per 1000; Guatemala, 40 per 1000).

Cuba's rapidly declining birthrate is especially significant when one considers that each of the above-mentioned Latin American countries conducts an extensive US government-assisted family planning programme that utilizes high

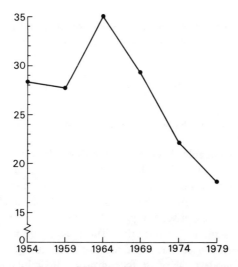

Fig. 2.2. Birth rate in Cuba 1954–79. (Sources: Government of Cuba, Junta Central de Planificacion. *Publicacion 5*, Direccion de Demografia, Sept. 1977. World Bank, *World Development Report 1981*.)

pressure tactics, including free services, hand-out 'incentives', extensive propaganda that verges on brainwashing, and (in Mexico at least) a quota system whereby health workers are required to 'recruit' a certain number of women for contraception or sterilization each month.

In Cuba, the situation is quite the contrary. Although the State does provide birth-control methods at low cost to those who want them, it conducts no public campaign or propaganda to promote family planning. In fact, the government officially states that it needs more people to fill the growing demand for labour. Nevertheless, the birthrate has fallen substantially since 1963, and continues to fall.

The fact that Cuba has experienced such a remarkable decline in birthrate 'without even trying', while other countries that have tried so manipulatively have failed, provides strong evidence in support of the argument that *only when people achieve a certain level of economic security will they choose to have fewer children*. Cuba has gone far towards providing all its people with such a guarantee. Although she remains a poor country, there is virtually no unemployment. People's basic needs for food, shelter, and health care are universally met. Hence the socioeconomic pressures for having many children have been mitigated and the many advantages to having a small family begin to outweigh the disadvantages.

THE STRUCTURE AND EVOLUTION OF THE CUBAN PUBLIC HEALTH SYSTEM

Health care as a top priority

Universal provision of health care has been one of the top priorities of the Cuban Revolution. Even before Batista's overthrow, Castro, Che Guevara, and their fellow guerrillas had begun to provide medical services to the mountain villagers of the Sierra Maestra, and in so doing helped win the people's affection and allegiance. Following the 1959 victory, the Revolutionary government determined to make the accessibility of free health and medical services to the entire population one of its immediate and major goals. The needs of the rural areas were to be put first.

The task was formidable. Even before the Revolution there had been a severe shortage of health personnel. In 1959, more than 60 per cent of the population had almost no access to modern health care. To make things harder, in the first five years following the Revolution in 1959, over half of Cuba's doctors fled the country. This was no surprise, for physicians had been among the most elite members of Cuba's privileged minority. The practice of medicine had always been a highly profitable career. Most did not take kindly to the prospects of accepting only a modest salary or to converting their lucrative business back into a public service, and so they left.

In an attempt to stem the mass exodus of doctors, the State compromised its commitment to equity and promised substantially higher salaries and special privileges to those who were willing to stay. Many were also offered high positions in the new health ministry, in spite of their privileged class background and ideological differences.

The Ministry of Public Health

Following Batista's overthrow, the new Ministry of Health at once set about re-forming and extending the health services. It nationalized all hospitals, clinics and other health facilities and began constructing new ones, focusing first on the more isolated and rural sectors of the country. Increased emphasis was placed on preventive measures, and on maternal-child health.

To implement some of the preventive measures, help was solicited from various community organizations, especially the Committees for the Defence of the Revolution (CDRs). With the help of these people's organizations, vacci-nation campaigns for polio were carried out throughout the entire country in as little as 72 hours! As a result, polio was completely eliminated from Cuba by 1963 – years ahead of the United States.

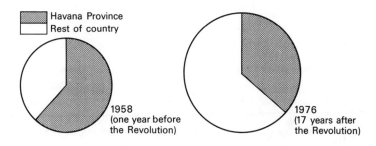

Fig. 2.3. Hospital beds: proportion in Havana Province and rest of country before and after Revolution (1959). (From *Cuba Review* **VIII**, No. 1, March 1978.)

Hospital services in Cuba were increasingly centralized (see Fig. 2.3). The health services were administratively organized into seven health provinces, each of about 1.25 million people. Today each province has a provincial hospital pro-viding tertiary (highly specialized) care, several regional hospitals providing secondary (specialized) care, and a network of 'polyclinics' providing primary care. These are arranged, geographically and in terms of referral, in a satellite formation (see Fig. 2.4). In the rural areas, provisional care, followed by referral to the polyclinics, is provided at community health posts. Where distances from a regional hospital are great, the polyclinic (out-patients only) is often replaced by a rural hospital (in-patients too).

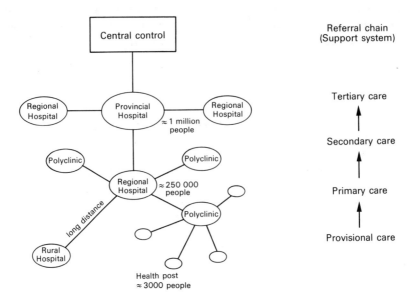

Fig. 2.4. Structure of Cuban Health Services

The polyclinic

The mainstay of the health system is the *policlinico*. Unlike primary care centres in many countries, the polyclinic is not run by general practitioners but by a team of 'primary care specialists' whose specialities are determined on a basis of the age and sex of patients – i.e., pediatricians, obstetricians/gynecologists, and internists. There are also social workers, sanitation officers, and a number of nurses, technicians, and other support personnel.

The polyclinic provides the chief link with the community. It coordinates school health services, 'multi health screening programmes', and prenatal home visits (primarily by nurses). It carries out vaccination programmes, sanitation activities, and other preventive measures, often in coordination with the local CDRs, the Cuban Womens's Federation, and other community organizations.

Medical manpower

The mainstay of health manpower in Cuba is indisputably the doctor. Unlike many other developing countries, Cuba has done relatively little by way of giving medical responsibilities to paramedics or community health workers, but rather has focused on training fully qualified MDs to handle every level and aspect of curative medicine.

This has not been an easy or inexpensive task. With the exodus of half her 6300 physicians after the Revolution, Cuba launched an all-out production of physicians. By 1971, 30 per cent of university students were studying medicine. In 1972, when the number of doctors reached 7200, the quota was dropped to 20 per cent. Today nearly half the practising doctors and over half the medical students are women.

An effort is presently being made to shift the training of medical students away from the provincial hospitals to the more modest regional hospitals. The revised curriculum focuses more on primary care, epidemiology, and preventive and community medicine. Senior medical students, interns, and residents must spend three four-hour sessions a week in the polyclinic.

In an attempt to bestow a higher value on the much denigrated field of public health, only the top 10 per cent of each class are eligible for public health residencies. Despite this unusual status and the increased exposure of medical students to community medicine, after their two years of compulsory rural service 80 per cent of doctors still apply for residencies in some branch of highly specialized, hospital-oriented, curative care. Evidently the prestige linked with classical Western medicine has not greatly changed with the Revolution.

The remarkable outreach of the health system

One of Cuba's accomplishments is the extent to which the government, in the short period of 20 years, has extended its social services, including health services, to virtually every corner of the island. Today more than 90 per cent of the population lives within one hour's travel from a polyclinic or rural hospital. Only a few people in the most remote mountain areas now live as far away from a health centre as three to four hours (usually on foot or mule trails).

To accomplish this remarkable extension of coverage has required the joint effort of different ministries and work forces: a full-scale programme for extension of roads into formerly inaccessible areas; the mining, manufacture, and transportation of building materials; the construction of scores of polyclinics and dozens of regional and rural hospitals.

In 1978 I was in a group which visited one such rural hospital in La Sierrita, a beautiful, remote area in the Sierra de Ascambray. It was a small, simply constructed 20-bed hospital tucked in a jungle clearing. The young doctor in charge was fulfilling his three-year stint of obligatory rural service. In marked contrast to the majority of graduating medical students from other Latin American countries, who often bitterly resent the interruption of their comfortable, urban, hospital-oriented careers caused by the compulsory term of rural service, this young Cuban doctor had eagerly accepted the challenge and expressed his commitment to bring the best health care possible even to the most remote parts of his country. (He did, however, admit he hoped to return to Havana as soon as his period of rural service was up.) We were informed that even in this remote area, where some of the population lives up to four hours away by trail, nurses make an effort to visit pregnant women for prenatal check-ups. We learned that virtually 100 per cent of babies are born in the hospital, and that 'the only babies not born in a hospital are those born on the way'.

We asked about the present role of traditional midwives and folk healers in Cuba, and were told that, in effect, they no longer existed. 'Modern, professional medicine has completely taken their place', the young doctor told us with pride. He also told us that use of home and herbal remedies was now completely a thing of the past. Nevertheless, as we all became more relaxed during our long conversation, the young doctor confided that even he occasionally prescribes *te de manzanilla* (chamomile tea) for stomach-ache – an old folk remedy. So apparently some of the old traditions have still survived the official policy that recognizes only modern medical science with its imported ideas.

LIMITATIONS OF THE CUBAN HEALTH SYSTEM

Over-dependency on professionals: rigid medical hierarchy

Recently, in many parts of the world, there has been a gradual awakening to the unhealthy situation that too often results when people become over-dependent on experts, and by so doing, fail to develop their potential for decision making and self-reliance. Ivan Illich, for one, has strongly criticized what he has called the 'expropriation of health' by institutionalized medicine. By empowering an elite fraternity of doctors with the sole, almost sacred, right to medical knowledge and skills, the health care institution has, in effect, placed the cost and accessibility of modern medical technology out of reach of the world's poor majority who need it most. In terms of basic coverage for an entire population, the closed professional monopoly imposed on the world by the western medical model is increasingly being recognized by regional planners as a major obstacle to health.

In many countries there has been a trend during the last few years toward the training of volunteer, part-time, community-based health workers, who assume an increasing number of responsibilities that have long been the coveted domain of the professional physician. In Cuba, however, the trend has been just the reverse. Non-physician health workers, while they are being trained in limited numbers, have been relieved of virtually all medical decision making, including diagnosis and treatment of even the most common and easily managed of ailments. Rather, people are instructed to make full use of the free professional services available. Self-care is actively discouraged.

For example, diarrhoea in children, regardless of how mild, in Cuba is always cause for professional intervention. At the first sign of 'gasteroenteritis', mothers are expected to take the child to the nearest polyclinic at once. The paediatrician in Guines told us, 'Any child who has had diarrhoea for two days is hospitalized. This is the only way we have been able to substantially reduce mortality in children with diarrhoea.' We were greatly impressed when he pointed out to us that only one child in the 'diarrhoea ward' was being rehydrated intravenously. 'That is because we begin intensive medical treatment *before* they become dehydrated', he explained.

Yet at times professional unwillingness to share the most basic medical knowledge seems to be carried to an absurd extreme. Quite wisely, mothers of children in the diarrhoea wards are given daily classes in hygiene, home maintenance, and the prevention of diarrhoea. We were permitted to review the standard list of topics covered and for the most part were impressed at their comprehensiveness. To our surprise, however, we found no mention about the importance of giving plenty of liquids in order to prevent dehydration. This is surely a grievous omission, in view of the fact that dehydration caused by diarrhoea is probably the number one killer of children in the world today. Many health programmes have found that infant mortality can be dramatically reduced simply by educating mothers to give lots of fluids to their children at the first sign of diarrhoea. It has been found that in well-nourished children, if mothers learn to prevent dehydration promptly when diarrhoea occurs, medication is seldom necessary, and hospitalization very rarely. Thus, most diarrhoeas can be successfully treated in the home, at no or little cost, without medication, and with no need for professional intervention.

We asked if, in fact, no instructions were given to the mothers about the importance of giving plenty of fluids to a child with diarrhoea. 'Definitely not', the doctor replied. 'We don't want to tell mothers anything that might lead them to put off getting adequate medical attention at once.'

This sort of concern by the state for protecting its people from 'dangerous' knowledge that might lead to self-care, would seem to conflict with the official policy that 'the people must participate actively to assure and maintain high health levels'. On the one hand, the people are required to 'participate actively' in prevention. On the other hand, they are instructed to depend passively upon professionals for even the most minor curative care.

Minimal responsibility given to community health workers

Of the visits that the Health Ministry arranged for us to observe different aspects of the Cuban health system, the great majority were to hospitals and large clinics. Only twice did we have a chance to meet community health workers. This emphasis on the professional end of the health-care spectrum unquestionably reflects the priorities of the Ministry of Health. Community health workers play a very secondary role.

We met one community health worker in the new 'agricultural community' of El Tablon in Cienfuegos Province. The new community, settled in 1971, consists of a line of box-like apartment buildings, a post-office, a store, a beauty parlour, a school complex, and a *posta medica*. The 192 families of the community are mostly former villagers who used to work as independent small farmers. Now they all work on a modern state-owned dairy cattle farm.

The medical post of El Tablon was run by a health worker — a young woman who had been trained one day a week for two years at the nearest polyclinic, seven kilometres away. We discovered, to our disappointment, that the health worker was mainly a communications agent between the distant polyclinic and the community. Her medical skills consisted, in the words of one of the doctors, of 'a few minimal concepts'. She was able to wash and bandage minor cuts and burns, give simple painkillers, fill out extensive forms, and refer patients to the polyclinic. She was permitted to inject certain medicines, but only when prescribed by a physician. A doctor came regularly from the polyclinic to inject diabetic patients with insulin – a responsibility that is apparently considered too great for the health worker.

The polyclinic, although not far away, was still too far in emergencies. We asked the health worker what she would do if someone who was stung by a bee went into allergic shock and lost consciousness. She replied, 'I would send him to the polyclinic'. That, of course, would probably be too late to save his life. Yet in five minutes she could easily be taught to combat such cases of allergic shock by injecting adrenalin. This, however, would entail an autonomous decision on her part to use a prescription medicine, and therefore was not permissible. As nearly as we could learn, the health worker was not permitted to make any significant medical decisions.

It was evident that the health worker filled a far less functional role than she could easily have done if her training and imposed limitations had been more in keeping with the needs of the people and with her potential.

Health education anti-educational

In Cuba today, a great deal of emphasis is placed on 'health education'. A large part of what is called education, however, consists of providing information that constantly encourages people to go to the doctor for even the most minor ailment. For example, a popular health education booklet, under the heading *Eliminacion* states:

'There are babies who urinate each time they are fed and this worries the parents; the correct thing to do is consult a doctor.'

The absence of educative content in this sort of popular informative material is often disguised by unnecessarily complicated language and typical medical-professional double talk.

This sort of health non-education serves to reinforce the image of medicine as a cryptic art decipherable only by an officially ordained minority – namely doctors.

Such mystification of, and professional control over, potentially basic information is standard procedure in many parts of the world. It is a form of social and intellectual exploitation, promoting subservience and dependency of the poor majority on a privileged few. Therefore, it is not only counter-educational, but also 'counter-revolutionary' – if one takes to heart the original vision of the Cuban Revolution, namely to put an end to the exploitation of the many by the few, and to work toward equilization of economic and social privileges.

Revolution, to be an ongoing process, means continued openness to fundamental change. Yet Cuba has become increasingly closed to change. True, the country continues to expand its public services, its housing, its industry, its education facilities. But in many respects it has ceased to evolve. It has ceased to doubt and question the basic premises and assumptions of its own institutions. Consequently, Cuba in many ways is ceasing to progress. In the field of medicine and public health there is already evidence that Cuba, which took a lead in many major advances from 1959–1963, has now fallen behind in a number of key areas.

One area in which Cuba has failed to keep up with international advances in health care in the last two decades is that of maternal-child health, although this is considered one of the Health Ministry's top priorities.

Cuban doctors are proud of the fact that 99 per cent of babies are now delivered by doctors in hospitals. The question must be raised, however, whether universal mandatory doctor-hospital delivery is the most healthy, appropriate or cost-effective approach to childbirth in a country as poor as Cuba – or even in a rich country. Comparative studies in many countries have shown that hospital deliveries by doctors are far more expensive, but not necessarily safer for babies of low-risk mothers, than are home births with competent midwives. In Holland, for example, where most babies are delivered by midwives, infant mortality is substantially lower than in the United States, where nearly all babies are delivered in hospitals by doctors. It should be strongly questioned whether, with its high psychological and economic costs, universal doctor-hospital delivery is not a disservice to Cuban women and their babies.

Of even more serious consequence is the mandatory requirement in Cuba that all newborn babies be separated from the mother for the first 12 hours following childbirth. This is ostensibly done in order to monitor and observe the infants better in case complications arise. While temporarily separating newborn babies from their mothers was common practice 20 years ago, in many countries this policy has now been revised. Studies have shown that, except for babies with a low Apgar score (those with conspicuous problems at birth), there is no evidence that early separation from the mother for observation provides any additional safeguard. On the contrary, there is overwhelming evidence that keeping the baby with the mother in the hours following delivery has beneficial physiological and psychological influence on both the mother and child.

I tried several times to discuss with medical personnel the policy of early separation of babies from their mothers, but almost no one seemed interested or willing to consider alternatives. At the Nursing School in Havana, after one of the instructors lectured to us about how, in Cuba, patients and people in general can influence and provide feedback to the planners and administrators of national programmes, I asked what would happen if a group of women got together and informed the authorities of the maternity hospitals that they did not want to be separated from their babies after childbirth.

'But the mothers would not want to change the present policy', the instructor insisted. 'They realize that the doctor knows and does what is best for them.'

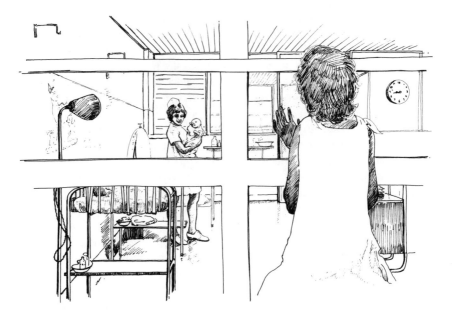

Fig. 2.5. In Cuba newborn babies are separated from the mother for the first 12 hours following birth.

'But let us suppose that in this case the doctors perhaps don't know what is best.' I asked, 'Could the mothers' collective concern effect a change in policy?'

The instructor looked at me hard. 'You must remember that here in Cuba doctors do not work to squeeze money from their patients or to take advantage of them in any way. Our doctors work in the best possible interest of the people. It is unlikely that mothers would know more about the health needs of their babies than do doctors who have devoted years of their lives to studying medicine.'

I wanted to say, 'But doctors are not omniscient. They, too, are human They too make mistakes They too get in ruts. . .' But I said no more. I was a guest. Besides, the instructor had already turned to speak with someone else.

Limited access by the people to non-approved information

As far as people gaining more control over different aspects of their own health care, here again Cuba in many respects has fallen behind progress made in other parts of the world. Perhaps if the people of Cuba knew more of advances elsewhere, they could be an important force in soliciting or demanding changes that could make health care services in Cuba more appropriate to their needs — changes which the medical profession is slow to initiate because they entail relinquishing and redistributing power. Unfortunately, however, in Cuba it is

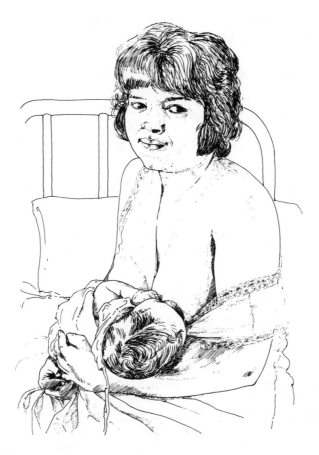

Fig. 2.6. There is overwhelming evidence that keeping the baby with the mother in the hours following delivery has beneficial physiological and psychological influence on both mother and child.

difficult for people to know what is going on in the rest of the world, other than via limited, carefully screened information publicized and broadcast by the State. If the mothers of Cuba had access to information about the medical and psychological evidence for not being separated from their babies following childbirth, they might very well petition for a change in policy – if they dared. But unfortunately, not even the obstetricians and paediatricians in Cuba today appear to be adequately informed on this issue. Even more disturbing, few we talked to showed interest in becoming more fully informed. It would appear that something devastating has happened to their innate curiosity as well as their values during their long years of institutional education. We were told that in each branch of science, a national committee exists to review and evaluate articles and new information appearing in major publications throughout the world. For anyone not a member of these committees, however, foreign journals are evidently extremely difficult to come by — except those from Russia.

The poor cost-effectiveness of Cuba's top-heavy health system

In many aspects of its development, Cuba has shown realistic and even Spartan concern for cost effectiveness — seeking and finding ways to accomplish the greatest benefit with the limited funds and resources available. Housing consists of large, low-cost apartment complexes. Transportation is to a very large extent public — mostly buses — with strict (although not altogether impartial) limitations on private ownership of vehicles. Food production concentrates on basic nutritious foods (with the exception of the major export crop, sugar).

In marked contrast, health care has taken what seems to be an unrealistic alternative in terms of cost-effectiveness. A cost-effective approach would be to facilitate a skills pyramid in which the bulk of simple, everyday health problems could be tended to by the people themselves with the assistance of modestly trained but readily accessible paramedics and community health workers. Such a system would reserve costly, more highly trained medical professionals for only those major problems that require their special skills. Cuba, however, has chosen to use highly trained professionals not only to cover every aspect of curative medicine, simple to complex, but also to oversee community and preventive health activities.

The State tries to justify its approach by insisting that a completely professional delivery-oriented system guarantees the best health care for its people. But is this the case? There are indications that both quality of care and cost effectiveness can be improved by partial deprofessionalization of medicine.

First, *quality of care*. Although services at the polyclinics are free of individual charge (except for medicines), the waiting lines are often long. Because of overcrowding, out-patient care is often hurried and impersonal. Pharmacies, on the other hand, are often closer to the people and the service is faster. Since the medicine prescribed at the polyclinic must usually be purchased in a pharmacy in any case, a great many people in Cuba do, in fact, 'self-prescribe' their own medication. Official policy emphatically discourages self-medication. The doctor at La Sierrita told us that ideally even aspirin would require a doctor's prescription.

Representatives of the Ministry of Health state that self-medication is now minimal, but this is simply not so. One pharmacist I spoke with told me that approximately 50 per cent of the medicines she sells are without prescription. The situation is complicated by the fact that there seems to be confusion as to which drugs can legally be sold over the counter and which by prescription only. I obtained contradictory information in different pharmacies. In any case — as is typical for Latin America — many more drugs are available over the counter in Cuban pharmacies than in the United States or Great Britain. For example, aminophylline and other anti-asthmatic medicines, including injectable adrenalin, can be purchased over the counter, at least in some pharmacies. It is ironic that trained health workers have less official access to medicines than completely un-trained people have in the pharmacies. (This, however, is typical of government-trained community health workers throughout Latin America.)

Given the fact that people in Cuba – like people everywhere – have persisted with a substantial amount of self-treatment and doubtless will continue to do so, it stands to reason that a partial deprofessionalization of medical knowledge could upgrade the net extent of health care people receive. In several countries (including China), this has been done by giving modestly trained community health workers greater medical responsibility in the management of common problems. Community health workers can be more quickly and easily approached than doctors in crowded polyclinics. They know the people they work with not only as patients but as neighbours and friends and often have greater insight into their problems and needs. Also, they are more likely to explain things in simple language that everyone understands. Most importantly, if the community worker is appropriately trained, he or she will share his/her knowledge with friends, neighbours, and those who come for consultation, so that little by little, the entire population is better informed. Thus, people will be more able to practise responsible self-care within rational, self-imposed limits. If this were to happen in Cuba, existing polyclinics would have less of a patient load, the waiting lines would be shorter, doctors could take time to be more relaxed and personal, and people would be more inclined to utilize professional services when they really needed them. Thus a partial deprofessionalization of medicine could result in better, more professional medical services when – but only when – they are truly needed.

Second, *cost-effectiveness*. Cuba takes pride in her universal free health care system. But, of course, there is no such thing as a free lunch – or free health care. Ultimately it is the Cuban people who pay for their enormously expensive, doctor-dominant health-care system. Cuba is a poor country, and is likely to remain so due to her intrinsic shortage of mineral, hydroelectric, and other re-sources. At present, food, shoes, clothing, and many basic goods are being strictly rationed. But is this necessary? Much of the fruit, meat, and leather that are presently exported could be eaten or used instead by the Cubans if the same level (or better) of health care that the people receive today were provided at lower cost by fewer doctors, more community health workers, and a medically better-informed public. More money could be put into food, clothing, shoe manufacture, housing, and other things the people still badly need.

To sum up: if a more economical, less dependency-creating health care sys-tem were devised, Cuba's perpetual economic straits could be somewhat eased, other needs of the people could be better met and the present rationing and centralized control over so many aspects of people's lives could be relaxed. Life could be less restricted.

THE POLITICS OF HEALTH IN CUBA

Founding principles

The founding principles of the Cuban health system are officially stated as follows:

1. The health of the people is the full responsibility of the State.
2. Universal coverage is guaranteed to all persons without discrimination.
3. The people must participate actively to assure and maintain the high health levels.
4. Preventive care is the primary goal of health care.

These principles may be highly idealistic. But on close inspection they are fundamentally self-contradictory – especially principles one and three. If health care is the full responsibility of the State, does this not entail restricting or depriving the responsibility of individuals and communities for their own health? And in the long run is such expropriation of responsibility healthy? If the State takes over full responsibility for people's health, yet insists that the people must participate in health matters, then in what irresponsible, subservient way are the people obliged to participate?

In several parts of the world, governments of diverse political convictions are discovering unhealthy repercussions that result from going too far in relieving people of responsibility for their own well-being. The United Kingdom, for example, has begun to realize the nemesis of a National Health Service that has focused on taking complete care of people rather than on helping people care more responsibly for themselves. As a result, the British health-care system is fast entering a state of crisis. Its facilities are overburdened and costs climb while public demand, dependency, and dissatisfaction steadily mount.

Medicine as a form of social control

As mentioned earlier in this chapter, in recent years not only in China, but in Tanzania, Venezuela, parts of Bangladesh, Sri Lanka, and other countries, it has been demonstrated that health care can be more effective, economical and humane when the completely doctor-dependent Western model is replaced by an approach that gives greater importance to the modestly trained, community level of health workers, and focuses on returning a large part of responsibility for health care to the people. The World Health Organization no longer believes developing countries can rely on doctors alone to bring health to their people. WHO and UNICEF have together drawn up a completely new strategy, which aims at increasing not the number of doctors, but the people's own capacity to fight disease. In the words of WHO's Director, Hafden Mahler, 'People should act to improve their own health rather than rely on doctors to do it.'

Why, then, should Cuba, which receives substantial support and advice from WHO, have taken a diametrically opposite approach, one that in typical Western fashion has involved the training of an ever-increasing number of doctors at unrealistically high cost and has systematically reinforced people's dependence on highly professionalized, State-controlled welfare?

Not only has Cuba's costly, highly professionalized health-care system resulted in growing dependency of the people on an influential minority of experts, but it has also perpetuated the dependency of Cuba as a nation on massive foreign aid. Without the enormous assistance of the USSR, there is no way that a country as poor as Cuba could afford the luxury of universal health coverage provided almost exclusively by doctors. (It is difficult or impossible to obtain the precise figure of the USSR's aid to Cuba, but it is known to be substantial.) Thus, Cuba's present health-care system breeds a double-edged dependency: first, that of the people on the State; and second, that of the State on foreign aid. It must be questioned whether such self-limiting dependencies are conducive to the optimal development or health of either a people or a state.

Cuba's economic dependency on Russia has undeniably given the Soviet Union a degree of more or less benevolent control over Cuba's national and international policies and institutions — including her health-care system, which closely resembles Russia's. In turn, the carefully nurtured dependency of Cuban people on the universal coverage of a highly centralized, state-run health-care system helps reinforce the state's more or less benevolent yet authoritarian control over her people.

Such creation of dependency is a well-known, long-established ploy of countries controlled by industrial powers. In such countries, it is to a large extent motivated by the selfish desire of the economically strong to perpetuate their material exploitation of the poor. But clearly this is not the case in Cuba, which, like China, has proved her 'anti-imperialist' commitment to egalitarian redistribution of wealth. Why has Cuba — whose government purports to be for (if not directly by) the people and whose first goals are equity and justice for all — found it necessary to resort to such coercive, and at times repressive, forms of social control?

The answer, I suspect, has to do with the nature of the human mind. Cuba's idealistic leaders have been so committed to re-creating man according to their own highly standardized, idealized image, that they seem to have lost sight of the fact that although all human beings are created equal, they are not all created the same. There is some essence in each of us that bitterly resents and resists our being put into a common mould and shaped according to a common plan — even if it be a benevolent plan, ideally designed for the common good. The thirst for a unique, autonomous identity and self-reliance is as basic to man as his need for air and food and love. No two of us are alike. People vary fundamentally from individual to individual. If they did not, we would never have evolved; we would all still be sea squirts. It is precisely the incorrigible individuality of man, for better and for worse, that has made, and makes, him human.

I came away from Cuba both deeply impressed and deeply disturbed. It was inspiring to at last see a Latin American country that, although still quite poor,

is without hungry or homeless children, without unemployment, without overwhelming untreated and unprevented disease, a country that has achieved relative
equalization of wealth, almost universal education, equitable social services, and
dedicated, honest leaders. Yet the more I saw of Cuba, the more uncomfortable
I became. I found myself asking over and over — 'At what cost equity? Does the
end justify the means? Are benevolent coercion and authoritarian enforcement
of conformity necessary to get people sharing and working to help each other,
rather than greedily hoarding and taking unkind advantage of one another? To
achieve greater fairness in human relations, to what extent must individual freedom to manage one's life and health and ideas be sacrificed?'

Ultimately — and ironically — it is this very dream of a free, sane, and just
society that has led the leadership of Cuba to compromise for their own people
the very liberation they fought for so courageously and won. Although Cuba's
leadership is theoretically committed to the idea that the people should participate in the decisions of the State, it is also determined to make sure that the
resulting decisions are 'right'; i.e. in the best interest of the people themselves
— according to the leaders' own definition. The end result is, of course, a para-
doxical denial of decision-making by the people. Thus, *poder popular*[2] becomes
an empty and deceptive facade and the CDRs (Committees for the Defence of
the Revolution) are reduced to instruments of political propaganda, and at
times, agents of almost police-like coercion.

By the same token, both the education and health systems of the country
have been solidified into institutions that serve the double purpose of both
providing universal coverage free of discrimination (the end) and also of facilitating a far-reaching, insidious mechanism of social control (the means).

Are such forms of social control necessary? Obviously the Cuban leadership
feels that they are. The State speaks of the Revolution being still in process, of
the nation being still only Socialist and not yet fully Communist. The country
is in transition, the 'new man' still imperfectly formed. When the final goal is
reached and the 'new man' is fully formed, the State can then begin to loosen
its authoritarian social control. When the people have learned to think the right
thoughts, and only the right thoughts, it can permit them freedom of press,
communication, and expression.

There is a dangerous paradox here. Who is so wise that he is entitled to be
the master of other men's values and other men's destinies? Is it not the ground-
work of new oppression? Are bread and a roof and schooling and medical care
alone enough for the health and well-being of people?

Cuba can rightfully pride herself on remarkable improvement in her vital
statistics — lower infant and maternal mortality, virtual elimination of malnutrition, fewer diseases, increased life expectancy. But vital statistics are not
the only measure of well-being. Are not self-determination, variety, individuality,
adventure, and an element of freedom just as essential? Had man been content
to live like the ants, the individual existing only to serve the colony with optimal
efficiency, he might have been more successful as a species. But he would never

have developed a mind of his own. He would still — for better or for worse — be an ant.

It is precisely the plight of the destitute in most of Latin America that makes the social structure in these countries humanly and ethically intolerable. The repressive — but egalitarian — restrictions imposed on the Cuban people seem minor when compared with the oppressive hunger and dire poverty imposed on the poor of other lands. Furthermore, the number of destitute in other parts of Latin America, the number of persons whose poverty is a cage with no forseeable escape, is rapidly growing. Throughout Latin America, the rich are getting richer and the poor poorer. The slums are growing, unemployment is growing, the incidence of violence and unrest is growing, and with it the incidence of repression, as well as dependency-creating paternalism by the rich minorities in control. The number of soldiers and security police is growing. The relative freedom of the poor in Latin America is like the freedom of wild animals that are being cruelly and methodically hunted. This must be remembered when evaluating the people's restricted freedom in Cuba.

Summary and conclusions

Cuba has successfully overcome the physical inequities and cruel exploitation of the poor by the rich and raised the physical living conditions of the entire population to acceptable levels. But the new autocratic minority, idealistic as it may be, is committing a more insidious — and in the long run, perhaps — even more crippling form of exploitation of the vast majority. In spite of the public facade of *poder popular*, there is little question that in Cuba the state controls the people far more than the people control the state. Government may be *for* the people, but it is clearly not *by* the people. Authoritarian, and at times repressive, social control is reinforced through the establishment of centralized institutions that encourage the people's passive dependency on the 'free' services and imposed decisions handed down by what amounts to a Big Brother — or a Big Mother — State. Thus, people are centrally both cared for and 'formed' — supposedly for their own good. In the process, however, one of the most invaluable parts of human nature is being suffocated: each person's innate need — and capacity — to find his own truths and to become a unique individual in his own right.

Notes

1. This apparent increase in birthrate is probably due to the fact that, before the Revolution, many children died in infancy, with no official record of either their births or deaths. In similar fashion, throughout most of Latin America, even today, unrecorded births and deaths of the 'forgotten poor' lead to highly misleading and erroneously optimistic statistics.

2. *Poder popular* (people's power) is the political organisation of the Cuban state. Established by the constitution of 1975, *poder popular* provides for elected representatives of the people at constituency, provincial, and national level.

3 The Community Health Worker Scheme: an Indian experiment

Ashish Bose assesses the achievements and weaknesses of the Community Health Worker Scheme launched by the Indian government in 1977 as a new means of providing primary health care services to India's rural masses.

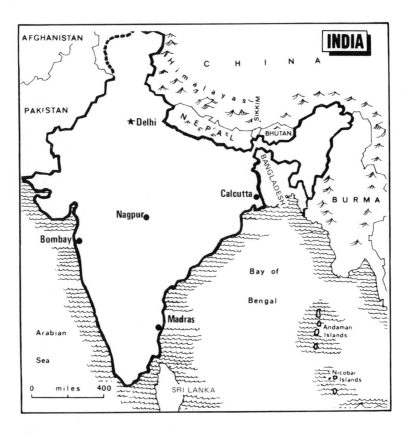

Ashish Bose, Ph.D., is Professor of Population Studies at the Institute of Economic Growth, Delhi University, Delhi. He is the author of several books on population, and for the past five years has been working on primary health care in rural areas.

Primary health care (PHC) is hardly a new concept in India. As far back as 1940, a Planning Committee of the Indian National Congress, chaired by Jawaharlal Nehru, called for the training of one health worker for every 1000 population with five years. It was followed in 1946 by the admirable report of the Bhore Committee, which proposed a national health programme bearing all the hall-marks of the PHC strategy now espoused world-wide by international agencies and national governments.

During the past decade a number of small-scale, experimental PHC projects have been initiated by voluntary agencies in various parts of India. Some of these schemes have made important contributions to international thinking on key issues such as community participation, the role of village health workers, and the evaluation of PHC programmes.

Yet now, 40 years after Nehru first called for one health worker for every 1000 people, the problems of PHC in India are still expressed in much the same way. With a few notable exceptions, India has failed to deliver adequate PHC services to the vast majority of its population of 700 million. The Community Health Worker (CHW) Scheme, launched by the Ministry of Health and Family Welfare in 1977, aroused high expectations in some quarters and scepticism in others. The working of the scheme during its first five years provides valuable insights into the problems of implementing PHC in a country like India.

HISTORICAL REVIEW: WHAT'S IN A NAME?

In April 1977, only a month after the general election which swept the Janata Party into power, the Minister of Health and Family Welfare, Raj Narain, issued a statement declaring that, despite 30 years work in the field of health since Independence, 'we have not made a significant impact on the health status of the rural population and the urban poor . . .' (Raj Narain 1977). Six months later, on 22 October 1977 – the 108th anniversary of the birth of Mahatma Gandhi – Raj Narain officially launched the Community Health Worker Scheme.

The modern medical profession reacted with a mixture of contempt and alarm. Typical was an editorial in the July 1978 issue of *IMA News*, the official journal of the Indian Medical Association, which dismissed the Scheme as 'a political eyewash and enormous waste of money'. By the time this editorial appeared, however, Raj Narain – a flamboyant, controversial political figure – already had lost the Health portfolio, which Prime Minister Morarji Desai was looking after on a caretaker basis. The editorialist advised the Prime Minister to 'take ample care while choosing an incumbent for the office so that the person has a scientific and realistic approach to the problem of health care and delivery to the teeming millions in this country and just does not go by fads'. This was an obvious reference to Raj Narain's enthusiasm for certain dietary and other fads and his espousal of traditional systems of medicine such as *ayurveda* and *unani*. He had been widely accused of gimmickry, and the CHW Scheme ridiculed for allegedly promoting quackery. So closely identified with the Scheme was the name of Raj Narain that it was virtually impossible to distinguish between the Scheme itself and the colourful politician who first had announced it to the country. Attacks on Raj Narain became, willy nilly, attacks on the CHW Scheme itself. This was the worst possible political context for the new Scheme, and its credibility suffered as a result.

One CHW for every 1000 population

The CHW Scheme aimed to provide adequate health care to rural people and to educate them in matters of preventive and promotive health care. Emphasizing the need for basic medical aid within the reach of every citizen, the Scheme planned to train one CHW for every 1000 population within three years. Each village community was to select from amongst its members one person to be trained as a CHW at a three-month course at the local Primary Health Centre.

The CHW would not be a government employee, but would be supervised by the local village council. Technical guidance and support, however, would be provided by staff from the nearest Primary Health Centre. During training the CHW was paid a stipend of 200 rupees per month. After training this payment was reduced to 50 rupees, since he was supposed to work only two or three hours a day as a health worker, spending the rest of his time in his normal job. He received a health care manual and a kit of basic medical supplies. A sum of

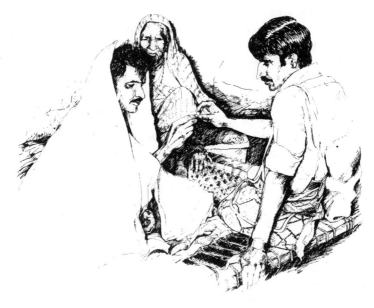

Fig. 3.1. The Scheme aimed to train one Community Health Worker for every 1000 population within three years.

50 rupees per month was allowed for the replenishment of drugs, to be supplied by the government through the local Primary Health Centre.

The CHW would have an important role in disease-preventive, health-promotive, and rehabilitative care. He would also treat simple ailments and refer more serious cases to a higher level of health care. The specific responsibilities of the CHW included the following:

- helping Health Centre staff in immunization programmes, the control of communicable diseases, family planning, mother and child health, nutrition, and mental health;
- arousing community interest in problems of environmental sanitation and personal hygiene;
- participating in health education activities;
- treatment of common ailments, giving of first aid in emergencies and referral of serious cases to the nearest Health Centre dispensary or hospital.

The CHW Scheme was also the first national programme to give due importance to indigenous systems of medicine such as *ayurveda* and *unani*, which can effectively treat certain conditions, especially those with psychosomatic origins. They also have the advantage of being cheaper than allopathic treatment which relies on relatively expensive drugs produced and massively promoted by multinational companies.

The Scheme was introduced in 741 Primary Health Centres (13 per cent of the nationwide total of 5686) in all States except Jammu and Kashmir, Tamil Nadu, Kerala and Karnataka[1] during the first year. Training of the first batch of CHWs began without delay in October 1977, and extended rapidly the following year. Early in 1978, however, there were reports that CHWs were dissatisfied with their modest honorarium of 50 rupees per month. They demanded the same payment as Multipurpose Workers (MPWs).[2] The government responded by emphasizing that CHWs were not government employees, but representatives of the people and social workers. They were paid only a small honorarium because their health work was only part-time. Yet the CHWs continued to agitate for higher remuneration and a recognized place in the health service itself. There were reports from different parts of the country of CHWs trying to form their own unions. The Ministry of Health rose to the occasion and in 1979 produced a curious administrative solution. They simply renamed the programme the Community Health *Volunteers* Scheme. The change of nomenclature from 'worker' to 'volunteer' was intended to disabuse recalcitrant CHWs of any notions that they were government employees or that they deserved anything but a modest honorarium for their work. Some improvements and modifications were also carried out in the running of the Scheme, but basically it continued as before, though under a slightly different name.[3]

Chopping funds and changing names (again)

In mid-1979 the National Development Council dropped an administrative bombshell by announcing a major change in the funding of the Scheme. Until that point the Scheme had been 100 per cent centrally financed, but henceforth the States would have to share costs with the Centre on a 50:50 basis. The States were shocked. They had agreed to the Scheme, they argued, on the understanding that it would be 100 per cent centrally financed. Yet after only 18 months they were being asked to pay half the bill, which seemed grossly unfair. Whatever the full reasons behind the government's surprising decision, it severely dislocated the implementation of the Scheme and caused its virtual collapse in several States.

Political turmoil at national level also had repercussions on the CHW Scheme. Charan Singh replaced Morarji Desai as Prime Minister in mid-1979, but the Janata government was toppled by Indira Gandhi's Congress Party in January 1980. The fate of the CHW Scheme hung in the balance while the new Congress government drew up a new Sixth Five-Year Plan (1980–85) to replace that of its predecessor. The Planning Commission and the Ministry of Health finally endorsed the Scheme, but retained the controversial arrangement of sharing costs 50:50 with the States. The Scheme continued to limp along until June 1981, when the government once again made a name change: the Community Health Volunteers Scheme became the *Health Guides (HG) Scheme*. The Ministry also issued new guidelines emphasizing and clarifying the responsibility of HGs to the community. Village Health Committees were to be established in order to better manage health activities. Mindful of the row about CHWs' honorariums and status three years earlier, the guidelines made it absolutely clear that the HGs were not government functionaries:

'The Health Guides and the Village Health Committees are to be treated and honoured as the representatives of the village community, who have come forward to assist the Government in the implementation of the Primary Health Care Programme. In no sense whatsoever are they to be treated as subordinate to the Health organization or subject to its commands and orders' (Government of India 1981.)

According to the new Sixth Five-Year Plan, some 220 000 CHVs would be trained between 1980 and 1985, bringing the total number to 360 000 by the end of March 1985. The Minister of Health and Family Welfare, however, stated at the end of 1981 that there would be a Health Guide for every 1000 village people by March 1984. This would amount to at least 494 000 Health Guides nationwide – far more than the estimate in the Plan.

Finally, to bring the wheel back to full circle, the government decided in December 1981 to make the Health Guides Scheme a 100 per cent centrally financed programme. This decision no doubt was popular with the States, especially by Bihar and Rajasthan, which totally abandoned the CHW Scheme in 1979. By January 1982 the Health Guides Scheme was operating in all States except the three with their own alternative schemes.

ASSESSMENT OF ACHIEVEMENTS, CONSTRAINTS, AND WEAKNESSES

Evaluating any health programme is a complex and difficult exercise, starting with the problem of methodology. While there is some general agreement on the evaluation of medical effectiveness in terms of reductions in morbidity and mortality, the methodology for evaluating social impact is still in its infancy. Qualitative phenomena such as community participation, behaviour, and perception are notoriously difficult to measure accurately. The exercise becomes even more difficult when one tries to take into account the wide range of demographic, socioeconomic, political, and environmental factors which interact with health variables. Some subjectivity and also criticism are thus inevitable in any process of evaluation. On both these counts, therefore, evaluation studies tend to be discouraged by official health administrators. Yet health planners and policy makers do accept the need for an *inbuilt* system of monitoring and evaluation right from the stage of project formulation through to implementation. As Professor Ramachandran writes:

'Evaluation is a complex process, involving both subjective judgement and objective measurements. In fact, there is no one unique way of performing an evaluation, since evaluation becomes judgement ultimately. However, as long as it is understood that the main purpose of evaluation is decision-making and not condemnation or approbation, unavoidable subjectivity is no impediment' (India Council of Medical Research 1980, p. 379).

In assessing the Indian CHW Scheme, we do not have available hard data on changes in morbidity and mortality on a State-wide or national basis, because adequate arrangements for evaluating the Scheme were not made. What we can attempt, however, is an analysis of the conceptualization and implementation of the Scheme. Much of our understanding is based on intensive fieldwork in rural areas and discussions with Health Ministry officials at all levels. Our focus is on non-clinical aspects of primary health care and the perception of the rural masses of their own health needs in relation to the Scheme.

Achievements

The basic philosophy of the Scheme — of placing 'the people's health in the people's hands' — was sound. Moreover, there is wide political acceptance of this broad principle. Yet, despite numerous exhortations for greater community participation in health care, the CHW Scheme was the first serious attempt by the government to delink the CHW from the medical bureaucracy. This was an important political step. Not being a government employee, the CHW could not be dismissed by the government Medical Officer. This relationship symbolized the supremacy of the community (represented by the village council) over the medical bureaucracy. The new guidelines for Health Guides underline and strengthen this policy.

There is evidence to suggest that the Scheme directly benefited women, children, and weaker sections of the community (harijans and backward castes) by providing greater access to curative care from the CHW and through referrals to higher levels of health care.[4]

To some extent the Scheme also made village communities more aware of the need for disease-preventive measures such as environmental sanitation. It also informed and educated some communities to demand better government health services as a right, rather than passively accepting the inadequate services provided. CHWs often proved to be a useful link between the health authorities and the community. Their successors, the Health Guides, have great potential for improving the effectiveness of health care by much higher coverage of, for example, services such as immunization and family planning.

Constraints and weaknesses

The turbulent political scene from 1977 until 1980 was a severe constraint on the CHW Scheme, and drastic changes in funding arrangements brought it to a grinding halt in several States. In short, the Scheme was never given a fair trial. There can be few more glaring examples of the way in which political events can adversely affect the people's health status.

The rural masses tend to perceive their health problems in terms of getting access to medicines, doctors, and hospitals. There is little appreciation of the part of village leaders or people in general of the health hazards created by bad sanitation, drainage and other aspects of environmental hygiene needing community action. The people therefore tended to judge the CHWs in terms of their limited competence in curative health care. CHWs for their part, were ill-equipped to overcome these prejudices: their own training emphasized curative care but gave them only the skills needed to treat the simplest of ailments. Though many tried to project themselves as the 'village doctor', their training in no way fitted them for this self-appointed role. As for disease-preventive and health-promotive work such as immunization, waste disposal, nutrition surveillance, and education, they were not trained (or expected) to handle any of these activities without strong leadership from the Health Centre — and that was usually lacking.

Even in cases where the CHW and the community were aware of a serious environmental health problem — such as the lack of safe drinking water — there was often little they could do about it without the backing of additional funds. A feeling of helplessness and frustration was the result.

The reluctance of the medical profession to view CHWs as partners rather than potential competitors in health care also was a severe constraint on the Scheme. Although the medical profession expressed grave fears about the danger of 'quackery' increasing as a result of CHWs working in rural areas, field studies have found these fears to be grossly exaggerated.[5] The uncooperative attitude of most health professionals stems from the system of medical education which trains them as a special elite oriented towards highly specialized, urban-based, westernized medicine. Unfortunately, however, little has been done to re-orientate health professionals through workshops, seminars, and training courses on the aims, strategies, and methods of primary health care.

The medical profession has been especially slow to allow village councils any meaningful role in deciding health priorities and implementing programmes. This reinforces a deep-rooted sense of over-dependence on government assistance, even when the community already has the financial and human resources to solve certain problems. In one village we met well-to-do villagers who proudly showed off their television sets and tractors, but right in front of their homes there were pools of stagnant water — perfect breeding grounds for malaria mosquitoes. When we mentioned this to the people, they replied that it was the job of the village council to get rid of stagnant water and ensure proper drainage. When we spoke to village council members, they said it was up to the government! The problem was certainly within the people's own capacity to solve. Yet, having never been allowed a meaningful role in solving their own health problems, the people were unable to conceive of taking any initiative themselves when the 'message' from the Primary Health Centre changed and they were suddenly expected to 'participate' in their own health care.

Health Centres often failed completely to communicate the content of the CHW Scheme to village councils. In many cases the block extension educators simply contacted the villages by letter and received in reply the names of CHW trainees selected by the councils, who knew virtually nothing about the programme and thought it was some kind of employment generation scheme. This misunderstanding obviously affected the CHW trainees themselves, many of whom thought they were entering government service and had totally unrealistic career and salary expectations.

Another weakness was that of inconsistency and overlap between the roles of multipurpose workers and community health workers. CHWs were supposed to work under the supervision of MPWs, who were full-time, salaried paramedics within the government health service. Yet, while the CHWs had their own medical kits, the MPWs did not. This diminished the standing and credibility of the MPWs in the eyes of the village people. There was also a tendency on the part of MPWs to pass part of their duties (e.g. distribution of chloroquine tablets) on to the CHWs, who ended up working far more than the expected two or three hours a day but were paid only a paltry fifty rupees a month for their efforts. These points of friction were not conducive to the smooth functioning of either the MPW or the CHW Scheme.

There was a striking bias in favour of selecting male CHWs: a mere 6.3 per cent were women. This seems curious, given that at least 70 per cent of the users of the CHWs' services would have been women and children, who comprise the most vulnerable section of the community. Granted, social customs in some parts of India might make it difficult for women to work effectively as CHWs, but women health workers in a number of small-scale PHC projects have demonstrated that even the most deeply entrenched social prejudices can be modified. (The December 1981 guidelines for Health Guides state that preference should be given to women in future.)

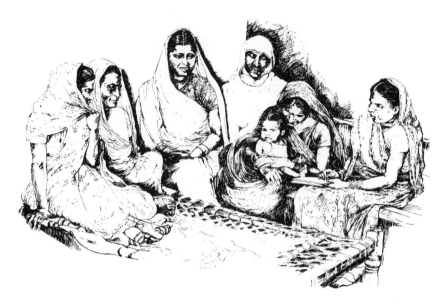

Fig. 3.2. At least seven out of every ten users of the Community Health Workers' services were women and children. Yet women CHWs like the one on the right (above) comprised only 6.3 per cent of the total.

The CHWs' medical supplies, worth fifty rupees a month and given away free, were often inadequate for the people's needs. This is a problem affecting not only CHWs but also Health Centres.

Finally, the CHW Scheme did not make adequate provision for concurrent evaluation, right from the start of the programme. This meant that many problems and weaknesses went uncorrected for too long, and also made it impossible to assess the effects of the programme on morbidity and mortality rates.

THE WAY FORWARD

We can draw certain lessons from the CHW Scheme to guide the future planning and implementation of primary health care in India. While the political and financial constraints on the Scheme were outside the control of health planners and workers, the weaknesses of the Scheme itself indicate the following lessons:

1. It is necessary to do a considerable amount of spadework to inform and educate the rural masses about the community orientation of primary health care, emphasizing especially the importance of disease-preventive and health-promotive measures. The block medical officer and the doctor in charge of the Primary Health Centre are not necessarily best suited for such spadework. Communications specialists and paramedics with direct experience of work in

rural communities should lead this important exercise in public motivation and education.

2. Selection and training of health guides should be organized by personnel with a background in education and management, with health professionals called on for specific inputs into courses.

3. Health professionals themselves are in need of training in communications and teaching skills through short courses, workshops, and seminars.

4. The training syllabus for health guides should be revised: new manuals of greater relevance to local conditions are required, and every trainee should prepare a simple health profile or 'community diagnosis' of his or her village as an obligatory part of the course. This not only will add to their own understanding of local health problems, but will also be an important learning experience for doctors and paramedics involved in the exercise. There are no shortcuts in such training. The only way is to go to the village and study conditions at first hand, with the people.

5. In order to meet the people's need for an adequate supply of low-cost drugs, the Health Department should establish fair price medical stores at all Primary Health Centres, where medicines would be sold on a non-profit basis.

6. Medical education must be restructured and re-orientated to take into account the government's commitment to primary health care. The present cadre of MBBS and MD doctors, who tend to be urban-orientated and not socially attuned to rural people's needs, is unlikely to prove effective in rural areas. The case for introducing a short-term medical degree and building up a new cadre of rural doctors trained according to the priorities of primary health care should be carefully examined.

7. Monitoring and evaluation of key medical and social indicators should be built into every health programme as a matter of course, making full use of the services of competent and independent researchers. The findings of particular studies should not be suppressed by the government, but acted upon to correct weaknesses, solve problems, and optimize the usage of limited public funds.

CONCLUSION

The past four decades have provided a wealth of experience on which India's health planners, administrators, practitioners, and people's organizations can build up a primary health programme meeting the needs of the country's whole population of 700 million. We must, however, be humble enough to learn from past experiences in order to build a better future for our people. Let us conclude by recalling the words of the Indian philosopher-poet, Bhavabhuti, who divided people into three categories:

The *lowest*, who do not begin for sheer fear of failure.
The *middle* ones begin but stop as soon as difficulties arise.
The *highest* begin and never abandon, in spite of repeated blows from difficulties, till success is won.

NOTES

1. Karnataka joined the national scheme two years later. Alternative schemes were operating already in the other three States.

2. MPWs were the key field personnel of a national health programme which began in 1975.

3. For the purpose of simplicity the term 'Community Health Worker (CHW)' is retained throughout this article.

4. See, for example, the evaluations by Bose *et al.* (1978), Dandekar and Bhate (1978), Demographic Research Centre, Patna (1978), Ghoshal and Bhandari (1979), and the National Institute of Health and Family Welfare (1978 and 1979).

5. See references cited in 4 (above).

REFERENCES

Bose, Ashish, Health Policy in India: 1947–1981. In *Policy making in government* (ed. K.D. Madan *et al.*) Government of India, Publications Division, New Delhi (1982).

Bose, Ashish *et al.* (eds.), *Social statistics: health and education.* Vikas Publishing House, New Delhi (1982).

Bose, Ashish *et al.*, *Limits to medicine, social dynamics of primary health care in India.* (In press.)

Dandekar, Kumudini and Bhate, Vaijayanti, Maharashtra's Rural Health Services Scheme: an evaluation, *Economic and Political Weekly, Bombay* Vol. 13, No. 50, pp. 2047–52 (1978).

Demographic Research Centre (Patna), *A report on evaluation of Rural Health Services Scheme in Bihar*, DRC Monograph Series No. 61. DRC, Patna (1978).

Ghoshal, B.G. and Bhandari, Vinod, *Community Health Workers' Scheme: a study.* Directorate General of Health Services, New Delhi (1979).

Government of India, Ministry of Health and Family Welfare, *Guidelines for the Health Guide Scheme.* New Delhi (1981).

Government of India, *Report of the Health Survey and Development Committee* (Bhore Committee) Vol. IV. New Delhi (1946).

Indian Council of Medical Research, *National Conference on Evaluation of Primary Health Care.* New Delhi (1980).

Indian Council of Social Science Research and Indian Council of Medical Research, *Health for All: an alternative strategy.* New Delhi (1980).

National Institute of Health and Family Welfare, *An evaluation of Community Health Workers' Scheme – a collaborative study.* NIHFW Technical Report No. 4. New Delhi (1978).

National Institute of Health and Family Welfare, *Repeat evaluation of Community Health Volunteers' Scheme – 1979: a collaborative study.* NIHFW, New Delhi (1979).

Raj Narain, *Policy Statement*, New Delhi, 20 April 1977.

4 'Prevention' is more costly than 'cure': health problems for Tanzania, 1971–81

Antony Klouda reviews Tanzania's health and development policies and concludes that — despite official commitment to 'Health for All' — the option of 'cure for the few' is still preferred by the government.

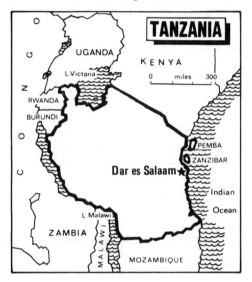

Antony Klouda, M.D., worked in Tanzania from 1978 until 1982 and is now Coordinator for Primary Health Care with the Private Hospital Association of Malawi.

According to conventional wisdom, the prevention of disease is cheaper than cure. This view fails to take account, however, of the many factors which determine the health status of an individual or a social group. Disease prevention is widely understood to mean specifically medical interventions such as vaccination, detection and care of 'high-risk' mothers and children, health education, hygiene, sanitation, and precautions against accidents. Yet these measures, unless supported by more comprehensive development strategies, will achieve only limited results.

Improved health for *all* the people also demands broadly based economic development, improved food production and distribution, specific anti-poverty measures, provision of safe drinking water, better housing, and universal education — a fact now recognized by international development agencies such as UNICEF and WHO. 'Health cannot be attained by the health sector alone' (WHO/UNICEF 1978, p. 11).

Disease prevention, in this broad sense, is one of the most complex functions of a modern state, since it involves a wide range of interlocking sectors, including Agriculture, Public Works, Education, Industry, and Health. It is therefore expensive.

The Government of Tanzania is well-known for its official commitment to providing adequate health care for all its citizens, as set forth in the Arusha Declaration of 1967 (Chagula and Tarimo 1975, p. 147). Yet the country's total development policies and specific strategies for eliminating poverty, ignorance, and disease do not adequately reflect this commitment. Furthermore, within the health sector itself, planning is unrelated to stated goals and the official allocation of human and financial resources does not match the needs of those groups suffering most from poor health. The overwhelming emphasis on hospital-based curative services maintains the popular illusion that health is provided by clinical intervention and knowledge. Curative care, rather than a broadly based attack on the real causes of poverty and disease, is still seen as the main 'road to health'. Any more radical strategy seems both politically and financially too expensive for serious consideration by a government which is most responsive to the demands of the country's urban elite. Cure for the fortunate few seems a cheaper option than comprehensive disease prevention for all.

BACKGROUND

Tanzania's major health problems

The pattern of Tanzania's health problems is similar to that of most African countries recently emerged from a long period of colonial domination: high prevalence of infectious and parasitic diseases; low nutritional levels; and problems related to pregnancy, childbirth, and infancy. The basic cause is poverty, with its associated inadequate food intake, low educational levels, lack of safe drinking water, poor environmental conditions, and inadequate housing.

The highest mortality level occurs around the time of birth and the first year of life, especially in low income groups. These deaths are due mainly to low birth weight, the poor nutritional state of the mother during and after pregnancy, and underfeeding of infants. Although children under five constitute only 18 per cent of the total population, they suffer 63 per cent of all deaths. About 200 000 under-fives die each year, with nutrition being the most significant factor in about half these deaths and diarrhoea in 10 per cent. With a national crude birth rate of 46 per 1000, both the size of this main 'at risk' group and the scale of the problem continue to grow at an alarming rate (see Table 4.1).

Local surveys also show high prevalence rates of infectious and parasitic diseases (see Table 4.2), which are generally well tolerated in adults but contribute significantly to deaths among children who are both underweight and poor.

Table 4.1. Estimated vital statistics of Tanzania, 1980

Crude birth rate	46 per 1000 population
Crude death rate	15 per 1000 population
Average annual rate of population growth	3.4 per cent
Infant mortality rate	103 per 1000 live births
Life expectancy at birth	52 years

Source: World Development Report (1982).

Table 4.2. Estimated prevalence of infections and parasitic diseases, 1979 (per 1000)

Hookworm	270
Malaria	220
Schistosomiasis	270
Filariasis	270
Tuberculosis	2
Leprosy	9

Source: Proceedings of 15th Post-Graduate KCMC Seminar on Community Health, October 1979.

Poverty, society, and ill-health

It is well known that the poorest groups in any society suffer most from ill-health. Poverty, however, is a very complex issue, dependent for its meaning on local conditions. In Tanzania the English word 'poverty' can be translated by two different Swahili words, both derived from a traditional form of tribal society which has largely broken down under the impact of modernization and the government's development strategies.

When Tanzania was composed largely of people living in groupings of a few large, extended families, the *maskini* concept of poverty referred to people who had suffered a loss or disaster. For example, if a mother and father had a malnourished child, members of their extended family would try to ensure that extra food was available for the child. In many tribes a milking cow would be lent or some of its milk given until the child's condition improved. In return, the parents would render some service or favour at a future time. For people who chose to live outside these closely knit social groupings, however, the laws of cooperation and reciprocity did not apply. Those who chose such a path but fell by the wayside were referred to contemptuously as *mafukara*.

Present-day poverty, however, is different. It stems from a socioeconomic system that has swept away traditional welfare mechanisms without putting anything comparable in their place. In today's Tanzanian economy individuals must earn money to survive, but those who fail have no support to fall back on —

either from the extended family or from the state. Loosely knit communities are springing up in cities as a result of the migration of young people from rural areas, while in the newly created villages families who are total strangers are thrown together and obliged to work out minimal ways of cooperation. In neither case have people been able to develop really viable structures for mutual support in times of need.

To many government and Party officials, however, people are poor either because of their own laziness, or a run of bad luck, or because of peculiar circumstances of some kind. Such are the present-day *mafukara* and *wamaskini* — though conditions have changed so much that these terms are hardly relevant today. What matters is that today's poor are caught in a trap from which, without help, they cannot escape.

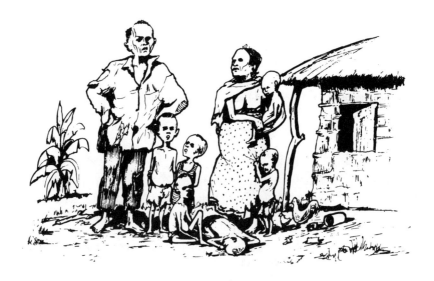

Fig. 4.1. Today's poor are caught in a trap from which, without help, they cannot escape.

This loss of 'room for manoeuvre' is associated in Tanzania (as in many other countries) with a rigid and yet ineffective bureaucracy subservient to a powerful political party demanding that all individuals conform to a set ideal of society. There are very few decisions an individual may make for himself — where he may live, farm, or run a business. Moreover, conforming with the Party's wishes may cost money — for example, contributions for a new stadium or a hospital. In rural areas the situation is even more difficult than in cities because of the demands of traditional village life. This contributes to the migration of village youth to cities, where life is much more independent of traditional ties.

GOVERNMENT STRATEGIES FOR COMBATING POVERTY AND ILL-HEALTH

The Government of Tanzania has often stressed during the past decade that its development policies will give highest priority to the following objectives:

— Equitable social and economic development.
— Reduction in the bias towards urban areas, by devoting more resources to the development of rural areas.
— Universal primary school education.
— Safe drinking water available to every person.
— National self-reliance in food.

In the Health sector the Government has emphasized the following:

— Universally available free health care.
— Stress on disease prevention rather than cure.
— A health facility within 10 kilometres of every person.

The strategies and programmes to achieve these aims and objectives were to be appropriate to Tanzania's situation as one of the poorest countries in the world. Let us consider what has happened in practice.

Government expenditure

The national budget for 1980/81 gives a reasonably accurate reflection of the government's perceptions of the country's main priorities (see Table 4.3).

Table 4.3. Government of Tanzania Budget Allocations, 1980/81

	Millions of Shillings	% of Total
1. Education	1896	11.6
2. Defence/national service	1511	9.2
3. Industries	1502	9.2
4. Agriculture/livestock	1099	6.7
5. Works/building	1044	6.4
6. Communications/transport	950	5.8
7. Public investment	940	5.7
8. Health	900	5.5
9. Water	647	3.9
10. Police/prison	603	3.7
11. Capital development	258	1.6
12. Others	5033	30.7
	16 383	100.0
	(= approx. US$1.9 billion)	

Source: Tanzania Ministry of Health (1980).

Education, Defence, and Industries get highest priority in government budget allocations. Expenditure on equipment and fuel for the Armed Forces is probably the greatest single drain on the nation's scarce foreign exchange reserves. (The impact of a transfer of only 1 per cent of the Defence budget to the Water or Health sectors could be considerable.) The Health sector is certainly not over-endowed, and its budget for recurrent expenditure actually declined slightly in real terms during the 1970s (see Table 4.4).

Table 4.4. Increases in recurrent expenditure

	1973/74-77/78	1977/78-78/79
Total government	+4%	+36%
Health sector	−1%	−2%

This does not necessarily mean that Health should be allocated more funds than, say, Education, Works, or Agriculture. If all sectors were targeted to have an impact on the country's major health problems, a relatively modest allocation to Health might well be appropriate.

Decentralization and people's participation

The Government of Tanzania has frequently emphasized that one of the corner-stones of its development strategy has been the involvement of the people in discussing, planning, and implementing their development. To make planning more appropriate to the needs of rural people, the government decentralized its administration so that the 95 districts within the 20 regions would have more responsibility for the development of their populations. Villages were to be enabled to make proposals to district administrations and to control their own finances.

Yet in practice attempts at independent planning at village level are not permitted and 'top down' planning remains the norm. Any proposal from a village must pass through several administrative screenings even before it reaches the desk of the District Development Director. By then the plans have been altered so much they are virtually unrecognizable, and the District Committee proceeds to add its own interpretation for good measure.

In the Health sector the people's 'involvement' is usually understood as their compliance with instructions in lectures, or contributions to the building of health facilities. Health workers rarely attempt to learn from village people, and the interdependency of Health and other sectors is largely ignored.

Villagization

A major development strategy of the government during the 1970s was the moving of the rural population into villages. This was done to enable the government to provide services more cheaply and easily, and also to collect agricultural produce for market. It was also envisaged that the planning process would be easier as a result. By 1980 just over 8000 villages had been formed, each with an average population of about 2000. Less than 5 per cent of the rural population of Tanzania currently lives outside villages.

Although many villages already were in existence before this programme and some of these were used as the basis for new, larger settlements, a very large number of small rural communities was moved to new villages established in previously unpopulated areas. Much of this was done in a rushed, forceful, and poorly thought-out manner. Siting was often difficult in areas without water or good farming land.

Village agricultural production was to be based mainly on the collective use of communal land: the communally owned and cultivated fields were supposed to support the entire village and enable it to be self-sufficient in food and cash. The pooled resources would be used to buy fertilizer, insecticides, farm equipment and seed. But too much was expected of the communal land. In many villages this land, lying close to people's homes, has been over-used, resulting in soil erosion, loss of tree cover and finally desertification. As communal land near the village has become exhausted, people have had to walk further and further to their privately owned plots. Poor families have been affected most, since their land is furthest removed from the village. As women do most of the field work, mothers who spend several hours a day walking to and from their fields cannot adequately feed and look after their younger children left behind at home. Pressure to stop breast-feeding early has also increased, since breast-fed infants have to be carried with the mother to the fields.

Urban bias

In 1981, after several years of officially attempting to help the rural majority of the population, the government formally reverted to favouring the urban areas. This emphasis results from an economic theory based on industrialization, economic growth, and increased agricultural productivity through mechanization. Only in this way, so it is argued, can the nation earn sufficient foreign exchange to pay for its fuel, armaments, fertilizer, spare parts, vehicles, and tractors. It is also hoped to increase food production and to establish an industrial base independent of imports.

The urban bias is clearest in the Water sector. Over 85 per cent of urban areas are served with a piped water supply, compared with only 15 per cent of the rural population. This bias will be reinforced by the campaign to provide 'Clean and Potable Water for All by 1990', which will allocate only half the expected expenditure to rural areas, where the needs are greatest and most of the population lives.

In 1981 the government introduced a Bill authorizing the formation of a National Urban Water Supply Authority. Defending the Bill against criticism that it was manifestly unfair to rural areas, the Prime Minister argued that most of the country's industry was in urban areas, and that rural development was heavily dependent on industrial production, which the new Authority sought to revitalise. In what could perhaps be regarded as a strange approach in a nation committed to 'Health for All', he pointed out that a fall in industrial production could reduce revenue from industries such as the Tanzania Cigarette Company (whose contributions to the Treasury equal the entire Health budget). He also reminded MPs that the 1980 election manifesto stated clearly that the urban base was crucial to the country's economic advancement and that it should be developed.

Urban areas are certainly developing, with an annual growth rate of 7 per cent (compared with 3.4 per cent for the country as a whole), mainly due to migration of youth from the villages. There is no doubt that urban dwellers are generally healthier than their rural neighbours. The results of the 1967 Census suggested that the infant mortality rate among families of white collar workers in urban areas was half that of rural families, and life expectancy was 10 years longer.

Food and money

The Tanzanian Food and Nutrition Council (1980) believes that the main nutrition problem in Tanzania is low food intake rather than a deficiency of specific nutrients. About 25 per cent of Tanzanian children do not get adequate food, and the problem is compounded when feeding is infrequent, as is often the case among the poor when the mother has to work long hours away from the home. Surveys in various parts of the country have found malnutrition co-existing with poverty in 90 per cent of cases.

The Council also noted that cash crops such as sugar, cashew nuts, coffee, and tea have received most government attention, while food industries of nutritional importance (flour-milling, meat and dairy industries, vegetables, oils, and fisheries) have been neglected. Though farmers are exhorted to grow drought-resistant crops, marketing and processing facilities are poorly developed and prices are too low to act as an incentive to greater production.

A well-researched study (Jakobsen 1978) in the Southern Highlands has attributed an increase in malnutrition to the growth of the monetary economy. The study found nutritional levels highest among families who had stayed out-side the monetary economy and still clung to subsistence farming. The author of the study drew a graph (Fig. 4.2) showing that it was only when monetary income exceeded a certain level that nutritional status rose again. Money intro-duced a new method of obtaining status — by buying beer, iron roofing, shoes, radios, etc. — and these purchases conflicted with the need to buy adequate food for the family.

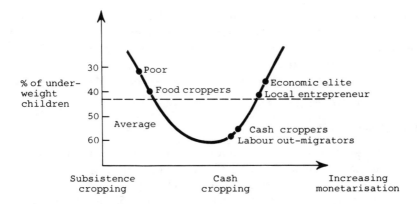

Fig. 4.2. The proportion of underweight children – and thus those with malnutrition – increases as farmers move from subsistence to cash cropping and monetarization.

Status of women

Although there is an official section of the Party for women, and women are supposed to enjoy equal rights with men, this is not the case for most rural women (especially those from poor families). Rural women are still expected to do most of the work in the fields and to rear the family. This has significant effects on health – poor maternal nutrition contributes to low birth weight, and a mother spending most of her working day in the fields finds it hard to devote enough time to feeding and generally caring for her young children. The fact that the husband controls the family purse strings makes it even more difficult for mothers to purchase adequate food for the whole family.

Education

Tanzania has made great efforts to ensure that every one of its citizens achieves at least a primary school education. Most villages now have a building that serves as a primary school. The main problem is the quality, quantity, and distribution of teachers. A major effort is also being made to ensure that every adult attains a certain minimum level of literacy. The effects on health of this commitment to education and literacy, however, lie at least a generation away, since the foundations have only just been laid and the significance of education for health depends mainly on the level reached by mothers.

Ideals far from realization

Despite the official commitment of the Government of Tanzania to achieving greater social equity and eliminating poverty, ignorance, and disease, these ideals are still far from being achieved. Perhaps in the longer term the government's policies and strategies will benefit the majority of Tanzanians. At the moment, however, the main thrust of the government's development efforts is favouring the better-off groups, especially those living in urban areas. This trend is also evident in the Health sector.

THE HEALTH SECTOR

Hospital and urban bias

The Health sector is no exception to the urban bias of the government's approach to development. Despite the relative success of efforts to provide a health facility within 10 kilometres of every person, the country's rural areas still have poor health services. Only one-third of the total of 8153 villages has a health centre, dispensary, or first-aid post. The other two-thirds have no health facilities at all. Although the number of rural health centres and dispensaries has more than doubled during the two decades of independence, the number of hospitals has also risen by 50 per cent (see Table 4.5).

Table 4.5. Development of health facilities in Tanzania, 1961-78

	1961	1965	1969	1971	1973	1978
Rural health centres	22	40	50	87	108	220
Dispensaries	975	1236	1362	1436	1515	2308
Hospitals	98	109	121	123	123	151

Sources: Chagula and Tarimo (1975); Tanzania Ministry of Health (1980).

In the early 1970s hospital services consumed almost 80 per cent of the Health budget. This figure fell to 60 per cent in 1974/75 but has shown no signs of declining any further (see Table 4.6).

Table 4.6. Total health budget, Government of Tanzania, 1970/71-1978/79, by sector (percentages)

	1970/71	1971/72	1972/73	1973/74	1974/75	1978/79
Hospital services	79.8	78.9	71.6	69.0	60.2	60.0
Rural health centres and dispensaries	9.1	10.9	18.3	19.3	19.1	19.0
Preventive services	5.0	3.9	3.9	4.7	12.4	11.0
Training	2.4	3.1	3.5	4.8	6.3	6.0
Others	3.7	3.2	2.7	2.2	2.0	4.0

Sources: Chagula and Tarimo (1975); Tanzania Ministry of Health (1980).

The concentration of Health sector expenditure on hospitals is doubly in-appropriate. First, hospitals serve mainly the relatively well-off urban popu-lation (14 per cent of the total) rather than the poor, who live mostly in rural areas. Second, hospitals provide mainly curative services rather than a service aimed primarily at disease prevention.

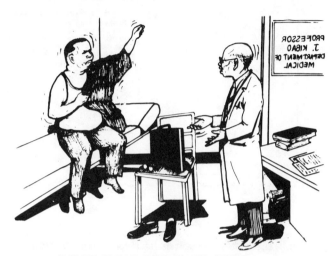

"I AM HAPPY TO SAY IT IS NOT YOUR HEART, MINISTER! ... BUT JUST INDIGESTION! ... HOWEVER, YOU KNOW WE HAVE NO CORONARY CARE UNIT IF IT HAD BEEN YOUR HEART! ..."

Fig. 4.3. Hospitals serve mainly the relatively well-off urban elite.

The cost of maintaining the expanding network of hospitals in Tanzania is crippling. For once a hospital is built, its recurrent costs become a large and permanent drain on the Health budget (see Fig. 4.4).

Some 45 per cent of hospital current expenditure goes on salaries, 25 per cent on drugs, and 13 per cent on food for patients. It is instructive to note that the main government hospital in the capital city, Dar es Salaam, consumed 14 per cent of the nation's total drug budget, compared with 15 per cent used by all the country's 220 health centres and 2300 dispensaries. The cost of treating an out-patient at a hospital is considerably higher than a health centre or dis-pensary (see Table 4.7).

The recurrent costs of one hospital seeing 137 000 out-patients per year are equal to those of 53 dispensaries which together see a total of 1 060 000 out-patients. The wastage incurred by heavy reliance on hospital services is indicated by a Ministry of Health Report (1980), which found that 27 per cent of all patients seen at hospitals could have been treated at a lower level or used self-medication. By comparison, 98 per cent of patients seen at health centres and dispensaries had gone to the appropriate level.

The heavy burden placed on the Health budget by hospitals means that rural

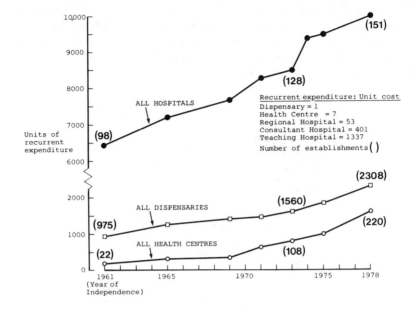

Fig. 4.4. The recurrent costs of hospitals have far outstripped those of dispensaries and health centres.

health facilities, where they exist at all, are often inadequately equipped and poorly maintained. Surveys of 2243 rural dispensaries in 1979 found that:

— 41 per cent had a working refrigerator
— 42 per cent had a working scale for weighing children
— 33 per cent had a working microscope
— 33 per cent had measles vaccine in store
— 37 per cent had an adequate supply of basic medicines
— 30 per cent had under-five growth cards.

Table 4.7. Recurrent expenditure and performance of various health facilities, 1978/79

	Recurrent expenditure per unit (Shillings)	Expenditure per out-patient visit (Shillings)	Expenditure per in-patient day (Shillings)	No. of out-patients per unit	No. of in-patient days per unit
Hospital (region or district)	2 800 000	4.6	53	137 000	36 400
Health centres	256 000	2.6	29	50 000	3800
Dispensaries	37 400	1.9	–	20 000	–

Source: Tanzania Ministry of Health (1980).

But apart from the question of the allocation of the Health sector budget, the government is genuinely handicapped by an acute lack of resources for the Health sector as a whole. For example, if the government tried to provide the 5497 villages that currently have no health facilities with at least one dispensary each, the recurrent costs alone would amount to 28 per cent of the 1978/79 Health budget – not to mention the capital costs in the first place. Such expenditure is out of the question at Tanzania's present stage of economic development.

It is therefore all the more surprising that the Government of Tanzania plans to construct two major consultant referral hospitals and several regional and district hospitals in the near future. These new facilities will only add to the recurrent expenditure burden and make little contribution to solving the health problems of the poor.

Village health workers

In an attempt to get around these financial constraints, the government has started another plan to place two village health workers (VHWs) in every one of the country's 8153 villages. Several attempts have been made, especially since 1971, to persuade villages to choose people for training as VHWs and to support them financially afterwards. The history of these efforts has been similar to that in other countries where health workers have been selected and trained in the absence of any fundamental changes to improve the position of the poor in society. Few VHWs have worked in their villages for long and in the few places where they have continued their work is mainly curative medical intervention, rather than disease-preventive support for those whose health is most at risk.

But given the ways in which these earlier efforts were organized, such disappointing results were inevitable. The selection procedure was badly handled; villages were sent a short letter demanding the selection of one or two people as trainee VHWs, without any description of their required abilities, potential duties, and responsibilities, and without any discussions between village people and health-service authorities. The feeling arose in many places that the VHWs were yet more government workers, placed in villages so the government would not have to meet the expense of establishing a large number of village dispensaries.

It is difficult to know whether the new proposals will differ radically from previous efforts to train VHWs. Some previous deficiencies are being patched over. Instead of expecting villagers to pay for their own health workers' salaries, the VHWs will receive a government allowance – totalling about 10 per cent of the 1978/79 Health budget (assuming all 8153 villages receive two VHWs). Recognizing that previous training courses were inadequate, the government is first training the trainers and drawing up a syllabus for a six-month VHW course. And to induce VHWs to work in their own villages, they will have automatic upgrading rights in return for a promise to work a certain minimum time in their own villages. International donor agencies have made substantial commitments to get this new programme started. It is quite unclear, however, how the Health budget can support these professional VHWs. They will need transport and medical supplies, which will cost as much as their allowances. If existing dispensaries and health centres cannot be maintained in satisfactory working order, it is difficult to envisage how this greatly expanded new system can function effectively. The possibility of substantially boosting the Health budget to meet these increased costs seems remote, with other sectors also clamouring for more money.

Pressure of political decisions

Despite these criticisms, the author has worked with many Tanzanians (at all levels and in every sector of society) who feel strongly about the plight of the rural poor, and who are seeking solutions to their problems of poverty and ill-health. They accept the constraints of the changes in society caused by modernization, they realize that no single policy is perfect for all the people, and – above all – they try to formulate plans that are within existing financial and institutional constraints. But despite all the efforts of these people, their logic and pragmatic commitment are often over-ruled in favour of local or national political considerations. The commonest example in the Health sector is that of hospitals. It is clearly against official national development policy and the people's real interests that more hospitals continue to be built. Yet, somehow, more get built. Many similar examples lie buried in the reports of meetings of District, Regional, and National Development Committees.

CONCLUSIONS

This article began with the assertion that 'prevention' costs more than 'cure'. In other words, the conditions necessary for *all* the people to enjoy good health – adequate food, employment, education, water supplies, housing, sanitation, welfare services, and health care – amount to much more than the expenditure on the Health sector alone.

Despite the Government of Tanzania's stated commitment to equitable social and economic development, there has been no effective reallocation of public resources in favour of rural areas, where most of the population happens to live and most poverty exists. Perhaps the political cost of such a radical step would have been too high. After all, urban dwellers are much better organized, more militant and better placed to exert pressure on government than their country cousins.

Even within the Health sector itself, 'prevention' has lost out to 'cure'. Most resources continue to be poured into hospitals concentrating on curative problems and serving mainly urban populations. Lip-service is still paid to the goal of 'Health for All' but this has yet to be translated into strategies and programmes that match up the people's basic health needs with the financial and human

resources available. The new Village Health Worker programme shows considerable promise, but whether it will be adequately funded for long enough remains
to be seen. The gap between rhetoric and reality in the Health sector in Tanzania
shows some signs of closing, but on present trends the promise of 'Health for
All' will take a long time to realize.

REFERENCES

Chagula, W.K. and Tarimo, E., Meeting Basic Health Needs in Tanzania. In
    Health by the people (ed. K. Newell). WHO, Geneva (1975).
Jakobsen, O., *Economic and geographical factors influencing child malnutrition
    — a study from the Southern Highlands, Tanzania*, BRALUP paper No. 52.
    University of Dar es Salaam (1978).
Newell, Kenneth (ed.), *Health by the people*. WHO, Geneva (1975).
*Proceedings of 15th Post-graduate KCMC Seminar on Community Health,
    October 1979*. Papers by K.N.M. Mtera, A.D. Chidua, E.S. Mwasha, F.D.E.
    Mtango.
Tanzania Food and Nutrition Council, *Food and nutrition policy for Tanzania
    for 1st Tanzania Nutrition Conference*, Report No. 483 (1980).
Tanzania Ministry of Health, *Evaluation of the Health Sector 1979* (1980).
WHO/UNICEF, *Primary health care*. WHO, Geneva (1978).

5 Social justice and the demographic transition: lessons from India's Kerala State*

John Ratcliffe explains how the Indian State of Kerala, despite low per capita income, has dramatically reduced mortality and fertility through emphasizing equitable socio-economic and political development.

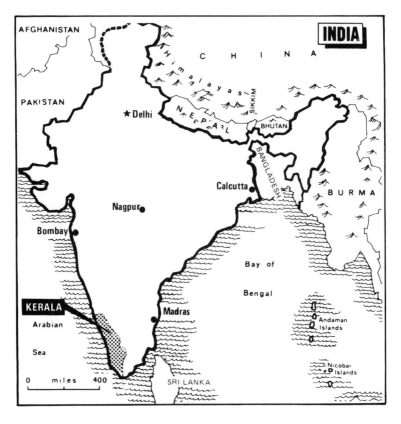

John Ratcliffe, Ph.D., is Head of Health Education in the School of Public Health, University of California, Berkley. He is also a consultant to the World Bank, UNFPA, and other international agencies.

*An earlier version of this article appeared as 'Social justice and the demographic transition: lessons from India's Kerala State' in *International Journal of Health Services* 8, No. 1, 123–44 (1978).

The small State of Kerala, located at the south-western tip of the Indian peninsula, gives little impression – at least on the surface – that it is playing a significant and exciting role in the Indian demographic context. It is a poor State, even by Indian standards. Its per capita income of US $135 is substantially lower than the all-India average of US $190. The daily per capita calorie intake is well below the all-India average. With a population of 25.4 million in an area of 38 864 square kilometres, the state is extremely crowded. The population density of 550 persons per square kilometre exceeds even that of Bangladesh. In addition, since its formation in 1956, Kerala's political history has been stormy, including a three-year period of Communist rule.

Perhaps because of its history of political turbulence, Kerala has not received much attention from Indian development planners. Expectations and inputs have been highest for Maharashtra State, the most industrially advanced State, of which India's premier city of Bombay is a bustling seaport, and Punjab State, the most agriculturally advanced State and home of the 'Green Revolution'. Nevertheless, Kerala has managed to surpass not only these States, but all the Indian States, in certain important measures of social development. For example, 69.2 per cent of Kerala citizens are literate, compared to 36.1 per cent of all Indians. Life expectancy at birth is 63.8 years, compared to 52.0 for all-India. The crude death rate for Kerala was 7.5 per thousand population in 1978, when the all-India rate was 14.5. Kerala has an infant mortality rate of 55, compared to 125 for all-India, and the rural crude birth rate in 1974 was 26.4 per thousand population in Kerala whereas it was 33.3 for all-India.

How did such a large population with levels of income and nutrition among the lowest in the world achieve levels of fertility and mortality substantially lower than surrounding populations with similar cultural backgrounds but higher incomes and caloric intakes? The answer to this question holds profound implications for all nations concerned with population, health, and social and economic development.

DEVELOPMENT STRATEGIES AND EQUITY CONSIDERATIONS

According to the social justice theory of demographic transition, demographic trends and levels reflect the degree to which existing political and economic institutions promulgate social justice. If this theory is valid, observed shifts in Kerala's demographic rates should be consequences of identifiable shifts from less to more social justice in Kerala's political and economic policies and development strategies. This analytical approach necessarily requires examination of a broader range of factors than those considered by conventional demographic theory to be relevant and explanatory. In particular, those factors that tend most clearly to distinguish Kerala's political economy from that of other Indian states require the most careful examination as opposed to those variables 'expected' to be causal given the assumptions basic to western demographic theory. Not surprisingly, Kerala's political economy contrasts most sharply with those of other Indian States in exactly those areas that, in other contexts, have been found to be associated with observed declines in fertility and mortality.

Income distribution

Mounting evidence indicates that agrarian reform is the most significant and effective approach to achieving a more equitable distribution of income in under-developed societies. Kerala, in sharp contrast to the rest of India, has success-fully implemented strategies to reform the land tenure system. The first attempts at land reform in Kerala took place in the southern-most region of Travancore in the late nineteenth century under the rule of a progressive Maharaja. However, land simply deeded to peasants with no experience in or knowledge of farming and in the absence of such supporting services as agricultural extension and credit tends to be relatively unproductive and to revert back to large landholders (either through sale or debt repayment) in bad years. Therefore, early attempts at agrarian reform remained largely ineffective for Kerala as a whole until the late 1950s.

In the 1930s the deteriorating conditions of tenants and agricultural labourers led to numerous mass movements demanding effective land reform. These move-ments were strengthened by the decision in 1956 to merge Travancore, Cochin State, and the district of Malabar and form the State of Kerala. This move drama-tically altered the balance of political power in these combined regions and resulted in a climate conducive to fundamental agrarian reform. Such reform was in fact the centrepiece of the development strategies espoused by the Communist Party of India (CPI), which was brought to power in the first general elections following formation of Kerala State in 1956.

The first legislative act passed by the CPI government made it illegal to evict agricultural tenants. In 1957 a set of proposals designed to accomplish radical and comprehensive agrarian reform aroused great opposition among the power-ful landholders in the State, resulting in a period of political turmoil and leading to the removal of the CPI from power in 1959 by means of an unconstitutional presidential decree. A coalition government was formed following new elections, but political pressures exerted by the citizenry made it necessary to continue pursuit of agrarian reform. As a result, some such reform was legislated and implemented during the late 1950s and early 1960s. A careful study of the impact of reform legislation in Kerala concludes that '. . . there is no reason to doubt that land reforms in Kerala taken as a whole have helped to reduce in-equalities in wealth and income, despite the limitations of the legislation and the impediments to its effective implementation' (Raj 1975, p. 70). Thus, land re-form, even though imperfectly implemented, has served to redistribute income within the state of Kerala. This experience is in sharp contrast with land reform measures legislated in the rest of India, where such reform either has not been implemented at all or has been implemented in such a way as to favour the privileged few.[1]

Factors other than land reform have also been operating in Kerala to reduce income disparities. Landholders in Kerala are relatively more dependent than elsewhere in India upon hired labour for the bulk of agricultural work, even on small holdings. As a result, a larger than expected number of landless labourers are absorbed into wage employment. In addition, an exceptionally large number of landholders report that their primary source of income is derived from a non-agricultural (i.e. service or industry) sector.

Wage rates are also extraordinarily high in Kerala, ranking second only to Punjab in all of India. Kerala's relatively high wage rates result, evidently, from a combination of factors. Tenant farmers have become less dependent upon wage labour to eke out their income; therefore, landless labourers enjoy an improved bargaining power. Activity in the industrial and service sectors, relative to other Indian States, appears to be more labour intensive than capital intensive in nature. It is therefore likely that a greater proportion of the labour force is participating actively and productively in the economy and therefore sharing in the overall distribution of income than would otherwise be the case.[2]

Recent legislation has also acted further to reduce income inequalities in Kerala. A bill passed in 1974 was designed not only to provide security of employment to agricultural labourers, a first in India, but also better terms and conditions of work, including welfare ('provident') and pension funds. In addition, some two million labourers now receive the benefit of a Labourer's Welfare Fund. Under this law employers contribute 5 per cent of the employee's wage, and the employee receives the money accrued at age 60. Employees who work in industry, services, and government receive pensions upon retirement (usually at age 54) under provisions of earlier legislation.

In sum, a number of factors unique to Kerala State in all of India are operating to reduce long-standing inequities among Keralites, even though average income remains low. That these factors have successfully reduced inequities is not in doubt. In all-India, for example, the decade 1961 to 1971 saw the highest income groups increase their proportional share of asset holdings over other income groups by some 5 percentage points. In only three states did the poorest income groups gain on the rich – Kerala, Maharashtra, and Jammu and Kashmir. Among these three States Kerala exhibited the largest recorded increase in share of asset holdings among the lowest income groups.

Education

One of the most telling differences that exists between Kerala State and the rest of India is the approach to education as a development strategy. Table 5.1 provides an indication of just how substantial that difference is. High literacy rates result directly from policy decisions taken in Kerala to skew educational inputs toward the poor majority instead of the privileged few. Free education at the primary level was introduced in Travancore in the first decade of the twentieth century, in Cochin during the second decade, and in Malabar in the third decade.

Table 5.1. Literacy rates in India, 1981

State	Total (%)	Male (%)	Female (%)
Andrha Pradesh	29.9	39.1	20.5
Assam	–	–	–
Bihar	26.0	37.8	13.6
Gujarat	43.8	54.5	32.3
Haryana	35.8	47.8	22.2
Himachal Pradesh	41.9	52.3	31.4
Jammu and Kashmir	26.2	35.5	15.3
Karnataka	38.4	48.6	27.8
Kerala	69.2	74.0	64.5
Madhya Pradesh	27.8	39.4	15.3
Maharashtra	47.4	58.9	35.1
Manipur	42.0	53.0	30.7
Meghalaya	33.2	37.0	29.3
Nagaland	42.0	49.2	33.7
Orissa	34.1	46.9	21.1
Punjab	40.7	46.6	34.1
Rajasthan	24.0	35.8	11.3
Tamil Nadu	45.8	57.2	34.1
Tripura	41.6	51.0	31.6
Uttar Pradesh	27.4	38.9	14.4
West Bengal	40.9	50.5	30.3
All-India	36.1	46.6	24.8

Source: Registrar General of India, Census of India, 1981, Series 1, *India*, Paper 1 of *Provisional Population Totals*, New Delhi (1981).

Middle school (higher primary) was made free only following the formation of the state of Kerala in 1956, and secondary education became free shortly thereafter, in the early 1960s. In terms of allocation of educational expenditure, fully 86 per cent of the total is expended on primary and secondary schooling.

Two consequences have arisen from this policy focus. First, there are relatively few college-trained persons in Kerala, for university-level education receives minimal government support and is therefore accessible only to a few. Second, universal primary education and mass literacy have become accomplished facts. Illiteracy among the 5–15 year age group is virtually non-existent, and functional literacy, even among the older adult population, is increasing at an incredible rate. In fact, a recent study of education in Kerala concludes:

'The limits to achievement, at least in terms of ensuring a minimum level of education to a great majority of the population, thus appear to have been reached in Kerala. Scope for further progress lies in improving the quality of education, particularly in terms of what is being taught at the primary school and beyond, and strengthening it with respect to its vocational content' (Krishnaji 1975, p. 126).

Thus, the Kerala experience confounds the notion, widely accepted among educational planners, that an acute shortage of investible resources makes it all but impossible to attain universal primary education in a poor society without diverting scarce resources from other more productive investments. In fact, the critical influence of deliberate public policy decisions becomes clear when the Kerala experience is contrasted to the rest of India.

In India as a whole, actual allocations of educational resources at both the State and central levels continue to subsidize the education of dominant castes and classes at the expense of the poor majority. While Kerala spends less than 12 per cent of its educational budget on higher education (all university, professional, and technical), in the rest of India fully 47 per cent of the total educational outlay (central and States) is allocated to university education — an education enjoyed by only 0.02 per cent of the population.

Political participation

Not coincidentally, Kerala State demonstrates a pattern of political development unique in all of India. Although the influence of Communism in Kerala has been substantial, relatively little has been written on this phenomenon. While the origins of the CPI movement in Kerala are somewhat obscure, the successes of the party were clearly rooted in its ability to organize lower class and caste peasants dissatisfied and frustrated by oppressive land-tenure systems.

The actual achievements of the CPI in its brief period of power were relatively small. However, even after it was removed from power, the CPI was able to maintain a position of considerable influence due to its popularity among the poor majority. Even though the CPI lost its legislative majority in the general elections brought on by the presidential decree in 1959, the party received over one million votes more than it had received in the 1957 elections. This wide popularity of the CPI and the development strategies it advocated during its brief reign have forced successive governments to pursue, often reluctantly, the policies initiated by their predecessor.

Many facets of Kerala's social, political, and economic context today are the legacy of a powerful Communist influence on the State. Kerala now enjoys a degree of social and economic mobility unknown in the rest of India except in the largest cities; yet in the recent past, Kerala had a caste tradition as powerful, rigid, and prevalent as anywhere in India. Recent analyses of Kerala politics conclude that these shifts are consequences of the period of strong Communist influence which imparted a dignity to and raised the political consciousness of the poor majority to such high levels that it is now believed that the poor will never again yield to suppression.

But other, more tangible evidence exists to demonstrate the Communist influence at work in Kerala. Following the election of the CPI, per-pupil expenditures on elementary education more than doubled, from Rs 35 in 1960-61 to Rs 80 in 1970-71. Other legislation affecting the distribution of income and resources within the State, such as land reform and health services, has already been mentioned. But land reform measures, while introduced by the CPI in 1957, were strongly resisted by the politically powerful landlord class, and serious implementation was not undertaken until the early 1960s — and then due only to 'the political environment which has kept up sustained pressure on this issue' (Raj 1975, p.59). Peasant organization, the strongest of any Indian state, has forced the government to act with relative alacrity on minimum wage and other progressive legislation. Job security and pensions to landless labourers have already been mentioned. And the pressure continues to increase. For example, of the 59 agricultural labour unions registered up to July 1974, 39 have been registered since January 1970. Unions and other peasant organizations have ensured that laws pertaining to labour, such as minimum wage and child labour laws, are enforced rather than ignored, as is the case in the rest of India. And, perhaps most importantly,

'... external capital, with the single exception of a midday meals (schools nutrition) programme provided by CARE, had nothing to do with Kerala's development; the basic factor was political action' (Raj 1976).

Health services

Kerala's health services provide yet another example of how education and political involvement can act to determine the success or failure of a development strategy. As Table 5.2 shows, Kerala enjoys the highest utilization rate of health facilities among the Indian States for which data are available, even though eight other States spend more per capita on health services.

The reasons for this situation may not be obvious to those without international field experience, so some explanation is in order. In all Indian States, there exists a clear bias in favour of central areas in the distribution of resources and the health care system is no exception. Medical practitioners with political influence receive the more desirable assignments to central areas (cities and large towns), while those without influence are assigned to the periphery (rural areas). And, due again to political influence, supplies and equipment officially allocated to peripheral areas are, in fact, diverted to urban facilities and, particularly, to large hospitals. Thus, there exists in virtually all Indian States an actual maldistribution of health supplies and equipment that favours the urban centres.

Further, even those health resources and supplies that do reach their destination are not equitably distributed among the population to be served. Health professionals in India, as in most developing countries, tend to distribute 'their' services and supplies in ways that are most beneficial to themselves; those among the dominant castes and classes who possess the power to influence present and future positions of health professionals have priority access to 'public' health services. The lower number of people 'served' in the Indian system of public health (as well as most other public and private systems supposedly designed to

Table 5.2. Utilization of health services, by Indian states

State	No. of beds per 100 000 population	Per capita expenditure on health, 1972–73 (Rupees)	No. of patients treated per 100 000 population
Andhra Pradesh	66.4	6.38	79
Assam	44.0	5.64	24
Bihar	33.5	4.89	10
Gujarat	58.6	9.17	165
Jammu and Kashmir	92.5	11.51	69
Karnataka	80.9	8.88	152
Kerala	84.7	8.64	210
Madhya Pradesh	40.3	7.26	10
Maharashtra	81.2	11.21	27
Orissa	44.5	6.77	44
Punjab	66.5	11.29	166
Rajasthan	61.9	8.97	61
Tamil Nadu	47.9	9.05	110
Uttar Pradesh	34.7	4.87	44
West Bengal	84.5	8.68	108

Source: *Poverty, unemployment and development policy; a case study of selected issues with reference to Kerala*, p. 139. ST/ESA/29, United Nations, New York (1975).

serve the many) exists apparently because of widespread ignorance and the absence of political organization among the poor majority. Those who lack a clear understanding both of their rights of access to public services and of the political process are easily manipulated and bypassed, and are thus powerless to enter or influence the system. While maldistribution of public resources in Kerala has not been eliminated, it has been much reduced due to a widespread understanding of both individual rights of access and political processes. Malfeasance and favouritism on the part of medical practitioners are not well tolerated by Keralites, who use the power of the press and the vote to force the system to be responsive to their demands. Because of these factors, Kerala's health system responds to a constituency considerably broader and more powerful than that in other Indian States.

Political action has thus been a critical factor in the successful implementation of any and all development strategies undertaken in Kerala. But the key to understanding Kerala's development experience is to recognize that the strategies themselves have been distributive and inclusive in nature. Political power and participation are not concentrated among the few, but have become widespread due to the deliberate actions of certain political groups. In terms of social and economic development strategies, Kerala's successes have been achieved not by the allocation of more resources, but rather through a more equitable distribution of existing resources, goods, and services. And the distributive political economy that distinguishes Kerala so clearly from other states has also been largely responsible for mortality and fertility declines.

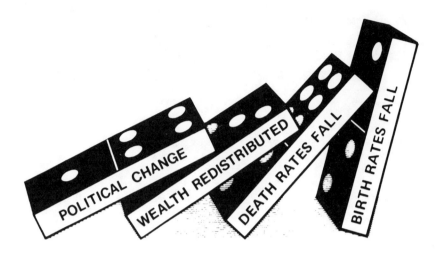

Fig. 5.1. The 'domino theory' of development: political action leads to more equitable distribution of resources, improved public health and lower birth rates.

Mortality declines

Mortality declines, like the spread of education, have been more rapid and substantial in Kerala than elsewhere in India, and it has been postulated (Panikar 1975) that these declines have resulted from a combination of the application of previous health measures and the spread of education. The role of education has been seen as one largely facilitating the application of modern technology. For example, it is felt that education served to minimize the extent to which measures such as smallpox vaccinations were hindered by traditional religious beliefs. While these factors may be important, they cannot fully explain the recent rapid decline in Kerala's death rates to the low levels shown in Table 5.3.

The Kerala experience is consistent with extensive research data (World Bank 1975, pp. 31-6) demonstrating that mortality rates are more closely associated with income, education and broad nutritional levels than with the spread of health services. Indeed, one investigation of Kerala's mortality decline (Panikar 1975) concludes that the extension of health facilities could not have significantly influenced observed mortality reductions, for mortality declines in much of the state occurred prior to the extension of such facilities. The observation that mortality declines occurred earlier in regions with higher literacy rates led to the conclusion that education interacted with preventive health measures in a strong, positive fashion to facilitate reductions in mortality. But other reasons also exist.

There now exists some evidence that the national study (Dandekar and Rath 1971) which claimed that 90 per cent of Kerala's citizens were malnourished in 1961-1962 may systematically have underestimated tapioca (cassava) intake

Table 5.3. Crude death rates (CDR) and infant mortality rates (IMR) per population for Kerala and all-India, selected years[a]

Year	Kerala		All-India	
	CDR	IMR	CDR	IMR
1941[b]	25.0	–	31.2	161
1952[c]	20.0	120	27.4	146
1956[d]	17.0	115	–	–
1961	16.1	90	22.8	134
1966	13.0	70	–	–
1971	9.2	55	16.9	122
1974	7.9	–	14.4	–
1976	–	55	–	132
1978	7.5	–	14.5	125

[a] Sources: *Demographic Situation in India*, pp. 65–9, National Institute of Family Planning (1974); *SRS/Sample Registration Scheme/Bulletin*, Nos. 2 and 3 (1974); *Pocket Book of Census Statistics* p. 92 (1972); *SRS Bulletin*, No. 4 (1975); *Sample Registration Bulletin*, Vol. 14, No. 1 (1980).
[b] Travancore State.
[c] Travencore and Cochin.
[d] Figures for 1956–78 are for Kerala State.

among the poorer classes. There also exists substantial evidence to indicate that nutritional levels have improved since that time (Krishnaji 1975).

Higher wages due to unionization and worker enforcement of labour and wage laws have acted to increase incomes for a substantial number of the landless poor. Land reform has affected at least 1.25 million households, with the demonstrable consequence of increased productivity (Raj 1975, p.69). This increased productivity from agrarian reform results not only from the new owners' increased motivation to maximize production, but also from the direct access, which ownership confers with one stroke, to such essential associated inputs as credit, fertilizer, seed and agricultural extension service.

Such increased productivity affects not only the nutritional levels of the new landowners and their families, but also the landless who benefit from any overall increase in food production and availability. And further increases in productivity were forthcoming in the 1960s due to the introduction of new high-yield (double that of traditional varieties) strains of tapioca. Tapioca production rose from 1.6 million tons in 1961–62 to 5.4 million tons in 1971–72 (Panikar 1975, pp.28–9). This factor is important for two reasons: the average per-hectare yield of tapioca is several times that of rice, and tapioca is the staple diet of the poor.

Another factor affecting nutritional status is the government ration shops that distribute food (primarily grains) at controlled prices. In most of India, such shops are available primarily in urban centres and, particularly in times of food shortages, are accessible only to the relatively advantaged classes; others are forced to buy food grains at uncontrolled, and often black market prices.

Widespread education and political participation in Kerala have resulted in a system of ration shops that covers virtually the entire population and, more importantly, is equally accessible to all social groups.

Kerala provides clear evidence that nutritional levels are influenced by educational levels. A diet survey of Kerala housewives at various income levels has demonstrated the positive influence education exerts upon caloric intake, at least above certain threshold levels. As Table 5.4 shows, the level of education makes no difference in the number of calorie-deficient persons seen in very low income households, presumably because there is simply not enough income to purchase food for all. But above the lowest income level, education apparently makes a substantial difference. In the Rs 100–250 category, for example, 98 per cent of those in illiterate households were found to be calorie-deficient, while in literate households only 70 per cent were so classified.

Table 5.4. Average per capita caloric intake per day and proportion of calorie-deficient persons classified by monthly income and education of housewife[a]

Education of housewife	Household income per month (Rupees)				
	Below 100	100 to 250	250 to 500	Above 500	All classes
Illiterate	1577 (93.9)[b]	1365 (97.7)	1575 (83.8)	– –	1471 (93.6)
Literate but below SSLC[c]	1432 (94.9)	1994 (70.5)	2213 (59.2)	2512 (43.2)	2108 (54.1)
SSLC and above[c]	– –	– –	2292 (35.3)	3062 (0.0)	2861 (9.2)
All classes	1513 (94.3)	1761 (80.6)	2088 (62.0)	2728 (26.2)	2010 (66.5)

[a] Source, Diet Survey, p. c–11, Centre for Development Studies. Trivandrum (1973/1974).
[b] Figures in parentheses are percentages of calorie-deficient persons to the total within each cell.
[c] SSLC = Secondary School Leaving Certificate (i.e. high-school graduate).

Kerala has the lowest average per capita caloric intake among the Indian states. Yet the intake of nutrients among pre-school children, a group particularly vulnerable to nutritional deficiencies, shows Kerala to rank above most other states, particularly at very low income levels. Clearly, as one investigator concludes:

'. . . given the level of income, the ability to allocate it in such a way as to meet minimal requirements improves with the level of education' (Krishnaji 1975, p. 39).

The Kerala experience thus provides further evidence that measures which affect the social environment are necessary to reduce mortality rates beyond the levels achieved by affecting the physical environment (e.g. through eradication of malaria-carrying mosquitos).

Fertility decline

Table 5.5 indicates that Kerala's crude birth rate has begun to decline in recent years in relation to the all-India average. During the period 1931–61, Kerala's birth rate appears to have remained fairly steady, beginning its rapid decline only after 1961. While there was little difference between the birth rates of Kerala and India during the 1941–50 period, the rates began to diverge noticeably after 1956. These data are consistent with the body of evidence (World Bank 1975, pp. 40–3) suggesting that declines in both mortality and fertility to modern low levels are demographic responses to broad improvements in economic equity and social development. Certainly, reductions in both areas of a magnitude such as to clearly distinguish Kerala's demographic trends and levels from those of the rest of India awaited the structural changes of the 1950s and 1960s in the political economy of the state that favoured the interests of the poor majority.

Table 5.5. Comparison of crude birth rates (CBR) per thousand population in Kerala and all-India[a]

Period/year	Kerala CBR	All-India CBR
1931–1940[b]	40.0	45.2
1941–1950[c]	39.8	39.9
1956[d]	39.8	–
1961	38.9	41.7
1966[e]	37.4	–
1967	36.3	–
1968	33.2	39.0
1969	31.3	38.8
1970	31.9	38.8
1971	31.3	38.9
1972	31.5	38.4
1973	29.9	–
1974	26.9	35.9
1978	26.4	33.3

[a] Sources, reference 3, p. 1205; Demographic Situations in India, pp. 65–69, National Institute of Family Planning (1974); *Sample Registration Bulletin*, Vol. 14, No. 1 (1980).
[b] Travancore State.
[c] Travancore and Cochin.
[d] Figures for 1956–78 are for Kerala State.
[e] Data for 1966–78 are for rural areas, where 90 per cent of the Indian population lives. Rural figures were unavailable before this time.

Indeed, fertility in Kerala appears to have responded largely to many of those same factors that were responsible for the more recent reductions in mortality.

Table 5.6. Per cent literate among those adopting sterilization in Kerala State[a]

Period	Males	Females
1961–62	93	72
1962–63	92	78
1963–64	74	75
1964–65	75	79
1965–66	81	77
1966–67	81	81

[a] Source: Demographic Research Centre, *Kerala Fact Book*, p. 28, Government of Kerala (1969).

The strongest association in the population literature for years has been the inverse relationship that exists between education and fertility. The Kerala experience again, presents no exception, as evidenced by Tables 5.6 and 5.7, showing the educational levels of those adopting programme contraception. But the effects of education go beyond merely facilitating the adoption of contraceptive technology. It is well known in India that:

'Illiteracy remains the greatest barrier to any improvement in the position of women – in employment, health, the enjoyment and exercise of legal and constitutional rights, equal opportunity in education, and generally in attaining the equality of status that our Constitution has declared as the goal of this nation' (Government of India 1975, p. 264).

Female literacy in Kerala has increased enormously since the 1950s. In 1961 the female literacy rate was 39 per cent; today it is 64.5 per cent (Registrar General of India 1981). The next highest state, Maharashtra, has a female literacy rate of only 35.1 per cent, just over half that of Kerala. And the all-India average is 24.8 per cent. While in the rest of India '. . . the education system itself is tending to increase social segregation and to perpetuate and widen class distinctions' (Government of India 1975, p. 10), in Kerala it is not. The status and social mobility of women in Kerala appear to be increasing directly with educational attainment. As one example, increasing numbers of women are entering the service sector, which depends upon literate staff for existence. The service sector has been expanding rapidly, but not at a pace which can absorb the increasing numbers of educated Keralites. Therefore, there has been substantial export of the educated, including women, to other States. For example, the majority of auxiliary nurse-midwives (women paramedics who are the mainstay of rural health delivery) in many Indian States, including north India, are Keralites.

Not only does education bring women into the labour force, but, because it remains at a relatively low level, such participation in productive economic activity evidently contributes to a more equitable income distribution. And female participation in the labour force, combined with more equitable income

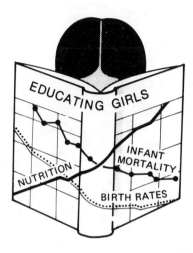

Fig. 5.2. Rising female literacy is closely associated with falling infant mortality and birthrates, and improved nutrition.

distribution, tends to be closely associated with fertility reduction. But the point is that alternatives to child-bearing become a real choice to an educated female. This is especially true, of course, in such a society as Kerala where social mobility has been significantly enhanced due to a weakened caste structure, also apparently a direct consequence of the spread of education. Yet in this regard, Kerala presents a sharp contrast to the rest of India where casteism (discrimination along caste lines) and communalism (Hindu–Muslim violence) are still rampant, where virtual slavery (compulsory unpaid labour to higher caste landowners) still exists, where bride-prices are on the increase, where women are still sent into prostitution to clear debts incurred by their own marriage expenses, and where those who dare to resist manipulation by politicians, police, higher castes, and landlords are commonly subjected to pillage, rape, and even being burned alive.

Increased educational levels also tend to be associated with increasing age at marriage for women. No exception to this rule, Kerala exhibits the highest female age at marriage in India. Census data reveal that the average age at marriage for females in India was below 15 years in more than one-third of the total number of districts. Yet 'No district in Kerala has below 15 as the average age at marriage, and only three districts (33 per cent) have an average below 20. In the case of Bihar, Rajasthan, and Uttar Pradesh, the picture is just the opposite, where 71, 65, and 48 per cent of the districts, respectively, have an average below 15' (Government of India 1975, pp. 319–20).

Moreover, fewer women in Kerala are marrying, evidently because of the attractive alternatives to marriage available to educated females. A recent study has found that fully 22 per cent of Kerala women never marry, while the com-

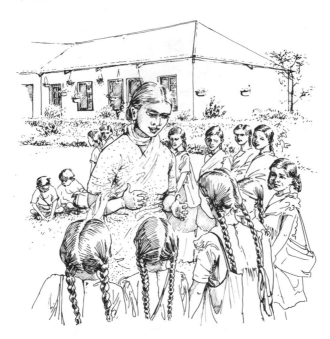

Fig. 5.3. Alternatives to child-bearing become a real choice to educated women.

parable figure for India as a whole is only 7 per cent (Krishnan 1976, p. 1209).

Other factors are also operating to reduce fertility in Kerala. Legislation providing for a more equitable distribution of goods, resources, and services no doubt has had a negative impact on birth rates. For example, land reforms have provided literally millions of couples with the opportunity to invest in land rather than children as a long-term security investment. Wages have been increased, job security for the landless has been legislated, and the need to rely upon children to fulfill welfare functions has thus been diminished. Finally, opportunities for child labour have been virtually eliminated due to worker enforcement of minimum wage and child labour laws. And when the value of children as employable economic assets declines, so does fertility.

SYNERGISM OF STRATEGIES

Many observers have suggested, after a cursory examination, that the critical factor in Kerala's development is mass education. Others have pointed to 'political will', claiming that the Kerala government has been more sincere and efficient in its efforts than those of other States.

An analysis of the historical context shows that Kerala's experience differs from that of the rest of India not because of a single factor, but because of a particular set of mutually supporting and reinforcing factors. Mass education has doubtless contributed to a heightened political consciousness and more effective political participation. Widespread political participation has resulted in a more equitable distribution of land, income, and services, including education. And a more equitable distribution of resources has served to reinforce political activism and to make schools and health services more accessible.

Kerala was for decades among the lowliest of Indian States, more 'over-populated' and possessing the fewest available resources to invest. But it has become the most socially developed State in all India. Its people are better educated, healthier, live longer, enjoy higher wages, are more secure in their jobs and personal lives – and have fewer children – than any others in India. In short, the quality of life has improved substantially for the broad majority – the espoused objective of all development plans. And because this objective has been achieved, Kerala's social, economic, and political problems, while not fully resolved, seem more amenable to solution, particularly when viewed in the broader all-India perspective.

Kerala's development experience differs from the rest of India's not because of some subtle cultural difference, or by accident. Development was achieved, purely and simply, through implementing development strategies based on equity considerations. The more just and equitable political economy that has resulted serves sharply to distinguish Kerala from other Indian States. And, therefore, so do its demographic characteristics.

The Kerala demographic experience is consistent both with research evidence drawn from other contexts and with the social justice theory of demographic transition. Significant reductions in mortality rates did indeed result from an early spread of education and the extension of preventive health measures. But fertility rates remained at high levels – and neither mortality nor fertility declined in response. As the political economy was transformed from one founded on exploitation of the many by the few to one which began increasingly to assume welfare functions traditionally fulfilled by children, fertility declined – and continues to decline – in response.

The Kerala example is an important one for a variety of reasons. First, it serves to refute the common thesis that high levels of social development cannot be achieved in the absence of high rates of economic growth and/or effective population control measures. Indeed, the Kerala experience demonstrates that high levels of social development – evaluated in terms of such quality of life measures as mortality rates and levels of life expectancy, education and literacy, and political participation – are consequences of public policies and strategies based not on economic growth considerations, but, instead, on equity considerations.

The Kerala experience also clearly supports the theoretical perspective that low levels of fertility result from public policies that effectively increase levels of social justice and economic equity throughout society. Of crucial importance in demonstrating this relationship is the fact that Kerala is not a nation but a State. Such Third World nations as Cuba, Sri Lanka, South Korea, the People's

Republic of China, and Taiwan have also recently experienced the demographic transition from high to low birth and death rates. But these observed transitions have not typically been explained as consequences of the social, political, and economic reforms implemented in those nations that preceded the transitions and which were based, in varying degrees, on equity considerations. On the contrary, alternative explanations abound. The transitions of Taiwan and South Korea are commonly attributed to some combination of their western-initiated family planning programmes and their high rates of economic growth. The transition of the People's Republic of China is frequently attributed to the fact that the people are of Oriental stock and culture. As for Cuba and Sri Lanka, their transitions are often attributed to their composition of 'island peoples', who, somehow, are more aware of the finite nature of their land mass and, therefore, of the limits to their expansion.

Perhaps the primary importance of the Kerala example lies in the very fact that it is *not* a country. It is functionally, geographically, linguistically, and culturally an integral part of India. Kerala's demographic transition occurred within the boundaries of a nation and culture noted both for its massive and long-standing attempts to achieve the demographic transition through the conventional western approaches of health care services, family planning, and 'beyond family planning' (including incentives and compulsory sterilization) as well as for its notable lack of success with these efforts. Thus the Kerala experience cannot be explained away in terms that seek to avoid focusing on the powerful demographic influence of a shift in the structure of political and economic institutions and the attendant changes in public policies regulating resource distribution. It is an undeniable fact that Kerala has achieved both the demographic transition *and* widespread social development. And, since Kerala State differs from the rest of India only in terms of the more equitable nature of its political economy and public policies, it is difficult not to assign these credit for observing developmental and demographic differentials. Political and economic reforms based on the interests of the poor majority apparently have resulted, directly, in an improved quality of life for most Keralites. And Kerala's successful demographic transition is evidently the direct consequence of that improved quality of life.

The Indian failure to resolve its population problem is commonly blamed on some combination of the irrational breeding habits of its impoverished and illiterate peasantry and the inefficient administration of its population control programme efforts. The Kerala experience suggests strongly that neither the fertility rates nor the impoverishment and illiteracy of the peasantry are independent of the structure of the Indian political economy and resultant public policies. The implication of the Kerala experience is clear: it is not the peasantry who are responsible for India's so-called 'population problem', but, instead, the socioeconomic development policies and strategies that systematically favour the rich over the poor.

The real causes of poverty, social underdevelopment, and high fertility are the unjust organization of Indian society and the unfair distribution of wealth. Actual responsibility for widespread poverty and illiteracy, of which high mortality and fertility rates are but symptoms, must lie with those who formulate and implement public policies designed systematically to channel available goods, resources, and services to the few instead of the many. To blame the impoverished peasantry for any observed population-resources imbalances is clearly to blame the victim.

The implications of the Kerala experience for other Third World populations, as well as for the western population control movement, seem clear and straightforward. *If* the reduction of population growth is indeed a priority, and *if* social development is more than merely an exposed goal of development strategies, then structural changes in the political economy are essential strategies. And, as the Kerala example points out, such changes must be based upon equity considerations rather than aggregate economic growth considerations. The task that faces those interested in reducing fertility levels is *not* the manipulation of human behaviour to suit the needs of out-moded and oppressive institutional structures; instead, it is to change those institutional structures to suit contemporary human needs. It is only through this approach that contraceptive delivery systems can be placed in their proper perspective: as programmes designed not to control aggregate fertility but to assist individual couples in achieving their desired family size.

NOTES

1. Agrarian reform measures in Kerala are not more radical than those legislated in other Indian States. The difference lies in the fact that, in Kerala, these reforms have been implemented, because '. . . Kerala happens to be the only State in India where political pressure based on mass organization and support has been a major factor forcing the pace of land reform and where such reform has constantly received sustained attention' (Raj 1975, p. 53).

2. Reported unemployment in Kerala is almost twice the national average. However, it appears that this relatively poor statistical position is due to the fact that there is less disguised unemployment (or underemployment) than in the rest of India. In Kerala the commercial crops of coconut, pepper, and tapioca require only seasonal care, and therefore the agricultural sector is unable to provide the semblance of continuous employment that characterizes the rest of India.

REFERENCES

Centre for Development Studies, *Diet Survey*, 1973–74.
Dandekar, V.M. and Rath, N., *Poverty in India*, Indian School of Political Economy (1971).
Government of India, Committee on the Status of Women in India. *Towards equality*. Ministry of Education and Social Welfare, New Delhi (1975).

Krishnaji, N., Nutritional norms and magnitude of undernutrition. In *Poverty, unemployment and development policy: a case study of selected issues with reference to Kerala*. ST/ESA/29. United Nations, New York (1975).

Krishnaji, N. Structure of education and the market for the educated in *Poverty, Unemployment and Development Policy: A Case Study of Selected Issues with Reference to Kerala*. ST/ESA/29. United Nations, New York, 1975.

Krishnan, T.N., Demographic transition in Kerala: facts and factors. *Economic and Political Weekly* (special number) (1976).

Panikar, P.G.K., Fall in mortality rates in Kerala. An explanatory hypothesis. *Economic and Political Weekly*, pp. 1811–18 (1975).

Panikar, P.G.K., Trends in the availability of food. In *Poverty, unemployment and development policy: a case study of selected issues with reference to Kerala*. ST/ESA/29. United Nations, New York (1975).

Raj, K.N., Land reforms and their effects on distribution of income. In *Poverty, unemployment and development policy: a case study of selected issues with reference to Kerala*. ST/ESA/29. United Nations, New York (1975).

Raj, K.N. Address made at the Overseas Development Council, Washington DC, 5 April, 1976.

Registrar General of India, Census of India, 1981, Series 1, *India*, Paper 1 of *Provisional Population Totals*, New Delhi (1981).

Sample Registration Bulletin. Vol. 14, No. 1 (1980).

World Bank, *Assault on world poverty: problems of rural development education and health*, Johns Hopkins University Press, Baltimore (1975).

Part II
People's participation

The key to the successful organization of PHC is community participation. Although this principle is almost universally acknowledged, it is interpreted in widely differing ways. Most commonly it is *mis*interpreted to mean simply the *mobilization* of the people's resources of money, labour, and materials for government-planned and -controlled programmes. Such contributions from the people are usually desirable, but they are only one aspect of participation.

A more sensitive approach is to view community participation as a process through which the people gain greater *control* over the social, political, economic, and environmental factors determining their health. By acquiring appropriate knowledge, skills, organizational capacities and a heightened sense of individual and collective responsibility, low-income communities can achieve remarkable improvements in health status.

The community must participate, not just in implementation, but in every stage of the health programme:

- initial assessment of the situation
- defining the main health problems
- setting the priorities for the programme
- implementing the activities
- monitoring and evaluating the results.

Here we present case studies of rural and urban communities in India, Sierra Leone, Indonesia, and the Dominican Republic, demonstrating the potential of poor, largely illiterate communities for active involvement in organizing primary health care. In each case the role of women is crucially important, not just in running the programme and managing family welfare at home, but in the wider role of breaking down traditional social prejudices and injustices.

Communities can also help make PHC programmes more appropriate to local cultural and socioeconomic conditions. One of the greatest handicaps of most health professionals in developing countries is their tendency to use a westernized, highly technical approach when training village health workers in the initial stages of a PHC programme. The experience of a voluntary agency in rural Nigeria, however, points the way to a more sensitive approach based on the local customs of imparting knowledge through stories, drama, and songs. In the Philippines, a young doctor relates how his westernized training left him, both culturally and professionally, ill-equipped to work in a rural area. The communities in which he worked, however, helped to re-train him as a more sensitive and effective community health worker. His experience also helped him to see beyond the narrow limits of medicine to the political and socioeconomic causes of hunger and ill-health.

Voluntary agencies, working within the community, have proven their ability to develop effective PHC programmes. Yet it is often argued that the success stories of voluntary agencies cannot be replicated on a large scale, because they depend on charismatic local leadership for their success. The experiences of two PHC programmes in Indonesia, however, appear to contradict this argument. In both cases a small, community-based programme was started by a voluntary agency and then successfully replicated on a larger scale by the government. The crucial factor in each case was political support at an intermediate level of the government hierarchy.

Yet the constraints on community participation should also be kept clearly in view. The scope of participation is limited by the community's own structure and composition. Many promising initiatives have been brought to grief by a clash of interests at local level. In an Indonesian village, for example, a group started a PHC programme and gained strong support from their fellow villagers. But the village head saw the programme as a threat to his own authority and status. He placed one obstacle after another in its way, until it gradually lost both momentum and direction. In a remote rural area of Peru, three communities with differing socioeconomic backgrounds reacted in quite different ways to the same PHC programme: one rejected it completely; one cooperated actively; and one demanded the right to participate and made a very substantial financial contribution. (Ironically, the third community has since become even more dependent on the governmental health system.)

A second factor influencing the scope for community participation in health is the attitude of the organization 'sponsoring' the programme. Governmental or voluntary agencies with a conservative orientation are unlikely to foster genuine involvement of the people in decision-making about health or any other activity. Rather, they will try to restrict the community to the role of providing labour, funds, and materials. This will ease resource constraints but will not help the people to understand or control the factors determining their health. On the other hand, 'sponsoring' agencies with a reformist or radical approach are more likely to involve the community in the programme from the start. Their scope, however, depends on a third factor — the overall political 'climate' created and sustained by the government at national level.

6   Evaluation in primary health care: a case study from India

Ashok Dyal Chand and **M. Ibrahim Soni** explain how the method of participatory evaluation has enabled the Comprehensive Health and Development Project at Pachod to match its programme to the needs of the most vulnerable groups — women and children — in a rural area of Maharashtra State.

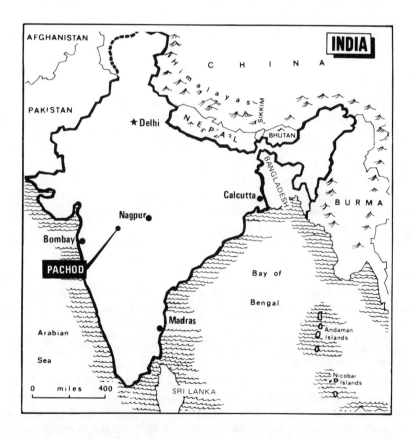

Ashok Dyal Chand, M.D., is Director of the Comprehensive Health and Development Project at Pachod.
M. Ibrahim Soni, a graduate of the International Institute of Population Studies in Bombay, is Project Demographer.

Evaluation, if its main purpose is to help a programme achieve its objectives, cannot be simply an isolated, terminal event. It must be part of a continuous process of two-way communication between health workers and the community, and be based on the routine monitoring of key indicators of personnel performance and programme effectiveness.

'Participatory evaluation' can be defined as a process of self-realization in which an organization, working with the community, studies the strengths and weaknesses of its programme through the participation of the community and all levels of health workers. The Ashish Gram Rachna Trust based at Pachod, in Maharashtra State, has followed this approach since the start of the Comprehensive Health and Development Project in July 1977. In the following article we shall present the results of our experiences during the first three years of the project, from July 1977 until June 1980.

BACKGROUND

The setting

The area originally assigned to the project by the government covered 72 villages and hamlets (reduced to 50 in 1980) in the southern part of Paithan development block, Aurangabad district, Maharashtra State. In 1977 the population numbered about 67 000 people living in 12 500 households. The area of 575 km^2 has low rainfall and only limited irrigation facilities. One in three households is landless, and half own less than four hectares. The main crop is *jowar*, a type of millet. Only one in five villages is serviced by buses; the remainder – far from the main roads – can be approached only by bullock cart or on foot and are virtually inaccessible during the monsoon.

The majority (70 per cent) of the population is Hindu, but there are sizeable Muslim and Buddhist minorities. Marathas comprise the dominant caste. Female literacy levels are low: only 16 per cent of women can read and write, compared with 45 per cent of males. In 1979 two out of every three households had an average monthly income of less than 200 rupees (US $18).

Health problems

The most prevalent health problems in 1977 included chronic malnutrition, xerophthalmia (night blindness), diarrhoea, and tuberculosis. Infant and maternal mortality rates were high, and only a small minority of mothers and children were immunized. Owing to the lack of safe drinking water and adequate sanitation, intestinal parasites and communicable diseases were high prevalence health problems.

Objectives

In 1975, when the project was being planned, the following objectives were set for the first four years:

1. Reduction in the crude birth rate from 36 to 25 per 1000 population.
2. 50 per cent reduction in the infant mortality rate of 128 per 1000 live births.
3. 50 per cent reduction in the child mortality rate of 48 per 1000 children under five.
4. 50 per cent reduction in malnutrition of under-fives.
5. Treatment of 80 per cent of existing blindness among patients with curable eye diseases, and 80 per cent control of xerophthalmia.
6. Effective ante-, intra-, and post-natal care and immunization against tetanus to 80 per cent of pregnant women.
7. Bringing under control 80 per cent of tuberculosis cases (15 per 1000 population).
8. Bringing under treatment 80 per cent of leprosy cases.
9. Training of traditional midwives (*dais*) in all project villages and training of Multi-purpose Workers (MPWs) for all the sub-centres.
10. Dissemination of health education through regular mass health education programmes in all villages.

As a result of rigorous self-evaluation from an early stage, however, some of these objectives were modified during the course of the first three years of the project.

Personnel

Project staff at the base hospital (20 beds) in Pachod consisted of two national doctors, one public health nurse, one nutritionist, one demographer, six auxiliary nurse midwives (ANMs), and various service personnel. Workers at 'grassroots' level comprised eight male MPWs, 20 women Community Health Workers (CHWs), and 37 dais — all recruited from within the project area and trained by the project staff.

COMMUNITY PARTICIPATION IN EVALUATION

A process of two-way communication with the community was initiated in 1976, before the implementation of any project activities had started. This process continued throughout the project, enabling the community to participate in evaluating the following aspects of the programme.
 — Setting priorities
 — Training traditional birth attendants
 — Implementation of activities

   — Health and nutrition education
   — Direction and emphasis of the programme.
Let us review each of these aspects in turn.

Setting priorities

In 1976 a 10 per cent systematic sample survey was conducted in 22 villages with a population of 20 000 to identify the priorities of the community. Health was ranked only eleventh, well behind priorities such as food and employment. The interviewers then tried to establish the community's highest priority in the field of health. In 21 out of the 22 villages the response was maternal care, because childbirth was usually the only time when immediate medical help was felt necessary, especially in villages situated some distance from the hospital.

The project proposal therefore was redesigned to give highest priority – at least during the first four years – to maternal care and midwifery services. The revised plan involved the training of a woman from within each village as a community health worker (CHW), with particular emphasis on midwifery. But as the project staff studied the role of the dais within the community, the revised plan also was called into doubt. Traditional birth attendants (*dais*) assisted at 6 per cent of all deliveries, with 8 per cent assisted by trained medical personnel and the remainder by mothers or mothers-in-law. Usually the dai was called only after serious complications had set in, by which time it was too late for her to take any useful action. To justify her involvement, however, she made some ineffective (and sometimes dangerous) efforts, such as massaging and stretching the woman's vagina. This resulted in further loss of time. When, in desperation, the dai referred the woman to a health centre or hospital, it was usually too late to save both mother and child. Yet despite the dai's lack of midwifery training, knowledge, and skills, people in the community still sought her help during emergencies. The project staff realized that this pattern of dependence on the dai would continue with many people even if the village CHW was given specialized training in midwifery.

The project was therefore revised a second time. The new starting point would be the training of village dais in maternal care and midwifery, with CHWs and MPWs to come later. But people's initial reactions to this plan were lukewarm. They had envisaged a sort of mini-hospital with a resident nurse in every village. What they were being offered instead was simply their own village dai – an illiterate woman of low caste who earned a meagre living as an agricultural labourer. This was far short of their expectations. The project staff therefore explained the impracticality of the people's hopes: the cost factor alone ruled out constructing a clinic and placing a nurse in every village. Gradually, though at first reluctantly, these explanations were accepted.

Three years after the start of the project, the dais had established themselves as key health workers in the community. Around 70 per cent of mothers were receiving ante-natal care from the dais; they conducted 56 per cent of deliveries and were rendering post-natal and neo-natal care to 77 per cent of mothers and children in the project area.

This example illustrates how community involvement in the early stages of planning a PHC project can make the project's priorities more relevant to the community's felt needs. At the same time, however, it shows how, through a process of two-way communication, the project can help the community to a better informed understanding of how their health needs can be met. The village dai today is a community-supported health institution — not dependent on the project for her survival — providing an effective and widely appreciated maternal and midwifery service helping to lower rates of maternal and infant mortality.

Training dais

This was essentially a process of *re*training, since most dais had been assisting deliveries by traditional means for 25 to 30 years. It involved changing a deeply entrenched set of values, beliefs, and practices. Simply telling the dais outright that their practices were harmful would have created serious psychological barriers and resistance to the acceptance of new knowledge and practices. We therefore adopted a problem-solving approach to the training process.

Each dai firstly was interviewed, using a 160-item questionnaire. We thus formed a detailed inventory of their attitudes, knowledge, and practices. We then designed a training programme aimed at changing harmful practices, encouraging beneficial traditional customs, reshaping attitudes and values, and adding new knowledge. Changing harmful practices required a very sensitive approach. We designed the training course so that participants were exposed to problems and hazards in midwifery and suggested solutions. One harmful practice, for example, was giving newborn babies two spoonfulls of castor oil in the belief that a catharsis was necessary to remove the fluids of the womb ingested by the newborn during birth. This often caused severe diarrhoea leading to dehydration and death. But instead of simply rejecting the harmful practice, we tried to modify it and render it harmless. Granted, we said, a baby needs a laxative, but castor oil is much too strong. Are there any alternatives sufficiently mild for a newborn baby? The dais suggested various traditional herbal laxatives. One suggested honey, which was readily available in all villages. Through concensus it was decided to recommend a spoon of honey as a laxative for the newborn, a practice now widespread in the project area.

We know, of course, that newborn babies need neither honey (though it does no harm) nor a laxative. But by helping the dais to modify their traditional practices rather than flatly rejecting them, we successfully discouraged a harmful health practice while avoiding the creation of psychological barriers to change.

Implementation of activities

In each village a health committee consisting of one person from each caste or each lane has been formed. Most committees are male-dominated, despite all the dais and CHWs being women, and 80 per cent of the project's services being directed to women and children. Nevertheless, the committees have generally played a useful role by giving official backing to the health project and over-coming logistical problems by providing a building, lighting, and other facilities for the mass immunization of children. The main point of delivery of health services, however, is the ante-natal clinic, held twice a month and organized mainly by the local dai and CHW in each village. This is also the forum in which women's attitudes, beliefs, and health practices are formed. Problems are aired and solutions proposed and discussed. One of the major problems with which the project grappled unsuccessfully for two years was accurate identification of the last menstrual period of new ante-natal women. Since most women are illiterate, they were occasionally 15 days to one month wide of the mark in their estimates. This in turn made it impossible for the dai accurately to calculate the expected date of the woman's confinement. Finally the dais and the village women developed their own solution: by comparing the data of each woman's menstrual period with the dai's every month, a very reliable estimate was ob-tained. While the project's professionally trained health workers had failed to solve this problem, a group of illiterate village women devised their own, dis-armingly simple solution.

Health and nutrition education

Rather than using a series of formal lessons, health and nutrition education take place in the informal atmosphere of the ante-natal clinics. For example, while examining a pregnant mother the dai asks questions such as:

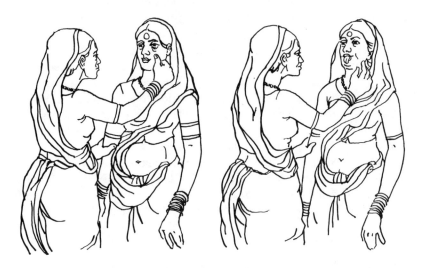

Fig. 6.1. Dai checks pregnant woman for anaemia.

'Why am I examining your eyes?'

'What is the cause of your anaemia, and how can it be overcome?'

'Why am I examining your abdomen? What do I find out? How can that help you?'

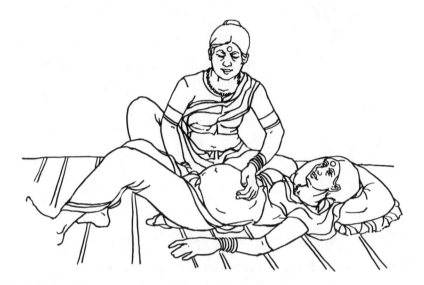

Fig. 6.2. Dai measures size of uterus to determine month of pregnancy.

After the dai completes her examination the pregnant woman moves on to the nurse for examination and vaccination. The nurse asks:

'Why are you having this injection?'

'How many more must you have?'

'Why am I taking your blood pressure? What can happen if your blood pressure is much above normal?'

If the newcomer cannot answer a question, women coming to the clinic for their second or third pregnancy take great delight in chipping in with the answers. This has become a kind of game played every second week at the clinic, and has established ante-natal care as a routine activity within the community. The same method of informal health education is also used for other components of the programme.

In this way the mothers become involved in an active learning process directly related to the factors influencing their own health and that of their children.

In nutrition education the people's questions and proposals have helped to eliminate weaknesses in the programme of which the staff had been unaware. For example, during the first four years of the project our village-based CHWs used to keep and maintain all the under-five children's growth charts. Every month they would weigh the children and explain the findings to the parents:

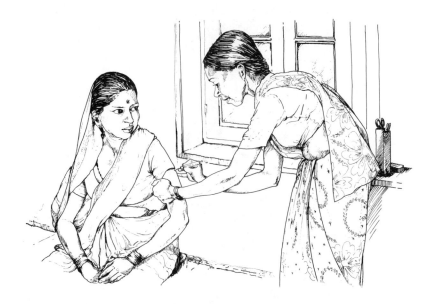

Fig. 6.3. Dai vaccinates pregnant woman against tetanus.

the child's weight, degree of undernourishment and what is needed to be done for the child to gain weight. If the child was severely malnourished the workers would give more intensive nutritional and health education.

During this whole four year period we explained undernutrition in terms of first, second, and third degree malnutrition. Then a chance episode made us realize that the message was not being understood by the people. In one village a grandmother who was always very particular about having her grandchild weighed commented to the CHW: 'What is this first, second, and third degree you keep telling me about? Tell me about the health of my grandchild in annas of a rupee.' The old Indian rupee had 16 annas and to this day a traditional form of expressing percentages in villages is:

100 per cent — 16 annas in a rupee
 75 per cent — 12 annas in a rupee
 50 per cent — 8 annas in a rupee
 25 per cent — 4 annas in a rupee

When we heard about this, we selected a random sample in all our villages to find out whether 'degree of malnutrition' had been understood by the majority of the parents or not. We discovered that, although the parents recollected the actual weight of their child, they could not recall the degree of malnutrition. This indicated that they did not understand the meaning of the word 'degree' in the vernacular.

We then instructed all our workers to tell the parents the actual weight of the child and to interpret nutritional status as follows:

normal   — 16 annas in a rupee
first degree malnutrition   — 12 annas in a rupee
second degree malnutrition   —   8 annas in a rupee
third degree malnutrition   —   4 annas in a rupee.

Today every parent throughout the project area can express the nutritional status of their under-five children in terms of so many annas in a rupee. Once we had established that parents could do this, we started giving them a copy of their children's growth charts to keep and maintain. The families of most villages in the project area now keep growth charts in this way.

Direction and emphasis of programme

The CHWs and dais have made a number of suggestions, based on practical experience, leading to significant changes in the direction or emphasis of certain aspects of the programme.

In the field of nutrition, for example, the emphasis has shifted from treating malnutrition to preventing it. From the start, the project has emphasized nutritional surveillance of under-fives and nutrition education for mothers. Good use has been made of locally available foods, rather than providing supplementary feeding with food brought into the region. The CHWs and MPWs used to visit severely malnourished children in their homes twice a month to monitor the children's growth and give nutritional demonstration to the parents. After three years the proportion of severely malnourished children was cut to one-quarter of its former level. But the CHWs also noticed that many children in the 'mild to moderate' category of malnourishment were failing to gain weight and some were even falling back into severe malnourishment. They therefore suggested that, in order to *prevent* malnutrition before it even started, the programme should give greater emphasis to educating the parents of children under the age of four months. This would better prepare them to feed their children adequately during the critical weaning period. The programme now incorporates this emphasis, though continuing the routine nutritional surveillance of all under-fives.

Changes have also occurred in the technology used to assist deliveries. Initially we provided the dais with blades, string, gauze, cottonwool, and iodine, all autoclaved (steam-sterilized) and sealed in polythene bags. Being autoclaved, the blades and string required no boiling before use. We instructed the dais, however, to teach families the importance of boiling these items before use if they conducted deliveries without the dais' assistance. We discovered in a survey that only one in five families was sterilizing their blades and string in this way. We reproached the dais for failing to educate village families about the need for sterilization, but the dais provided us with a more convincing explanation. Village women, they said, only saw the dais break the seal of the polythene bag, remove the blade and use it. 'They never see us boiling it.' They suggested that the project, instead of giving them autoclaved equipment in sealed polythene bags, should simply provide unsterilized materials similar to those used by village women. They then would boil them in people's homes, explaining the importance of doing so to the family. Several dais now work in this way, and we are evaluating the experiment before recommending its wider application.

EVALUATION AS A CONTINUOUS PROCESS

Evaluation takes place concurrently with other routine programme activities. The project staff meet the dais, CHWs, and MPWs every week to assess and discuss one another's performances, based on data collected by a detailed health information system. Much effort has gone into designing this system, which is convenient for health workers to maintain and for supervisors to follow up. All levels of health workers keep records on a daily, weekly, monthly, half-yearly, and annual basis. The basic sources of information are as follows:

- Household records maintained by multi-purpose workers.
- Ante- and post-natal records maintained by auxiliary nurse-midwives.
- Village files maintained by project supervisors.
- Records of vital events maintained by CHWs and MPWs.
- Growth charts for under-five children, kept by families.

This health information system enables the systematic evaluation of changes brought about by the health programme in three main areas:

- The knowledge, attitudes, and practices of health workers.
- Health awareness and practices in the community.
- Certain key health indicators.

Measuring change

After the programme had been running for three years an evaluation of the 22 villages covered showed significant changes in maternal health care (see Table 6.1).

These results indicate a marked improvement in the health awareness and practices of people – especially mothers – in villages covered by the project. The sharp decline in the maternal mortality rate is particularly striking.

The same evaluation also found a 33 per cent drop in the infant mortality rate (IMR) (see Table 6.2).

During the same period the IMR among children born to women in villages in the project area where maternal care services had not yet started fell only slightly, from 128 to 120. This marked difference suggests that the programme had a significant influence in lowering the IMR in the villages which it covered.

Another significant indicator of the well-being of infants and children is the nutritional status of under-fives. The evaluation found a 75 per cent drop in the number of children suffering from third degree malnutrition (see Fig. 6.4).

One cause of concern, however, was the continued inferior status of girls compared with boys (see Fig. 6.5).

Table 6.1. Changes in maternal health care among mothers

Item	1977 (Before Project)	1980 (Three years Project implementation)
1. Pregnant women covered by ante-natal services	Only in rare, complicated cases	70% of total pregnant women
2. Detection of pregnancy by trained dai	Nil (no trained dais available)	5th month of gestation period
3. Pregnant women vaccinated with two doses of tetanus toxoid	1.5%	55%
4. Pregnant women receiving iron tablets for at least one month	Not known (but probably negligible)	55%
5. Pregnant women attending ante-natal clinic at least twice	Nil (no ante-natal clinic available in village)	76%
6. Recently delivered women receiving post-natal services	Negligible	67%
7. Women attended by dai during delivery	6.0%	56%
8. Women referred to hospital (Ante- and post-natal cases)	1.5%	8%
9. Maternal deaths	12 per 1000 live-births	4.5 per 1000 live-births

Table 6.2. Infant mortality rate in project area

Year	No. of villages	Population	Live births registered	Infant deaths	Infant mortality rate per 1000 livebirths
1977/78	12	15 145	203	23	123.2
1978/79	19	26 015	508	53	104.3
1979/80	22	30 230	589	48	81.5

Although the nutritional status of girls did improve during the three years, their position is clearly still inferior to that of boys: twice as many girls were severely malnourished and considerably fewer were in the normal range. These findings have important social implications.

Immunization coverage was low before the programme started. Our baseline data survey showed that in 1978 only 8 per cent of children in the project area had received three does of DPT and only 17 per cent had received any vaccinations at all. The evaluation showed a great increase in coverage achieved by our mobile vaccination team, which began giving DPT and BCG vaccinations in 22 villages only nine months before the evaluation in June 1980 (see Table 6.3).

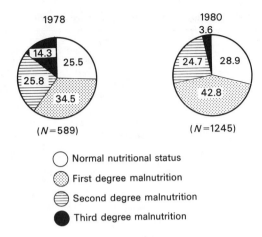

Fig. 6.4. Nutritional status of under-fives (both sexes).

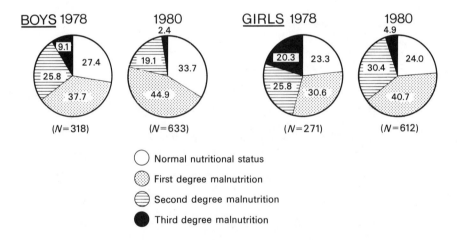

Fig. 6.5. Nutritional status of under-fives, according to sex.

Table 6.3. Immunization status of children, June 1980

No. of villages	No. of under-fives	Under-fives 3 doses of DPT		Under-fives BCG	
		Number vaccinated	% vaccinated	Number vaccinated	% vaccinated
22	2639	1729	65.5	1755	28.3

Family planning, which can contribute to improving the health of mothers and children through spacing births at wider intervals, has not yet been actively promoted by the project. (Even the words 'family planning' still stir up negative associations for many people.) But a modest number of men and women came voluntarily to the base hospital for vasectomies or tubal ligations in 1979, and the numbers increased in 1980 (see Table 6.4).

Most of the men and women coming to the hospital for sterilizations were referred by CHWs and dais, although they received no encouragement from the project staff to promote family planning.

Table 6.4. Family planning acceptors

	Method	
Year	Tubectomy	Vasectomy
1976	387	71
1977	187	121
1978	149	0
1979	244	13
1980	395	25

CONCLUSION

Participatory evaluation has helped us match our programme's priorities with the people's felt needs and to design training methods suitable for local cultural conditions. It has guided us in implementing activities appropriate to the special needs of women in rural Indian society, and in fostering health education for women. It has also enabled us to review the knowledge, attitudes, and practices of our health workers, to assess health awareness and practices within the community, and to measure the effectiveness of the programme using a set of key indicators. It is important to use the method as a routine part of the programme rather than simply as a special, isolated activity at the end of a certain period. We have found participatory evaluation to be an invaluable tool for correcting the methods, emphasis, and direction of our health programme.

Postcript, October 1982

Since the evaluation in 1980 we have been reconsidering some of the concepts underlying our health programme. We feel that terms like 'community participation' and 'participatory evaluation' too often mean in practice that the community participates in activities designed for it by outsiders. Despite our efforts to involve the people in decision-making, implementation, and evaluation of the programme, they still did not feel sufficiently responsible for implementing activities independently in their villages. We wondered whether 'health by the people' could be made a reality in a Third World country, where health has low priority.

We therefore decided to start work in 12 villages not previously covered, but without making any prior assumptions about the form or structure of any future programme. The people elected representatives from each caste and section of the villages, and we helped them organize a survey to identify their most urgently felt needs. The representatives then took part in processing the information collected, and held meetings with sections of their communities to discuss the results and propose ways of overcoming the problems. We believe this approach is helping us avoid the need for large corrections and modifications to the programme. It is an improvement on our approach in 1977, when we had sociologists and medical students from Aurangabad carry out the initial village survey.

Each village also selects a traditional birth attendant and a community development worker for training by our staff. After training, these village level workers initiate and guide the development of health-related activities within their own communities, to whom they are accountable. This has created a situation in which the community, once mobilized into action, implements its own programme with technical advice and training from our staff.

This more sensitive approach to community participation resulted from careful evaluation of the first three years of our programme. We are confident that lasting improvements in health status can be achieved through the community not only demanding health services, but providing some of these services itself and carrying out intensive self-education. 'Health by the people' need not be a Utopian dream.

7 Community assessment: a tool for motivation and evaluation in primary health care in Sierra Leone

Nancy Edwards and **Mary (Hilary) Lyons** explain why 'community assessment' is the key to starting, implementing, and evaluating health care services in a rural area of Sierra Leone.

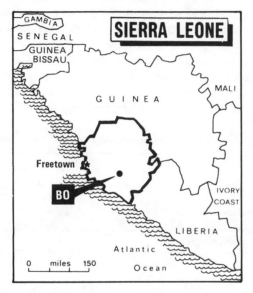

Nancy Edwards is a public health tutor who worked at the Serabu Hospital in Bo, Sierra Leone, from 1978 until 1981.
Sister Mary (Hilary) Lyons, M.D., is Head of the Serabu Hospital and has worked in Sierra Leone for 30 years.

A key factor in initiating and sustaining Primary Health Care programmes is the participation of the whole community in planning, implementing, and evaluating health services. Health planners and fieldworkers, however, are still experimenting with various methods of developing effective community participation. The Serabu hospital in southern Sierra Leone has designed and tested a method known as *community assessment*, which serves as a stimulus to community participation and also as a means of evaluating programme effectiveness and and impact. We believe this method may have potential for wider application.

Community assessment may be defined as a process in which health professionals and community members assess the people's health needs and evaluate the effectiveness of health programmes in meeting these needs, guided by certain key indicators of health status and community organization. We should like to present an account of our experience of community assessment since 1976.

BACKGROUND

Our health programme is centred on a 125-bed hospital in Serabu, a small town of 2500 people in Bumpe chiefdom in the Southern Province of Sierra Leone, near the coast of West Africa. With a population of 30 180, Bumpe is one of the largest chiefdoms in Sierra Leone. It is divided into eleven sections, each under the authority of a chief living in a section town, each section being further subdivided into a number of subsidiary villages. The population consists of low-income farming communities growing crops of rice, cassava, coffee, and green vegetables. The climate is tropical, with high average rainfall and two distinct seasons — the wet and the dry. Farming is a hazardous business: pest and rodent infestations destroy crops and the rains may be irregular. Demographic features and vital health statistics reflect those of the country as a whole (see Table 7.1), with high birth rates, high infant and child mortality, and low life expectancy.

Table 7.1. Demographic features and vital health statistics of Sierra Leone

Population	3.4 million
Birth rate	46.0 per 1000 population
Death rate	19.0 per 1000 population
Annual rate of population growth	2.5%
Infant mortality rate	200 per 1000 live births
Life expectancy at birth	47.0 years

Sources: World Bank, *World Development Report* (1981); Kandeh, H.B.S., *Infant Mortality in Sierra Leone*, Ford Foundation (1978).

HEALTH COMMITTEES — THE STARTING POINT

In 1976 the staff of Serabu hospital decided to conduct a survey of 669 people from seven villages to determine what medical care people sought when sick. Although the hospital had provided medical treatment and operated mobile under-five and ante-natal clinics for the previous 15 years, hospital records and the staff's own observations suggested that disease patterns in the villages had remained largely unchanged during this period. We wanted to know the extent to which the existing static and mobile health facilities were being utilized by the population. People interviewed were asked two questions:

1. Have you been sick during the past 12 months?
2. If 'yes', what was your *first* line of action?

The results (Table 7.2) showed that only a small minority went first to the hospital or mobile clinic for treatment.

Table 7.2. First action taken when ill (August 1974–July 1975)

Action	Proportion of sample (%)
Buy drugs from shopkeeper or trader	36
Take indigeneous (mainly herbal) medicine	35
Go to hospital or mobile clinic	17
No action	10
Visit fortune teller	2

We concluded from these results that health knowledge and care needed to be available within village communities themselves. The method by which we hoped to achieve this was through training a group of local people, selected by the community, to deal with common health problems. The group would work on a voluntary basis and would be known as the health committee. Three pilot villages, all within a five-mile radius of the hospital, were selected for the new approach. After evaluation of the results, the approach was extended to all eleven section towns, each of which has spread it further — in a 'ripple effect' — to nearby villages.

The health committee concept aims at the realization of the potential of every person, family and community to take greater control of the factors influencing their own health and lives. Our initial efforts, however, soon ran into difficulties. Village meetings, though apparently showing great enthusiasm for forming health committees, sometimes failed to produce any follow-up action. In one case the village chief appointed the health committee without even informing the members. Hospital staff visited people at home to explain the health committee idea, but often it was difficult to distinguish between courtesy to the visitor and real understanding of the issue.

We became especially concerned that members of the health committee tended to hold themselves accountable, not to their own communities, but to the hospital staff. As far as the great majority of the community was concerned, health care still remained a peripheral activity. Moreover, we, the health professionals, had helped create this situation through:

- *pedantic teaching methods*: phrases like 'were taught' and 'had learned' kept recurring in the written reports of the health committee members;
- *failure to delegate responsibility*: rather than encouraging local health committee members to carry out home visits, we did these ourselves;
- *over-emphasis on scientific methods*: to collect data on the people's health status a doctor and a team of nurses carried out full physicals on every person in three villages — but with absolutely minimal community involvement;

— *frequent staff changes*: as a result, many staff were unable to form close working relationships with committees;

— *placement of student nurses*: the tasks of the committee members tended to be taken over by student nurses doing practical training.

By the end of 1979 it was clear that health committee members somehow had to be turned around to face, not the hospital, but their own communities. They had to take their 'Stop'/'Go' signals from fellow villagers, with health professionals called in only as consultants on particular problems. They had to be responsible for collecting relevant information about health in their villages and explaining its implications to others. The people thus would look first to their own health committee members for health care rather than to shopkeepers, herbalists, and the hospital. The method of community assessment was thus designed as the means of bringing about these changes in attitudes and practices.

COMMUNITY ASSESSMENT — INITIAL SURVEY

At the outset, hospital staff approach community leaders and explain that they would like to learn with the people about their particular health problems. Since the leaders know the people better than do the hospital staff, they are best placed to gather this information. The staff explain the background to their approach:

'Even though Serabu hospital has existed for many years, still we see the same diseases over and over again. Many men come saying they are too tired to do their farm work. Infants die from tetanus, toddlers become seriously ill and often die of measles and malnutrition, and some of the young women are dying in childbirth. We do not understand why this is, and so we want to learn with you how to find out the causes. Perhaps then we can work together to try and eradicate the diseases.'

Staff then explain the need to determine how great the health problems are. This is done by asking a series of questions. How many children died in this village last year? What is the main cause of death of school-age females? The difficulties faced by the leaders in trying to answer these and other questions help them realize that there are many gaps in their own understanding of the people's health. At the same time, staff stress that the information to be gathered is for the *community*, not for the hospital or the government. After the staff have studied the information, they will share it with the people and together they will plan action to solve their health problems.

The assessment consists of several components, mainly:

— a *sanitation* survey, to determine primary and secondary water sources, methods of refuse and sewage disposal, laws for maintenance and protection of water sources, and local beliefs related to the water sources.

— *a village map* showing the location of homes, latrines, water sources,

markets, mosques, churches, and housing compounds; this eventually is pasted up in the house of the health committee clerk.
- *an interview* with community leaders to ascertain their perspectives on health-related problems such as food storage, common illnesses, methods of transport and communication, utilization of existing health facilities, population mobility and education. Leaders explain the history of the village and the origins of its name. They also identify traditional health workers (midwives, herbalists, etc.) in the community.
- *an agricultural questionnaire*: the community selects prominent and re-spected farmers to obtain their views on farming methods, pest control, marketing of crops, types of crops grown, and farming cooperatives.
- *traditional midwives* are interviewed about their delivery practices, beliefs related to nutrition in pregnancy, ways of dealing with obstructed labour, their understanding of patient referrals and the problems they experience in carrying out this voluntary service to other mothers.
- *a house-to-house survey* is conducted to make a census determining the nutritional (based on weight for age) and immunization status of under-fives; the number of births; the number and causes of stillbirths and infant deaths during the past 12 months; as well as the parity and total number of stillbirths and neo-natal deaths to all women aged 14 years and over in the household.

While carrying out this initial assessment, the health workers explain what they are doing and why, and encourage people to regard their health problems as being within their own capacity to solve. Traditional leaders and any local volun-teers available accompany the health workers and reinforce their explanations during discussions. Schoolchildren are asked to explain the purpose of the team's visit to their parents, so that when the team reaches them they already have some understanding of what they will be asked and why. As children tend to be naturally curious and lively, they are invited to help draw the village map.

Traditional midwives are also part of the survey team. They help explain to women the importance of giving accurate information about their obstetrical history. (This is a delicate subject: childless women raising adopted children are unwilling to admit that the children are not their own.)

The results of the initial survey are shared at a village meeting. Since everyone takes part in the survey, there is a lot of interest in the results and attendance at the meeting is invariably high. The survey results give the village its first image of itself. To stimulate greater community involvement in the meeting, the health worker uses a question-and-answer technique to present the results. How many houses with latrines are there in the village? How many women of child-bearing age are there? How many under-fives have had their full course of immunizations? As the correct answers emerge, the community assessment method takes on a motivational function. As more emotional questions — e.g. 'How many infants died last year?' — are posed, the people feel more and more drawn into the assessment exercise. Although most families have known the trauma of an infant or child death, the community as a whole never views these events collectively, against a time frame. Quantifying this information for a certain period gives a startling new perspective, and stimulates both traditional leaders and ordinary villagers to start asking what they can do to prevent such deaths. This is the first, tentative step towards greater community control over some of the causes of disease and death.

At this point the health worker may introduce the idea of a health committee. It is entirely up to the community, however, whether they decide to form a committee. Before returning to Serabu, the health worker suggests that the community should meet again later and decide for themselves, informing the hospital when they have made their decision. The health worker leaves the community assessment report in the village. Though few people can read it, simply having a document depicting their own health status seems to reinforce their new sense of optimism and growing self-confidence.

When a village informs the hospital that they want to form a health committee, a health worker attends another community meeting to explain the functions of each committee member and describe the sort of person ideally suited to fill each position. The committee generally consists of the following:

- a chairman: the village chief or his assistant;
- a curative health worker: he or she should already have some knowledge of medicine, either indigenous or western;
- someone responsible for water and sanitation: preferably the person already appointed to ensure that weeds do not overgrow the paths and water collection points in and around the village;
- all the village's traditional midwives: these are elderly women, usually heads of a secret society called the *Bundu* (or *Sande*);
- a woman responsible for child care: a mother with healthy children of her own;
- a clerk: a literate person, usually in his or her twenties or thirties.

The community then selects people to fill these places, and training starts in the village itself. The course makes extensive use of the results of the initial community survey: subjects covered and skills taught are targeted at the main health problems of the community. The training team consists mainly of auxiliary nurses, and stresses disease-preventive and health-promotive activities.

After the course is completed, the committee organizes another village meeting to reconsider the results of the initial survey and to try and establish realistic objectives for their work. Gradually the group begins to function as a unit seeking out, implementing and integrating all preventive and promotive activities such as sanitation, immunization, agriculture, water supply, housing, endemic disease control, mother-and-child health care, and social welfare. The committee is visited twice a month by an auxiliary nurse who gives technical guidance and encouragement.

COMMUNITY ASSESSMENT — THE ANNUAL STOCKTAKE

After the health committee has begun its work, hospital staff explain that there is certain information which it is useful to collect every year in order to assess what progress is being made. An annual community assessment is thus made on the basis of the following data:

— weight for age of under-fives;
— immunization status of under-fives;
— number of infant deaths;
— number of deaths from neonatal tetanus;
— number of wells, and latrines, and their condition;
— number of births and deaths during the previous 12 months.

The committee itself collects and analyses this data during periods when farming needs are least pressing. Nurses and auxiliaries from the hospital give technical guidance when requested. Finally the committee presents the information to a village meeting attended by a health worker who takes careful note of the people's opinions and occasionally gives advice and guidance. This annual meeting is the focal point of the community assessment method. It symbolizes the people's increasing capacity to understand and control some of the factors affecting their health, and breaks down feelings of fatalism and helplessness in the face of seemingly unsolvable health problems.

MEASURING RESULTS

We began introducing health committees in 1976 but it was not until 1978 that we had extended the system to all 11 section towns. The community assessment method enables us to measure the medical effectiveness of the programme, expressed by changes in a number of health indicators. Monitoring the health status of under-five children between 1979/80 and 1980/81, for example, gave the picture shown in Table 7.3.

Table 7.3. Infant mortality rate in 11 Section Towns

	1979/80	1980/81
Number of livebirths	403	262
Number of infant deaths	123	45
Infant mortality rate	305 per 1000 livebirths	171 per 100 livebirths

The infant mortality rate was thus almost halved in the 12-month period — a very encouraging result. The main reasons seem to have been sharp drops in deaths from neonatal tetanus and measles, and a decline in deaths from diarrhoea, as shown in Table 7.4.

Table 7.4. Causes of infant deaths in 11 Section Towns

Causes of Death	1979/80		1980/81	
	No.	%	No.	%
Tetanus	29	23.58	3	6.66
Diarrhoea	20	16.26	6	13.33
Fever	23	18.7	12	26.66
Measles	10	8.13	0	0.00
Pneumonia	3	2.44	0	0.00
Meningitis	2	1.63	2	4.44
Whooping cough	0	0.00	1	2.22
Other	36	29.27	21	46.66
Total	123	100.00	45	100.00

These results were due in part to improved immunization status of under-fives, as indicated in Table 7.5.

Table 7.5. Immunization status of under-fives in 11 Section Towns

	1979/80		1980/81	
	No.	%	No.	%
Fully immunized for age (1st, 2nd, and 3rd DPT, measles, smallpox, BCG)	418	36.70	322	55.90
Not fully immunized for age	719	63.29	254	44.10

There was also a significant decrease in the proportion of severely malnourished under-five children during the 12-month period, as shown in Table 7.6.

Table 7.6. Nutritional status of under-five children in 9 Section Towns

	1979/80		1980/81	
	No.	%	No.	%
Above 3rd percentile	336	72.57	500	77.16
Below 3rd percentile	127	27.43	148	22.84

Nutritional status is a complex problem, depending largely on factors which are only partly within the scope of a health programme, such as the quantity, acceptability, and quality of whatever food is available; the accessibility of safe water supplies; and the effects of social customs such as the widespread practice of adoption of children by relatives. Changes in nutritional status are thus more gradual than in other health indicators.

HUMAN DEVELOPMENT

The community assessment approach has led to some attitudinal and behavioural change among both villagers and professional health workers. Such change is difficult to analyse and quantify, but we have observed several interesting developments.

Attitudes towards doctors

Previously a hospital doctor could not enter a village without people rushing up and asking for medication and injections. Now, however, the people's needs for curative care are being met by the local volunteer member of the health committee or by referrals to the health centre or hospital. A doctor can go to a village for a meeting with the health committee or the traditional leaders and never be asked to treat a patient. The people have learned that health care does not start and end with the doctor.

Role of health committees

By bringing health concerns into the mainstream of village activities, the health committees have helped create a heightened community understanding of how people can organize themselves to prevent disease and improve their health. Sometimes this has involved bringing health matters into the conflict areas of village life. In Yengema village, for example, the clerk of the health committee resigned because the chief would not cooperate with the committee. The chief, on the other hand, insisted that the clerk had insulted him. The case was finally decided in the village court, and created great public interest and discussion. The court ruled that the clerk had to apologize to the chief and the elders, and then could be reinstated in his position. Though this was somewhat of a humiliating process for the clerk, the dispute threw the spotlight on the health committee. By the time it was resolved, everyone knew about the role of the committee in improving health care in the village.

In several cases the committees have had to use their data in self-defence. The local schoolteacher of Yengema village once accused the committee of having achieved nothing worthwhile. The clerk, who was a school dropout, whipped out his notebook. Citing statistics from the previous four years, he proved decisively that neonatal tetanus — once the main killer of the newborn — had been eliminated completely! The teacher was forced to make a humble apology.

Attitudes and skills of traditional midwives

Initially uncooperative and distrustful of our hospital staff, traditional midwives have come to value the knowledge and skills which we have brought them. Far from taking away their 'clientele' and lowering their status in the community, we have helped increase their popularity and prestige. Groups of midwives visit the hospital and attend operations such as Caesarian sections, and this often leads to lively and informative discussions about maternal care.

In dealing with midwives, hospital personnel must exercise great tact and sensitivity. It is often advisable to make only the most discreet initiatives and allow opinion-forming processes within the community to do the rest. In one village a young woman attended by a midwife in childbirth died in a most deplorable and unnecessary way. A formal investigation by hospital staff would have risked alienating local midwives from both the hospital and local mothers. Yet to allow such an incident to pass and therefore risk it happening again would also have been unacceptable. The matter therefore was handed over to the local village leaders and the health committee of the section town. After two weeks the hospital received a message asking for a nurse to come and train the midwives involved in the incident, so that they could do a better job in future. When other midwives in the vicinity heard this, they also wanted to join the course, and 25 from 10 villages finally took part in the full six-month course. It was never revealed publicly which midwife was responsible for the tragic death of the young woman which set in motion the whole train of events.

Attitudes of hospital staff

Our own health personnel have learned to care more about what local people think about their health problems, to ask more questions and to listen to the responses with respect rather than indulgence or scorn. They also have a deeper, better-informed understanding of the people's economic hardships. This has tempered their (sometimes unrealistic) expectations of how much time, effort and money the community itself can raise for projects such as communal water supplies and latrines.

CONSTRAINTS AND PROBLEMS

Although community assessment has raised community involvement in planning, implementing, and evaluating health care, there still remain a number of constraints and problems. These can be categorized according to whether they arise in the community as a whole, the leaders or the professional health workers.

The people

Traditionally, people in the area believe that sickness is thrust upon them by someone who has received the power to inflict evil. Sickness is only one possible form of such evil: others include bad fortune in farming or in business. In its extreme form such evil may cause death. People able to inflict evil may be members of one's own family (for example, a jealous mate in a polygamous household), or they may be neighbours. Though they may live in the same

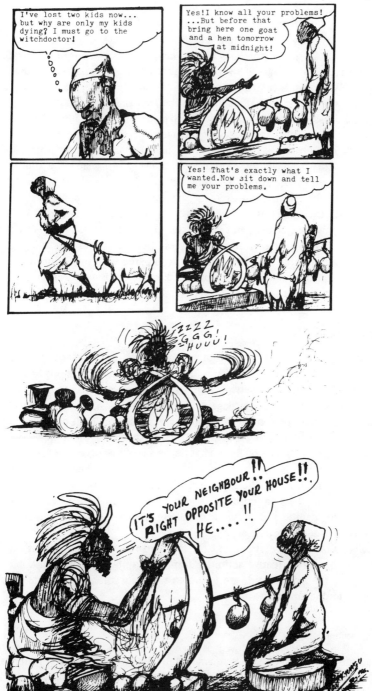

Fig. 7.1. 'Who put the virus on my child?'

community, they are extremely difficult to identify. At certain times, therefore, the community may hire a witch 'detector' or 'hunter' to identify just who is responsible for all the misfortunes in the village. Western theories of causality — virus, bacteria, etc. — may be accepted but still leave unanswered the basic question: 'Who put the virus on *my* child?' (Western medicine has no satisfactory answer either!) What may seem like tremendous apathy towards combatting the causal organism is merely the flip-side of immense and frantic activity to get to the root cause — the bewitched person.

A witch hunt (our staff have attended many) is an expensive affair, and no village can afford to have one more than once every few years. The 'hunter' and his or her entourage are wined and dined in grand style, and the local chief also takes his 'cut' for giving permission for the hunt to take place. Night after night the centre of the village is packed with men, women, and children, while the witch hunter dances, chants, and points the finger. It may take a month or two before guilt finally is pinned on some hapless victim, allowing the village to feel purged of evil and able to start life afresh. Compared with this colourful, deeply ingrained traditional way of combatting disease, an immunization campaign may well seem like a prosaic and unexciting alternative.

Local leadership

For local village leaders, health is but one concern — and a relatively minor one — among many important (and often lucrative) matters such as power struggles, collection of house tax, receiving important visitors and handling court cases such as land disputes and marriage problems. While some chiefs have taken a more active interest than others in health care, this often boils down to requesting handouts — cement for latrines, a new health centre, or a well — without understanding how the use of these facilities can be fully maximized.

Another problem is that traditional leaders tend to rely heavily on the authority of their position to elicit community 'participation'. Lacking the knowledge to explain the relationship between latrines and better health, and not being used to 'democratic' ways of decision-making, they tend to fall back on old habits of ordering people around.

Finally, all chiefs are appointed for life, and many are so old that they are unable to take any effective action to improve community organization. Their deputies, on the other hand, are afraid to take any initiatives in case they are accused of undue ambition.

Health workers

The training of all types of professional health workers tends to emphasize curative care, which is a totally inadequate preparation for primary health care work. Initially our staff tended to view 'the patient' as an entity quite separate from his or her family or community. They had little understanding of how a rural community functions and did not even understand how to elicit this information. With no training in communication skills, they were awkward in their dealings with community members and leaders. Being fairly young and with no direct experience of solving health problems through community action, they felt uncertain in the role of community motivator and teacher. The people tended to doubt the credibility and even the sincerity of some young health workers. This led to tensions and frustrations. For example, a dejected health worker once returned to the base hospital after a trip to a village and said disgustedly that he had been unable to hold a health meeting the previous evening because a professional storyteller had held the villagers enthralled until 1.30 a.m., completely ignoring his presence. Such situations call for careful handling and generous support from more senior health workers. (The storyteller has since joined the health team!)

CONCLUSION

Community assessment is the most effective method we have yet devised of stimulating and maintaining community participation in planning, implementing, and evaluating health services. It also has helped us, as professional health workers, to overcome the curative bias of our training, to appreciate the real health needs of rural people, to understand how rural communities are organized and to help people work out appropriate preventive, promotive, and curative health care services. The method certainly demands sensitivity, patience, and a willingness to discard preconceptions and learn new communications skills. The results so far, however, are encouraging, both in terms of medical effectiveness and human development. Although it may need further modification and refinement, the community assessment method seems certain to remain a central, integrating theme in our approach to primary health care.

8 Nutrition education and social change: a women's movement in the Dominican Republic

Lindsey Hilsum describes how a nutrition project developed into a strong women's movement aiming at fundamental social and economic changes in society.

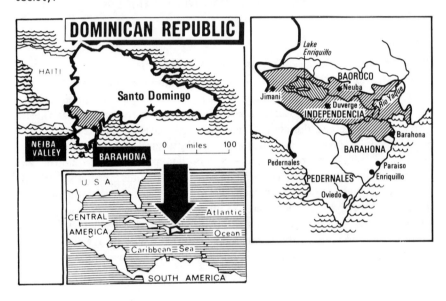

Lindsey Hilsum is a journalist who has worked in the Caribbean and Central America. She now works for UNICEF in Kenya.

'Mothers must be well-trained in home economics to feed their families adequately on a small monetary resource. Obviously nutrition education is a requisite to achieving the country's goal of well-nourished families within economic means.'

'The transfer of technical information (for example, nutrition) is not an entirely neutral or uninfluential process. Information is conveyed within a particular society. Above all, educating malnourished people about nutrition is not an apolitical activity.'

Both the above statements refer to the same nutrition project in the Dominican Republic. The first expresses the aims of the funding agency in 1973, and the second the attitude of local women eight years later. The project — Women of the South[1] — has evolved from a number of mother-and-child health feeding centres into a women's movement; from an attempt to teach mothers to be good housewives into an association of poor rural women determined not only to feed their children better, but also to understand and attack the roots of malnutrition. To appreciate what these women are doing, it is necessary to know something about their country and their position in society.

THE DOMINICAN REPUBLIC

The Dominican Republic shares an island in the Caribbean Sea with the poorest country in the western hemisphere, Haiti. It is the Dominican Republic which seems to have most of the advantages — it has twice Haiti's area but only a slightly larger population; it has mineral resources including bauxite, nickel, and gold, and rivers to irrigate its arable land. Yet despite these advantages, 70 out of every 1000 Dominican babies die before they are one year old, 40 per cent of the labour force is under- or unemployed, 33 per cent of the population is illiterate, and 45 per cent do not have access to safe drinking water. The Dominicans may be a little better off than their Haitian neighbours, but the majority still live in poverty.

Since 1965, when US marines landed to put down an attempt at constitutional reform, successive Dominican governments have favoured United States investments and export-oriented economic policies. The Dominican Republic now supplies the United States with nickel, coffee and cocoa, and — most significantly — sugar. Sugar normally accounts for half the country's export earnings, and the United States-based corporation Gulf and Western controls one-third of all production. During the past two decades the area planted to sugarcane has doubled, and now occupies around a quarter of all cultivated land. The rapid expansion of sugarcane cultivation, however, has been at the expense of staple food crops such as rice and corn.

Less than half the country's arable land is used to produce food for domestic consumption. Of the land currently producing food, about half is used to graze beef cattle, mainly for export purposes. (Few Dominicans can afford to buy beef.) Patterns of land tenure are similar to many other Latin American countries. A small number of *latifundistas* own large, plantation-type farms, while the vast majority of the rural population are relegated to tiny plots — the *minifundios*.

In the south-west of the country, where Women of the South works, the imbalances in land tenure are particularly acute, and land use is heavily oriented towards cash crops. Sugar takes up 40 per cent of the arable land, most of the remainder being devoted to coffee, cotton, and food crops consumed outside the region. Research undertaken by the Women of the South in 1980 showed that 90 per cent of cattle produce from the region was eaten elsewhere, as was 80 per cent of fish, 92 per cent of bananas, and 80 per cent of grapefruit and kidney beans. Government credit, irrigation, and desalination schemes are directed almost exclusively into export crops. In the Neiba Valley, over 80 per cent of the land planted with sugarcane is irrigated by the Sabana Yegua dam, which also produces hydroelectric power. Yet the land in the rest of te region is so dry and salty that farmers are lucky to harvest one meagre food crop a year. Few farmers own the land they cultivate, but rent it on a share-cropping basis. As the sugar kingdom expands, an increasing number of rural families are landless.

Every year thousands of Haitians slip over the border to work on the sugar plantations. Their desperation keeps wages low and conditions appalling. Haitian workers are cheaper than Dominicans and can be deported if they organize or protest.

Poverty, the most extreme and widespread in the country, characterizes the south-west. As the men tramp the region looking for work, the women often are left to support and bring up the children. When women manage to find work, it is usually as small traders, domestic servants, or farm labourers. They fight a never-ending battle against poor housing, lack of sanitation, ill-health, and malnutrition. It is these women who have been organizing to reduce infant-and-child malnutrition and to improve their general situation. Their story shows they have the potential to make significant changes in Dominican society.

FALSE START WITH FEEDING CENTRES

In 1969 a team of nutritionists led by Dr W.H. Sebrell conducted a survey of 5500 people in the middle to low-income bracket in the Dominican Republic (Sebrell 1972). Their findings painted a picture of ill-health and economic deprivation. Some 75 per cent of under-fives were found to be malnourished, and infant mortality averaged 85 per 1000 live births. Vitamin and mineral deficiencies were common among adults and children alike. Women of reproductive age were in especially bad health, with many suffering from anaemia, goitre, bone rarefaction, and low serum albumin.

Children in the south-west of the country showed the highest levels of malnutrition. Second- and third-degree malnutrition were found in one-third of under-five children, 5–7 per cent higher than in other parts of the country. Sebrell did not make a regional study of infant mortality, but statistics compiled by Women of the South in 1976 showed levels of around 115 per 1000 in parts of the south-west.

Although there are few reliable statistics on nutrition earlier than 1969, the nutritional problems of the Dominican Republic had been noted already by the US food aid agencies. Catholic Relief Services (CRS) started a programme using PL 480 Title II food in feeding centres in 1962. Church World Service (CWS), and the Co-operative for American Relief Everywhere (CARE) were – and CARE still is – operative throughout the country.

In 1973 CRS decided to step up its activities, working through the offices of CARITAS Dominicana – the official agency of the Catholic Church responsible for handling food aid in the Dominican Republic. CRS and CARITAS planned a three-tier nutrition programme on national, regional, and local levels, concentrating on children under six and pregnant and lactating women. Highest priority was given to the south-west, as the region most severely affected by malnutrition. The population of the four south-west provinces at the time was approximately 250 000 people.

The programme began in 1974 with a budget of US $9.6 million over three years for staff, transport, equipment, medical and other costs, plus US $6.5 million worth of Title II food aid. Aiming 'to lower infant mortality' and 'to improve dietary habits, childcare, and sanitation', the programme consisted most importantly of feeding centres where mothers and children received meals prepared from food aid – oat meal, bulgur wheat, flour, corn-soya blend, and wheat soya blend – sometimes mixed with locally bought sugar and cocoa. The centres had no money for buying local staple foods such as rice, beans, and plantains. By dispensing foreign foods which poor families could not afford to buy, the programme aimed to train mothers in ways of feeding their children within the limits of their own economic means. The inherent contradiction in this approach meant that the educational goals of the programme were unachievable, while the benefits of the feeding centres were short-lived. Malnourished children fed by the centres remained malnourished because their mothers were neither trained nor encouraged to feed them at home. A system of dependence on the feeding centres had been established and malnutrition in the region showed no signs of decreasing.

Yet one element of the programme eventually demonstrated how poor families could break out of the cycle of malnutrition – though in a way which had not been envisaged by CRS or CARITAS Dominicana. From the start, it had planned that some nutritional research would be done at community level, working closely with local women. This work began in 1974, when groups of local women worked with the programme's nutritionist in weighing pre-school children, carrying out surveys of local food habits, and also starting small kitchen gardens. Dissatisfied with the lack of educational and social activities at the feeding centres, the nutritionist and a group of women began casting about for alternative means of making a significant and lasting impact on the problem of infant and child malnutrition. By December 1974, they were ready to start a Nutrition Education and Recuperation Centre (CERN) in a poor section of the provincial capital of Barahona.

CERNS AND FOOD AID

The CERN was envisaged as a place where children weighing 60 per cent or less of their standard weight-for-age could be recuperated, and where mothers could learn about the causes of malnutrition and disease by participating actively in recuperation activities. CARITAS Dominicana and CRS agreed to provide the necessary funds and Title II food.

Local women, however, had not yet been trained to organize nutrition-improvement activities of any kind. So in February 1975 a women's nutrition training course began on a scale never before seen in the region. Some 62 women started attending the course – structured along Paulo Freire's lines (Freire 1972) – which examined nutrition not only in technical terms but also in the social, political, and economic context of the women's lives. Many local people doubted whether the women would leave their homes for more than a single afternoon. But in the event, the majority attended the full course for three days every month over ten months. They studied the nutritional situation of their own region, and of the entire country. They also made surveys in their own neighbourhoods to assess the nutritional problems of their families, friends, and neighbours, and to work out ways of dealing with them. Finally, after 12 months theoretical and practical training, 42 of the original 62 women 'graduated' to become *promotoras* – local promotors of nutrition and social education.

The *promotoras*, by this time, already were working with groups of women in 40 communities. These women's groups were to become the backbone of the movement, which at this time still used the name *Educacion Nutricional Caritas*. Meeting twice a month, they discussed nutrition-related topics, composed motivational songs, and tried out new recipes using low-priced local foods for optimum nutritional value. Discussion topics were worked out in advance by the *promotoras*, who introduced them to the meetings and enlivened the discussions. The topic of 'drinking water' was chosen in 1976. The groups examined health-related questions such as the necessity for boiling water, agricultural problems such as drought and salty lands, and social issues such as who had access to water for household needs and irrigation.

In early 1976 a second CERN was set up, again supported by CARITAS and CRS. Both CERNs worked closely with local women's groups. Mothers brought severely malnourished children for recuperation using only food and deworming medicines over a three-month period. The CERNs were run on a strict policy of admitting only those children whose mothers were prepared to participate by coming for a half day every week over the whole period of the child's recuperation. Though this may appear a harsh policy, the women knew from their previous experience of feeding centres that there was little point in recuperating children whose mothers were not trained to feed them adequately afterwards.

Mothers attending the CERNs became actively involved in the recuperation of the children by regularly weighing them and taking anthropomorphic measurements. They also participated in lively learning sessions where they discussed topics such as oral rehydration therapy for diarrhoea, the nutritional value of local foods, infant feeding (especially the importance of breast milk), vaccination against preventable diseases, treatment of common child illnesses, and environmental and personal hygiene. Over the three months that the child was being recuperated, the mother was being educated so that she could control some of the factors influencing the wellbeing of her children.

Meanwhile, the *promotoras* continued to carry out nutritional surveys in the region. Their growing doubts about the efficacy of dispensing Title II food aid were reinforced by the results of weighing children over two years in various communities. Results showed that malnourished children receiving food aid from the local feeding centres failed to gain weight except at three distinct times of the year – the mango season (May), the avocado season (October), and also in December – the only month of the year when the food aid actually *stopped!* Far from averting malnutrition, Title II food aid, so it seemed, actually contributed to it. The women set about trying to solve this mystery. They found that food aid was being used, not as a supplement to local foods, but as a re-placement. The free foreign 'wonder' food was thought to be sufficient in itself, which was far from being the case. Moreover, it often was shared among the whole family, or some of it sold for cash, so that malnourished children did not consume the recommended amounts. Yet during December, when no food aid was available and mothers had to feed their children with local foods, they managed to do this successfully.

The *promotoras* then looked into the high cost of transporting, storing and distributing food aid, and decided it would be more economic and nutritionally effective if the donor agency ceased to supply food aid and instead gave their organization a cash grant for agricultural and animal husbandry projects. This was not acceptable to the donor agency, which then ceased to provide further support to the CERNs and the women's groups. This sequence of events was a major turning point in the development of the women's movement.

CERNS REDUCE MALNUTRITION

The women were determined to continue the two CERNs using local food rather than Title II food aid. They were also determined to expand the number of local women's groups, which now numbered more than 50 in the Neiba Valley. Yet to spring from heavy dependency on foreign funds and food to total self-sufficiency in money for running costs and food to recuperate malnourished children was impossible. Two European agencies therefore agreed to provide funds for running costs, while CARITAS in Holland agreed to provide the organization with free powdered milk.

Milk had the advantage of being familiar. But although locally produced, milk was above the means of ordinary people, and often contaminated. It was decided to use a small proportion to supplement the diets of malnourished children at the CERNs, and to sell most of it made up in liquid form at 'milk posts'. Simply giving away milk powder not only would have created dependence, but would have been irresponsible, few mothers having access to adequate amounts of safe water. At the milk posts, therefore, a few women from the local group used boiled water to make up liquid milk in sanitary conditions. The product was sold cheaply (about half the market price), but the costs of transport, storage, and administrative overheads were still covered.

The women defined their aims specifically: to reduce third-degree malnutrition by 75 per cent and second-degree by 25 per cent. Their strategy had four main components: first, recuperation of malnourished children, using mainly local foods, in CERNs; second, nutrition and social education for mothers in CERNs and women's groups; third, projects to increase family incomes and food availability; and fourth, projects to increase the income of the organization itself.

The CERNs differed from the food aid-supported feeding centres in important aspects. While the CERNs worked closely with local women's groups, the feeding centres had no comparable community support system. Whereas CERNs involved mothers actively in weighing children and checking their growth, the feeding centres allotted mothers merely passive roles. And while the CERNs used mostly local foods purchased and prepared by the mothers themselves, the feeding centres used imported Title II foods, too expensive for most families to buy (if available at all).

By mid-1977 a third CERN had joined the programme and 1800 women were active in 74 groups throughout the Neiba Valley. The combination of CERNs and women's groups had a marked impact on nutritional levels. In Vengan a Ver, a community of about 3000 people, 147 severely malnourished children were recuperated over a 12-month period in 1977/78. Four years later, in 1981, neither the original children, nor their younger siblings, had suffered malnourishment (see Fig. 8.1). Similar results were obtained in other communities. The CERNs linked with mothers' groups succeeded in breaking the cycle of malnutrition in these communities.

By the end of 1978 less than 1 per cent of under-fives in the whole project

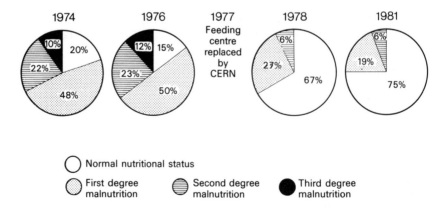

Fig. 8.1. Nutritional status of under-fives in Vengan a Var, 1974–81.

area were found to be severely malnourished (see Fig. 8.2). The CERNs there-fore were closed, and two were converted into nursery schools for about 300 children. ·

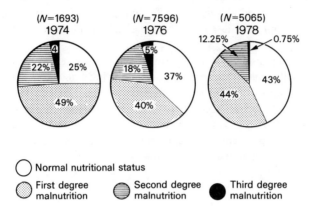

Fig. 8.2. Nutritional status of under-fives in project area 1974–78.

At the same time as the CERNs and women's groups were reducing severe malnutrition in the project area, feeding centres in the nearby communities of Fondo Negro and Las Baitoas continued to reproduce the familiar pattern of malnutrition and dependency (Fig. 8.3).

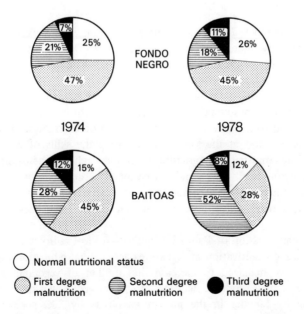

Fig. 8.3. Nutritional status of under-fives in Fondo Negro and Baitoas 1974–78.

Fondo Negro has been called the 'economic miracle' of the Dominican Republic because of heavy government investment in local agricultural export industries. Yet in 1978 some 11 per cent of under-five children suffered severe malnutrition, an increase of 4 per cent from 1974. In Las Baitoas, another community with a food aid-supported feeding centre, the proportion of under-fives suffering from second- and third-degree malnutrition rose from 40 per cent in 1974 to 60 per cent in 1978.

The contrasting results of food aid-supported feeding centres on the one hand and CERNs with women's groups using mainly local food on the other, have been noted by outside observers. A survey done for CRS in 1980 'found malnutrition in all of the dioceses where there are MCH feeding centres with the exception of Barahona. This diocese, the poorest in the country, has long rejected the food programme as detrimental to the beneficiaries and has designed their own programme based on the value of local food' (CRS Dominican Republic 1981, p. 5).

ECONOMIC PROJECTS

Most of the economic projects started by Women of the South have aimed to increase food availability and incomes of individual families. Some projects have also been designed to contribute income to the organization itself.

Vegetable gardens

These were started in 1974 and two years later several women were growing vegetables regularly under the auspices of CARITAS Dominicana. In 1976 there was a drought and several gardens faltered through lack of water and technical assistance. As they had been cultivated individually, there was no community effort to overcome the problems. In 1977, however, several women decided to cultivate vegetables communally, partly for home consumption and partly for sale. They aimed to increase family consumption of vegetables, thereby raising nutritional levels, and at the same time learning the skills of cultivation and marketing. The Ministry of Agriculture offered technical assistance, but the government agronomist visited only occasionally, the seeds provided did not germinate and the promised pesticide and wire to guard against insect and animal damage never arrived. Once more, the women were thrown back on their own resources.

With the participation of Radio Enriquillo — a local radio station which produces booklets on cultivation and features agricultural education broadcasts — the women have managed to increase the number of vegetable gardens and market some of their produce. According to the project's own surveys, vegetable consumption by families in the project area rose by 200 per cent between 1975/76 and 1981.

Livestock

An early attempt at breeding rabbits failed because the animals sickened and died. A pig-fattening project was wiped out by swine fever in 1979. The chicken project, however, was successful for a few years. The aims of the project were to sell chicken meat cheaply, thus providing additional employment and income, while also increasing consumption of locally produced animal protein. Several women took a chicken-rearing course run by the Ministry of Agriculture. Groups of five women bought chicks, which they fattened, killed, and sold. By 1979, in Pueblo Nuevo alone, there were three groups of five women with 6000 chickens per group.

The hurricane of August 1979 brought production to a halt. It was impossible to obtain chicken feed or replacement chicks. Entrepreneurs blocked attempts to buy chicks locally because they benefitted from steep prices for scarce chicken meat. Eventually, with the help of the Ministry of Agriculture, the women bought hens. The competition, however, was fierce and the Ministry refused to give extra financial and technical help. Whereas before the hurricane the women all had been selling US $100-200 worth of chickens per month, now they were losing money. The final blow was dealt by the government itself: INESPRE, the official price control body, set up a large chicken project nearby. This received the technical and financial assistance the women had been denied, and their small project was unable to compete. The poultry project thus owed its demise to big business control of prices and supplies, lack of government support, and the women's own commercial inexperience.

Milk posts

The sale of milk has been the best source of steady income for the project. By 1978 there were 30 milk posts selling 4000 litres of milk per day. Hurricane David in 1979 created a need for more, so another 20 were established selling 10 000 litres a day. This was reduced in June 1980 to 41 posts selling 9000 litres per day.

The main disadvantage of using imported milk powder is that it signifies dependence on a foreign product — something which the women want to avoid. But milk has been an important factor in reducing infant and child malnutrition, so the women believe it important to replace it with a locally produced protein product as soon as possible. Currently the women are investigating the feasibility of establishing a soya bean processing plant, raising dairy cattle or goats, or buying milk locally.

Community shops and restaurants

The first CERNs had small grocery shops and food stalls attached. These have continued to be a success: in mid-1982 there were five grocery shops and two food stalls. They sell food cheaply and where possible buy direct from producers rather than middle-men, thus under-cutting competition. The food stalls sell bean soup and rice, yucca leaf soup, milk, fruit juices, and fresh fruit. Fuel costs are so high that some people find it cheaper to eat at a food stall than at home, and the stalls have thus become popular meeting places. The grocery shops sometimes have difficulty obtaining sufficient stocks of basic foods such as rice and sugar, due to hoarding by local entrepreneurs and the unhelpful policies of government agencies. Despite these problems, the shops and the food stalls continue to prosper and provide a valuable service to many people.

Priority for collective efforts

In early 1980 the women took part in a self-evaluation of the whole programme, including the economic projects. When questioned about the economic projects, many women expressed concern that most of these benefitted only a few individuals rather than the whole community. The 'project holders' were seen by many as ambitious and self-seeking rather than community-spirited. 'Before they were cats, now they are tigers', said one woman. Another said: 'It resolves the problems of the project holders, but it doesn't touch the big questions'. Another placed her objections in a wider context: 'The government must take more responsibility'.

Yet attitudes to the economic projects were not entirely negative. Several women felt that the measure of economic independence they enjoyed through the collective projects was important for their strength: 'It helps to defend ourselves against the exploiters'. The evaluation concluded that the economic projects tended to benefit only a small number of people, did not always answer the community's needs, could cause conflict, could not always compete with other businesses, and were often badly administered. Most importantly, 'it is possible to confuse educational success with material success'. In other words, sometimes it was the economic potential only of projects which attracted women to join a group, and this tended to undermine the educational purpose of the group as a whole.

The women therefore decided not to start any more projects such as chicken-raising until there was adequate protection from local governmental and legal structures. It was also decided to define clearly the line between educational work and economic ventures. The *promotoras* should not have a personal economic interest in any project. The primary motivation of the groups must be educational, with economic projects being a secondary concern. Every economic project would be subject to strict criteria. Does it raise or lower 'consciousness'? Does it help organization or cause conflict? Does it promote independence in the face of exploitation? Does it benefit many or only few? Any *collective* economic activity such as milk posts, food stalls and shops which satisfied these criteria would receive group support, but no *individual* economic ventures would be supported in any way.

GROUP ORGANIZATION AND OPERATIONAL METHODS

When the women decided to discontinue the use of Title II food aid in CERNs in 1976, they also began a process of restructuring the organization and operational methods of their own groups. It was decided that the *promotoras* would continue to hold twice-monthly meetings with local women's groups and also organize one day meetings for the 12 or so groups in each zone three times a year. The *promotoras* also would attend twice-yearly three-day courses at the Popular Education Centre to assess their work. Every two years there would be an *Encuentro de la Mujer* — a mass meeting of all women involved in the movement to consolidate their work and establish themselves as a united movement of 'Women of the South'. Nutrition would be the central theme, but treated as a socioeconomic problem rather than simply a technical matter.

Another significant decision taken at this time was to select six of the most able *promotoras* for further training, so that they could take over the running of the programme from the end of 1978.

The first series of one day meetings took as their theme 'The Situation of Women in the South'. They discussed family planning and sex, prevention of disease, and the promotion of good health in low income communities. To enliven the discussions and emphasize certain points, the women made collages from newspapers and magazines, composed and learned songs, and carried out a kind of role play which they call *sociodrama*.

Sociodrama has become an important part of the women's regular activities. A group chooses an everyday situation exemplifying a particular theme and acts it out. The scene presents ideas rather than preaching a set message. The songs on the other hand are more explicit:

>Let me tell you, my friend
>These days we can't cope,
>Rice costs 34 cents,
>And it's 40 cents for soap.
>
>In the neglected slums,
>We're tired of having to say:
>'Light costs too much
>And we can't afford to pay'.
>
>*Chorus:* Onward, women, onward!
>   Together we must strive,
>   Let us unite
>   To better our lives.
>
>In the schools, my friends,
>There's neither chalk nor blackboard,

> But the teacher just sits there;
> The omission is ignored.
>
> After so much exploitation,
> Hear the people cry:
> 'Those who are in power
> Are squeezing us dry'.

The women's groups have become quite renowned locally, contributing their songs, sociodramas, recipes, discussion topics, and health-care suggestions to the radio station *Radio Enriquillo*.

At the end of 1978, as planned, the six *promotoras* who had received further training took over the running of the programme. They became *encargadas* (organizers), each responsible for a zone containing about 12 women's groups. There were five such zones, and the sixth *encargada* was in charge of the CERN and nursery school programme. The *encargadas* are full-time, salaried employees of the organization.

In 1979 the women took the Year of the Child as their theme. First they looked at childbirth, then at the principles referring to children in the United Nations Human Rights Charter. They asked whether all children in the Dominican Republic enjoyed those rights, and what could be done to improve the lot of those who did not.

> A child shall enjoy
> The Rights in the Charter
> They can now be fulfilled
> In the Year of the Child.
> How can a child grow
> Without milk, without meat?
> When the fever comes and goes
> And leads him to death?
> Some are born lucky
> And experience their Rights.
> Others are born poor,
> And their Rights are denied.
> The child in the slum
> Asks his father 'Is it true
> That this is the year
> When something will change?'
>
> But they say the year has ended,
> And yet they are wrong.
> The Year of the Child
> Has only just begun

Women of our group,
We will fight on,
The children of the South
Need us for years to come.

On the last day of August 1979, the programme was severely disrupted by Hurricane David, which wreaked heavy damage throughout the Dominican Republic. It was followed by Hurricane Frederic, which caused further destruction in the south-west. Thousands of families lost their homes and their livelihoods. All land communications were cut, food stocks and crops destroyed, hunger and starvation threatened tens of thousands of families. It was in this emergency that the women's groups demonstrated their organization and unity for the benefit of the whole community.

With emergency food rations from the government and World Food Programme (WFP) not reaching the people of the south-west, the women decided to act. Through the local Catholic Bishop, they contacted WFP in Haiti and Rome and CARITAS in Holland, asking that food in keeping with local customs be sent directly to them, not via the national capital Santo Domingo. Their requests were met swiftly, and supplies of rice, beans, fish, milk, and maize began arriving at the docks in Barahona. But the men unloading the food started diverting much of it for their own use, either to eat or to resell. The women quickly intervened to stop this, but the men retaliated by refusing to unload the boats. As the men sat on the docks, the women themselves started unloading the sacks of food and guarding them, frightening off would-be robbers with wooden staves. The men finally gave in and resumed unloading the boats, but the women maintained their guard on the unloaded supplies.

On returning to their communities, the women worked with branches of the Farmers' Association to distribute the food rations for the duration of the emergency, which was three months and three weeks. People were asked to contribute $1 towards their ration, to cover transport and distribution costs, and local committees were set up to guard against corruption. The women also established stocks of some basic commodities so local entrepreneurs could not create false scarcities by hoarding, and so push up the prices. Finally, the women organized the collection of fruit from trees which had been blown down by the hurricane, and made jam which they sold to finance some of their work during the emergency.

When the groups met again they naturally discussed the effects of the hurricanes. Whereas houses in the south-west had been flattened, those in wealthier (especially urban) areas had withstood the high winds. They discussed housing standards and the effects of bad housing on children's health.

Despite the disruption of the hurricanes, the women still managed to organize a massive *Encuentro de la Mujer* at the end of 1979. They addressed themselves to the issue: 'Analyse the rights of the child and whether they are fulfilled, taking into account the economic situation'. Their conclusions were

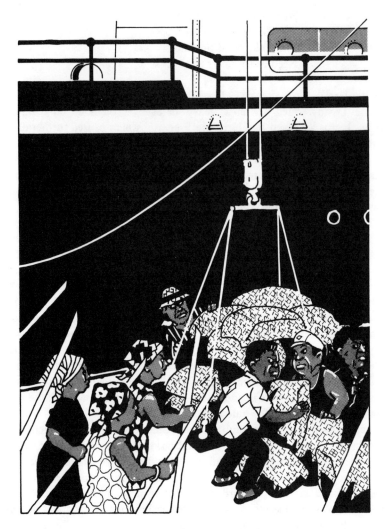

Fig. 8.4. Emergency food supplies arrive at Barahona docks: women intervene to stop pilfering.

summarized in an open letter signed by 1783 women, published in six daily papers. The letter listed the women's concerns about the state of children in the south-west: their low nutritional status, the appalling school system, totally inadequate health services, poor housing and sanitation, and widespread child labour because of their parents' poverty due to lack of resources, employment, and income. The women concluded: 'Given this situation, we see that, despite the government's promises, the International Year of the Child has been the same as, or even worse than, other years'. The women demanded that the government should:

- fulfill the United Nations Charter for the Rights of the Child;
- keep its promises to the south-west region;
- create more employment for both men and women;
- take into account their denunciation, made by women concerned for the better future of their children.

This public statement, with its obvious political overtones, was an important milestone in the development of the women's movement. Their own report on their activities from July to December 1979 made the following observation on the changing orientation of the groups:

'The groups are orienting themselves increasingly towards becoming a movement to demand the rights of each person, which the government should fulfill, and to impress upon the authorities that they must provide at least basic services to communities.'

By 1980 the movement involved nearly 3000 women in about 100 groups throughout the Neiba Valley, but at least 20 000 women listened to the weekly radio broadcasts on Radio Enriquillo. Their activities for the year fell into two main parts. First, an evaluation of their work over the previous four years — what had they achieved and learned, and what should they do now? Secondly, in conjunction with a people's education centre from Santo Domingo, an analysis of the wider political context of the Dominican Republic, Central America, and the Caribbean. The report for January to June 1980 explains the thinking behind this year of understanding.

'Since January our situation has worsened. This can be explained partly by the hurricane; but every day the country gets more chaotic and without a doubt harder for the poor — in our case, the most marginalized women. Because of this, each of our activities has been increasingly oriented towards an *understanding* of the situation, in the hope that through such an understanding we will see more clearly the way to a fairer and more humane way of life.'

The women continued to examine the effect of the hurricanes of 1979 on their lives. Poverty had prevented many people from rebuilding, sanitation and hygiene had deteriorated, so health problems had increased. Many women and children were ill, and some had died. The groups worked on immediate and practical measures to cope with food contamination and curing the sick; they also tried to develop preventive measures. They asked what the government had done to limit the effects of the hurricanes on the poorest sections of society. Later in the year they showed an audiovisual presentation about the effects of the hurricanes to youth groups, farmers' associations and other community organizations and discussed issues raised. Reaching out to other organizations, 'conscientizing' them, was now a high priority.

October 1980 brought Hurricane Allen, which severely damaged the south-west. Once again, the women's groups became the focus of the community mobilization in the emergency. Now established as local leaders and with good contacts with other organizations, the members of Women of the South often acted as catalysts for effective local relief efforts.

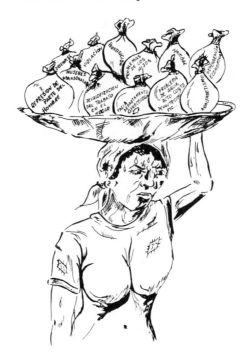

Fig. 8.5. 'Every day the country gets more chaotic and without a doubt harder for the poor': poster designed by Women of the South.

The evaluation undertaken in early 1980 also brought about important changes within the women's organization itself. In order to further decentralize and democratize decision-making, the organizational structure was simplified and reduced to a council of management and nine operational teams (see Fig. 8.6).

The Council of Management consists of representatives from the various teams, and is designed to ensure that no one person or group has absolute authority over the others.

As the women were becoming increasingly outspoken in their demands on both local and central government, they felt a need for the protection of a legally registered body. It therefore was decided to become *Promocion de la Mujer del Sur, Inc.* – a legally registered association.

LIMITS TO NUTRITION EDUCATION

In 1981 over 3000 women living in 76 villages and towns scattered throughout the valleys of the Neiba and Yaque rivers (see map, p. 114) were active in 106 groups belonging to Women of the South. Though the programme is intended to cover all four provinces of the south-west, its activities to date are confined

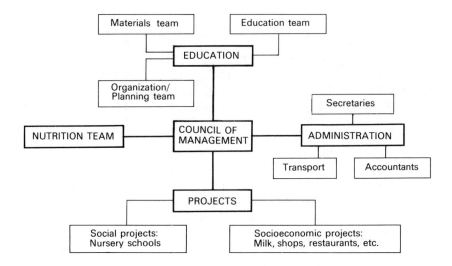

Fig. 8.6. Administrative structure of *Promocion de la Mujer del Sur, Inc.,* 1981.

to only three provinces. Of the 28 000 low-income women in the south-west, only about 11 per cent are active in the women's movement, but at least 70 per cent are in regular contact with it through the weekly broadcasts on Radio Enriquillo.

The two former CERNs now function as nursery schools for around 300 children, with teachers' salaries paid by UNICEF through the Ministry of Education. A child psychologist works with the teachers, and the children are learning about their region through visits to different places. Except for the imported powdered milk, the only food consumed by the children is locally produced and made with recipes which mothers can easily learn. Each mother pays a small weekly fee for her child, and meets the teachers once a month to discuss the child's progress and the running of the school. A nurse carries out systematic nutrition surveillance of the children.

Yet the nutritional status of many children in the region remains precarious. A nutrition survey of under-fives in the programme area in 1981 found no improvement on the situation three years earlier. The dramatic improvements between 1976 and 1978 could not be sustained largely because of sharp increases in food prices. According to statistics compiled by Women of the South, basic food prices in the south-west rose by an average of 54 per cent between February 1978 and February 1980, while wages rose by only 10 per cent.

Analysing these inflation statistics, the women are relating the problem of malnutrition to the export-oriented economic policies of the government. Recipes using locally grown foods are accompanied by a cost analysis. How much did the ingredients cost this year compared with last? Who grows the food, who markets it, and who makes the profit? In this way the women are addressing the question of how they can combat the economic system which raises prices irrespective of the poverty of most Dominicans. They see Women of the South as a movement to conscientize members of the community and as a pressure group to influence the media and the government. Over six years they have built up the confidence and unity needed to assert themselves within their own society, and they are achieving increased recognition on both a local and national level.

CONCLUSION

Over the past six years the members of Women of the South have increased their knowledge of nutrition, health, and food production, enabling them to reduce the prevalence of malnutrition in their communities. Many of them also have gained administrative and financial skills, which they have demonstrated by organizing local communities in emergency situations caused by natural disasters. Their realization of the limits of nutrition education has led them to analyse the socioeconomic and political structure of their own society and their own role within it. They have become truly *conciente*, aware of themselves and their role, and their first question when faced with any problem is: 'What can we, as women of the South, do?' They believe in their own power to instigate a social change, and to work with other organizations to create conditions in which children will be well fed, clothed, housed, and educated. The slogan of the 1979 *Encuentro de la Mujer* expresses their determination and their aims:

Women of the South – it is time to awake!
Fight for the Future of your children!

NOTE

1. *Promocion de la Mujer del Sur*, literally 'Association for the Advancement of Women of the South'.

REFERENCES

Catholic Relief Services, Dominican Republic, *Summary of Interpretive Report on the evaluation of the Title II Food Program in the Dominican Republic*, September (1981).
Freire, Paulo, *Pedagogy of the oppressed*. Penguin, Harmondsworth (1972).
Sebrell, W.H. *et al. Nutritional status of middle and low income groups in the Dominican Republic*, Archivos Latinoamericanos de Nutricion (1972), 22 (Numero Especial). Institute of Human Nutrition, Columbia University, New York.

9 Human development through primary health care: case studies from India

Maitrayee Mukhopadhyay argues that effective primary health care programmes are largely the result of the human development of village health workers and their communities.

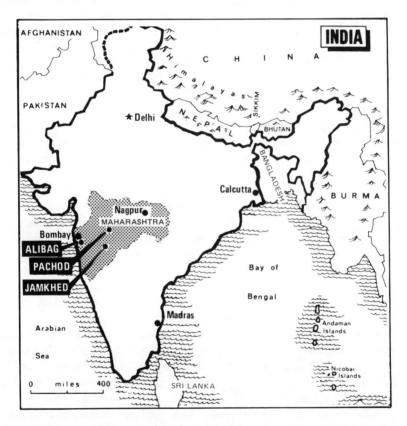

Maitrayee Mukhopadhyay, a graduate in Sociology from Bombay University, is a rural development consultant based in Calcutta.

Primary health care programmes generally give high priority to training a cadre of village health workers (VHWs)[1] as the first point of contact between the people and the health care system. Living and working within their own communities, VHWs have certain advantages over health professionals: they have close cultural and social affinities with the people, besides being relatively inexpensive to train, equip, and maintain in the field.

In a highly stratified society such as India, the conscious decision to train ordinary people and give them responsibilities for health care can represent an important investment in *human development* at two levels: the individual VHW on the one hand, and the community on the other. Indeed the effectiveness of PHC programmes depends critically on such human development — transforming the attitudes, knowledge, health practices, and organizational capacities of VHWs and the communities in which they live and work.

Yet merely selecting and training large numbers of VHWs is no guarantee of their effectiveness in a PHC system, as shown by the experience of India's Community Health Worker Scheme (see Chapter 3). Government-sponsored PHC programmes in India generally have made little headway in promoting the sort of comprehensive human development essential for long-term improvements in public health. It is often forgotten that thw VHW concept is based largely on the experience of the 'barefoot doctor' in China. The socioeconomic and political structures of post-1949 China, however, are very different from those of post-1947 India. Transplanted into the Indian context of hierarchical and exploitative structures, the VHW concept has often become a cheap, gimmicky means of mobilizing 'community participation' in health programmes planned and implemented in top-down fashion and of little or no benefit to the vast majority of the people.

By contrast, various small-scale PHC programmes sponsored by voluntary agencies in India during the past decade have demonstrated a distinctive type and quality of human development accounting largely for their relatively high degree of medical effectiveness, and distinguishing them from programmes of the Ministry of Health. It would be unrealistic to expect these small-scale programmes to be replicated on a national scale. Yet they do provide valuable experience of the conditions determining the effectiveness of PHC programmes. Official health planners and administrators, however, still seem unable to draw appropriate conclusions from this experience.

Nowhere are the dimensions of human development through PHC programmes in India more noticeable than in projects involving women VHWs. This may be because Indian women, who traditionally have very low social status, are potentially more responsive than men to the unaccustomed recognition they receive from performing socially productive and relevant roles. It is essential, however, that their trainers and mentors assign them real responsibilities rather than treating them as lackies to the health professionals.

In the following discussion of the dimensions of human development through PHC, examples will be cited from three projects sponsored by voluntary agencies in Maharashtra State of Central India. Since most disease-preventive and health-promotive work is closely related to women and children, all three projects decided to recruit and train female VHWs — traditional midwives (*dais*) and community health workers (CHWs). The first and best known, the Comprehensive Rural Health Project at Jamkhed, began in 1971 and ten years later covered 62 villages with a total population of 100 000 (Arole 1978). The second project, begun in 1973 by the Foundation for Research in Community Health, covers 30 villages with a population of 35 000 in Alibag district, across the harbour from Bombay (Battiwala 1981). The third project, the Comprehensive Health and Development Project based at Pachod, began in 1976 and now covers 50 villages with a population of 67 000 in Aurangabad district (see Chapter 6).

HUMAN DEVELOPMENT AT COMMUNITY LEVEL

Three dimensions of human development at community level were observed in the three projects:

- health knowledge and practices;
- decision-making processes;
- attitudes towards women, caste, and VHWs.

Health knowledge and practices: de-elitism of health care

In a hierarchical society such as rural India, the local elite generally monopolizes health services. Health professionals, being mostly of high social status themselves, tend to relate to their own peer group in the village. Low-status, underprivileged groups cannot easily avail themselves of health services, and they have only limited knowledge of the causes of ill-health and disease. When VHWs of low social status were recruited into the three programmes, however, the bias was turned in favour of the underprivileged groups. A study of the Alibag project (Mukhopadhyay 1974) found that 90 per cent of the VHWs' clientele consisted of low-caste, low-income people living within half a kilometre of the VHWs' homes. The services provided by the VHWs were valued highly: 80 per cent of the clients stated they had received attention within 20 minutes, compared with one to five hours if a doctor had been called. Nine out of ten respondents claimed a significant improvement in their health after receiving attention from a VHW – the same proportion as for treatment from a doctor.

Similarly at Pachod, where the emphasis has been mainly on maternal care, VHWs (mainly retrained traditional midwives) working within their own peer group of low-status, low-caste women, have had a marked impact on the patterns of health practices and knowledge within the community. Over 80 per cent of the women attending ante-natal clinics are employed as agricultural labourers, construction site workers, or marginal farmers. Despite the inconvenience of having to fit attendance at the clinic into their otherwise busy lives, they attend regularly and participate actively in running activities at their clinic. They are not merely consumers of a service, but have acquired much of the knowledge and skills needed for organizing community-based, disease-preventive and health-promotive health services.

Similar examples could be cited for Jamkhed. In all three projects a process of 'de-elitism' of health care has taken place: low-status, low-income groups are delivering and utilizing health services which previously had been the almost exclusive preserve of a small elite of health professionals and their peer group of village notables.

Decision-making processes

A second dimension of human development at community level is that of organizational capacities. In all three projects more effective health services were associated with shifts in decision-making processes away from people at the centre of power towards those on the periphery.

In Pachod, for example, health matters were officially the responsibility of health committees consisting of all-male village authority figures. But after female VHWs were trained and began working with local women, decision-making and opinion-forming powers on health issues shifted subtly to the informally organized ante-natal clinics, attended only by women, who previously had virtually no voice in village affairs. Granted, the men's health committees have served the limited but useful purpose of neutralizing opposition to the Pachod health programme by putting the full weight of their authority behind it. The changing of attitudes and health practices and decision-making on practical problems, however, has been carried out entirely by the women's ante-natal clinics. Organized originally to make fortnightly check-ups of pregnant women, the clinics now play a large role in community affairs. They still provide ante-natal care, but also function as under-fives clinics where mothers bring their children for nutrition surveillance and take part in health education. A large number of older women with grown-up children also attend. These are the mothers, mothers-in-law, or 'good neighbours' who act as a sort of chorus encouraging those attending to undergo examination, explaining why this is necessary, citing instances of women who had difficulties because they did not avail themselves of ante-natal care. These older women comprise a powerful lobby group in favour of the programme.

The atmosphere of a typical ante-natal clinic in the Pachod programme is lively, cheerful, and occasionally chaotic, as women discuss their experiences and exchange opinions. Discussions cover a wide area apart from purely health topics – the prices of basic foods, money-lending, means of exploitation of poor villagers by the rich, and ways of resisting these. The auxiliary nurse, CHW, and dai present at each meeting have developed skilled techniques to spread information and form opinions and habits. Health education is thus not a sterile, pedantic activity but a dynamic process affecting practical decisions. Whether a mother will try a suggested diet pattern for an under-nourished child, whether or not she will adopt family planning, how she treats a child with diarrhoea – these are the sorts of decisions shaped by the group norms prevalent in the forum of the ante-natal clinics.

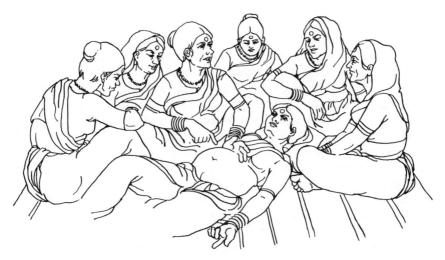

Fig. 9.1. Dai conducts ante-natal clinic.

In the village of Thergaon in the Pachod project for example, a woman with an extremely serious problem found a solution with the help of the local ante-natal clinic. She was pregnant for the sixth time, was suffering from tuberculosis, and wanted to terminate her pregnancy. Her husband, however, refused to allow the hospital to carry out the operation, even though having the child would entail a grave risk to her health. To complicate the situation still further, she was a wage labourer and because of her family's grave economic circumstances had to continue doing heavy manual work in the fields. The women at her local ante-natal clinic discussed her problems and eventually thrashed out solutions. Two women were charged with the responsibility of persuading her husband and relatives to agree to the operation. They also agreed to accompany her to the hospital. Similar examples of group solidarity and mutual support among women in the other two projects suggest that the process of devolving decision-making power upon the group most directly affected by a health project — mothers — is a meaningful indicator of human development at community level through PHC.

Attitudes towards women, caste, and village health workers

In traditional, male-dominated Hindu society, women are assigned a subordinate role and caste discrimination rigorously upheld. In the field of health care, female VHWs such as dais are generally denigrated as inferior to fully trained male health professionals. Yet experience from the three projects studied illustrate how the attitudes of a whole village community towards low caste women health workers can undergo a dramatic transformation.

Pimpalgaon is a village with a population of about 100 people, eight miles from Jamkhed (Arole 1978, pp. 129–31). In 1973 it was a very caste-ridden community. The *harijans* ('outcastes') lived outside the main village, and were not allowed to enter the temple or any non-harijan homes. It was at this time that Lalanbai Kadam was chosen as a community health worker. She is a harijan and a widow, probably the most unfortunate status that a human being in India could have. Every week Lalanbai came for training, mostly out of curiosity. She was hearing things she had never heard before: all people are 'equal'; women have as many rights as men; disease is not due to the gods but to germs or lack of food. The nurse showed a child with kwashiorkor and explained that this condition was caused simply by lack of food. Lalanbai came a little closer to the nurse and started listening with greater interest. By the time she had completed the course, Lalanbai was determined to start breaking down the old prejudices which stamped her as a virtually worthless human being.

Lalanbai started walking boldly around the village, attending public meetings (previously all-male occasions), and entering people's homes to make suggestions for health improvement and development. Though there were murmurings about her 'audacity', nobody publicly opposed her. Then disaster struck. A young man in the village died of a cerebral haemorrhage. The whole village panicked. They felt it was God's curse because they were allowing a harijan widow to enter their homes, they were listening to her advice and taking medicines touched by her. Many people wanted to chase her out of the village. On the advice of the project staff, she stayed in the village but stopped her health work. That same day, one of the village women went into labour, and Lalanbai was called. She refused to attend the delivery, however, on the grounds that the villagers had asked her to stop working. Mothers brought children for medicine, but were obliged to go to the CHW in the next village because Lalanbai could no longer dispense medicine. Within two days the whole village realized the importance of the role played in their lives by Lalanbai. She was presented with a petition pleading her to resume her health work. Finally, after a public apology for the shabby way she had been treated, Lalanbai was formally reinstated. A total transformation in the attitude of the whole community to this poor, 'outcaste' widow had taken place.

HUMAN DEVELOPMENT AT INDIVIDUAL LEVEL

At the level of the individual village health worker, five dimensions of human development were observed in the three projects:

— development of professional skills and attitudes;
— growth of a positive self-image;
— desire for self-improvement;
— breakdown of cultural prejudices;
— growth of leadership qualities.

Development of professional skills and attitudes

A learning process took place enabling women with little or no previous health training to acquire a high degree of proficiency in certain areas of health care. The dais at Pachod, for example, achieved impressive results in the field of maternal and neo-natal care. Previous to being trained at Pachod hospital, they were giving a totally unprofessional service often detrimental to the health of mothers and infants. With no knowledge of ante- or post-natal care, their role was simply to assist deliveries after the baby's head appeared at the introitus. They never washed their hands before assisting a delivery, and also practised harmful techniques such as stretching and massaging the vagina and pulling out the placenta, which not infrequently caused puerperal sepsis. Severing the umbilical cord was done with an unsterilized instrument such as a piece of glass, a sickle, a kitchen knife, or a sharp stone.

The situation changed dramatically after the dais had been trained. A survey of their knowledge, attitudes, and health practices three years after the initial training course found that all 37 dais were in the habit of visiting mothers in their homes to teach them about ante-natal services, identify pregnancies, and carry out an initial examination before bringing them to the village ante-natal clinic and referring high-risk cases to the visiting nurse or the hospital in Pachod. During deliveries they sit with the mother right through her labour pains, and visit her at least three times within the first ten days after delivery. Washing their hands with soap and water before assisting delivery has become standard practice. Harmful practices such as stretching and massaging the vagina and pulling out the placenta have ceased. All the dais use the safe delivery kits

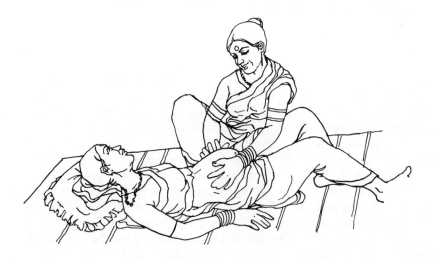

Fig. 9.2. Dai checks position of baby in womb.

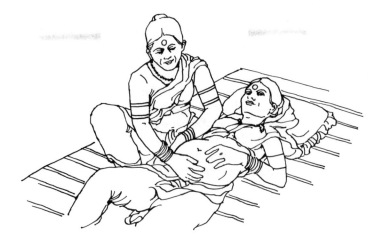

Fig. 9.3. Dai examines head position of baby.

provided by the project. Whenever the supply of kits is exhausted, the dais ask the mother's family to provide a blade and string, which they boil before using. In short, the dais have become competent paramedical workers providing effective maternal and neo-natal care to the community. They are confident of their professional skills and aware of the importance of their role in the community.

Growth of a positive self-image

The experience of acquiring new knowledge and practising socially useful skills has greatly boosted the self-esteem of the CHWs and dais in the three projects. Before training, they behaved as typical low-caste women in Hindu society: extremely self-effacing and reticent towards men and authority in general, they reflected the culture of oppression and silence of which they were part. But after training and working in the community, they are able to relate to people of higher social status with much greater frankness and openness.

The case of Patilbai of Mankhule village in the Alibag project is a good example. A middle-aged, illiterate widow of low caste earning her living as a farm labourer, Patilbai had worked as a CHW on the project since its inception in 1974. Her village was virtually inaccessible during the monsoon season, when the two streams between which it was situated were in full flood. It was during the monsoon that many young children in the village died from dehydration caused by diarrhoea. Families sank into indebtedness to pay doctors' fees whenever such an emergency arose. On Patilbai's suggestion, an auxiliary nurse was placed in Mankhule village during the monsoon, and the two women succeeded in greatly reducing the number of deaths from dehydration. Some time

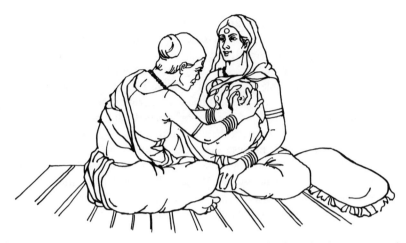

Fig. 9.4. Dai examines woman's breasts to check whether nipples are normal.

afterwards a State Government Minister visited the project area. All the CHWs were assembled and the Minister spoke to them. He commented on how little they were paid and asked what their motivation was for doing such lowly paid work. Patilbai, normally a very reserved person, shot up from where she was sitting on the floor and retorted: 'I do not know who you are and what you work for. I am Patilbai of Mankhule village and I work not for fifty rupees but for the people of my village!' Before her health worker training, Patilbai would never have dared address even a minor government official in this way, let alone a powerful State politician.

Another example is Anjanabai Bahir from Nahuli village of the Jamkhed project (Arole 1978, p. 131). She had to walk ten miles every week to come to the health worker training classes. As the teaching went on, she became intensely interested in leprosy. Previously she used to spit any anyone who had leprosy and pass on the far side of the road. But as she learned more about the disease, she realized how prevalent it was, and that something effective could be done to treat it. She conducted a house-to-house survey in her own village, where she discovered 22 previously unrecognized leprosy cases, and quickly arranged for treatment to start. After some time a group of well-dressed health professionals visited her village and asked whether she was satisfied with the payment she was receiving for her service to the community. She replied, with quiet dignity: 'You educated people wearing fashionable clothes work only for money, but we village health workers get far more out of our work, because we see change in our village – the mother's joy when her child gets well, the satisfaction of preventing a child going blind for life. It is enough to have sufficient to eat and clothes to wear, when all around you there are so many with much less.'

Desire for self-improvement

Becoming a VHW is often the first step in a process of self-improvement enabling an individual to take advantage of opportunities previously open only to the rich, educated, and powerful. The dais at Pachod, for example, participate in a literacy programme because gradually they have come to realize the economic benefits of being able to read and write. Initially the Pachod project staff informed the dais that banks were obliged to provide them with loans if they saved enough money. All 37 of them soon opened bank accounts. Then they realized that, in order to operate their accounts without depending on others, they had to be literate. Otherwise they had to bribe the bank clerks and risk being duped because they did not understand the procedures. Several dais have since received loans for small-scale cottage industries, while others have used their savings to pay for seeds, goods for trading, or traditional festivals. Previously they would have contracted crippling debts for these purposes.

Breakdown of cultural prejudices

The prevalence of caste prejudice is a powerful constraint on development efforts aiming to promote a more equitable social order in India. Training a cadre of health workers at village level, however, can help lower caste barriers.

The case of Malanbai, a dai from Thergaon village in the Pachod project, illustrates how caste prejudice can gradually be eroded. A 45-year-old mother of nine, Malanbai belongs to the Marathas — the dominant caste in her village.

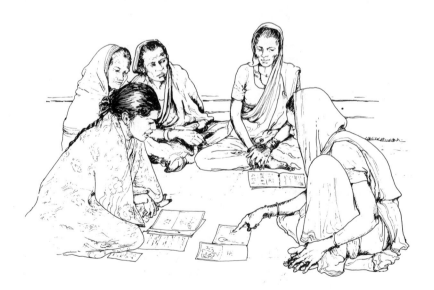

Fig. 9.5. Dais learn to read in order to operate own bank accounts.

Despite their high-caste status, she and her husband have only a small plot of dry, infertile land, so they often have to look for work on other people's land. When she started coming to the dai training course, Malanbai had many problems, all stemming from her prejudice towards women of lower caste. She had brought her own supplies of food and utensils for cooking, drinking, and eating, and refused to share with anyone else. She sat apart from the other women – all of low caste – during the training sessions and meals. Malanbai's strong adherence to the principles of 'untouchability' also meant that her usefulness as a trained dai would be very limited. Though she had practised as an untrained dai for 25 years, she had never assisted women outside her own caste.

Yet close contact with project staff and frequent interaction with the other dais during training began to weaken her prejudice. Gradually Malanbai realized that she could not fulfill her professional role of delivering maternal and neonatal services to all women in her village unless she dropped her caste prejudices. A recent survey revealed not a single instance of caste discrimination in Malanbai's work with the women of her village. (Indeed, if questioned today, Malanbai would say she cannot remember whether she *ever* discriminated against lower caste women!)

Growth of leadership qualities

Training a villager to become a health worker often releases latent leadership qualities which otherwise might never have come to light. The case of Gangubai from Harshi village in the Pachod project is illuminating. A 35-year-old mother of five, Gangubai inherited the role of village dai from her mother-in-law. She and her husband own a small piece of infertile land, and are forced to work as agricultural labourers on other people's land in order to make ends meet. Four years ago, when Gangubai began attending the dai training course, she was habitually depressed. Her husband, an alcoholic with venereal disease who frequently failed to do his share of work, used to beat her so badly that she sometimes was unable to come to training sessions.

Today Gangubai's situation is virtually unrecognizable. Her performance as a dai has been outstanding. Even more importantly, she has assumed leadership among the women of her own village. She heads a women's labour cooperative which takes contracts on building sites and shares the payment among its members. Extremely tough and resourceful, Gangubai also led a movement to force a road-building contractor to pay women labourers the government-approved wage rate. Within her own household the leadership roles have been reversed. Gangubai is now the *de facto* household head. Her husband stays at home minding their youngest son while she carries out her work at the clinic or makes house-to-house visits. He is unable to do contract work without her because he needs her help. Gangubai's life and circumstances have undergone an immense transformation.

CONCLUSION

The expectations and attitudes of project staff and community members help shape the self-image and therefore the performance of VHWs. The highest compliment the community can pay VHWs is to regard them as selfless workers for the welfare of all. VHWs, for their part, emphasize that they are not performing a service for personal gain but for the good of the whole community. In an environment of caste and class division such as rural India, doing something selflessly for the greater good raises the doer above the humdrum, everyday level of life. Indeed the virtue of selfless service to the people has been predominant in Indian legend and folklore, and still occupies an important place in the Indian consciousness. It has been reinforced by the Gandhian movement – the major sociopolitical force in India this century.

When VHWs earn recognition from the community for their work, the human development occurring on an individual level makes them someone special. At the same time, the attitudes and values of the community itself start to change. This is particularly striking in the case of women. A woman previously regarded essentially as somebody's mother, mother-in-law, daughter, or daughter-in-law is seen as an individual with knowledge and skills of value to others in the community. No longer categorized according to the accident of her birth, she is valued in more rational terms by what she is capable of doing for the community.

It is often observed that VHWs are as good as the technical support they receive from health professionals, yet it is also true that a PHC programme itself is only as effective as its grassroots health workers – the midwives and CHWs living and working within their own communities. In planning, implementing and assessing PHC programmes, it therefore is important to give greater consideration to the human development of village health workers and the communities in which they work.

NOTE

1. The term 'village health worker' (VHW), as used in this article, refers to all types of full- or part-time paramedical workers trained in some aspects of basic health care who live and work in a rural community. It includes traditional midwives trained in maternal health care and community health workers (CHWs), who have received more comprehensive training.

REFERENCES

Arole, Mabelle, Village health workers and community involvement in health care in India. In *The changing roles and education of health care personnel worldwide in view of the increase of basic health services* (ed. R.W. McNeur). Society for Health and Human Values, Pennsylvania (1978).

Battiwala, Srilata, *The foundation for research in community health, our story 1975–1980*, Bombay (1981).

Mukhopadhyay, Maitrayee, An evaluation of village health worker medical practice in Alibag District, unpublished paper (1974).

10   'Tell us a story': health teaching in Nigeria

David Hilton describes how stories, drama, and songs have become an essential feature of a community-based primary health care programme in north-eastern Nigeria.

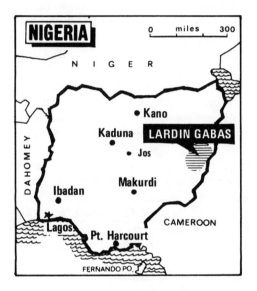

David Hilton, M.D., was medical consultant to the Lardin Gabas Rural Health Programme for four years. He is now Clinical Director for the Seminole Indian Tribe in Florida, USA.

Once there was a village surrounded by hills where there lived many bandits and thieves. When villagers travelled outside the village, they often were beaten and robbed. The elders used to prepare a stretcher and send two men out to bring victims back to the village. As time went on, the banditry increased, so more and more stretchers and bearers were needed. Finally someone said, 'Why not do something about these bandits?'. So a posse was formed which went out, captured the bandits and put them in jail. There has been no more trouble ever since from bandits in the area.

This story illustrates by its form and content the approach of the Lardin Gabas Rural Health Programme in north-eastern Nigeria. The main objective of the programme is to assist the population in preventing disease and promoting better health, through training local people in basic health care.

A unique feature of the programme is the extensive use of stories, drama, and songs in training village health workers (VHWs), who in turn use these methods to motivate and educate people within their own communities to take more responsibility for their health.

BACKGROUND

Lardin Gabas, which literally means eastern diocese or district, is an area of about 10 000 square miles and 900 000 people. The area of the health programme covers over 1000 villages with average populations of 300–500. The villages have round, earthern-walled huts topped with conical thatched roofs. A family's huts and granaries are encircled by grass mat fences which afford some privacy for the family. In this enclosed compound area, the family often gathers around the evening fire to share riddles, stories, and jokes or to pass on advice from one generation to the next. The Lardin Gabas farmers cultivate guinea corn, a type of sorghum, which provides the flour for the meals eaten twice daily. Meat and vegetable sauces are used to provide variety in the diet. Though affected to some extent by urbanization and the expanding cash crop economy, most people continue to relate directly to the soil for their sustenance. Their living patterns and beliefs are still shaped largely by their physical surroundings.

At the time the programme began in 1974, health services were sparse and limited mainly to towns and large villages. Few health personnel were from their area of work. Most had been trained for curative care in an urban setting, and had little understanding of the need for preventive medicine in a rural area. Morbidity and mortality rates were very high. Life expectancy at birth was 40 years. Waterborne diseases were responsible for many deaths. Latrines were uncommon and, if they existed at all, were rarely used.

The most commonly treated diseases of children in the Lardin Gabas area include malaria, gastroenteritis, pneumonia, malnutrition, and intestinal parasites. Malaria and schistosomiasis are common among adults. In addition, tuberculosis and leprosy are relatively high prevalence health problems.

Hospital facilities originally established at Garkida and Lassa by the Church of the Bretheren Mission (CBM) have been integrated into the government health-care system. In 1973, however, in response to the unmet needs of the area, the CBM decided to shift its emphasis from the institutional approach to community-based health care. The Rural Health Programme thus stresses the necessity of educating people to change behaviour patterns related to health. Furthermore, the educative process itself is based on the traditional oral means of learning in the local culture.

SELECTION AND TRAINING OF VILLAGE HEALTH WORKERS

Each village joining the programme forms a Village Health Committee (VHC) which organizes community meetings and manages health-care activities on a daily basis. One of the first tasks of the Committee is to select six candidates (three men and three women) from the community as potential VHWs. The Committee looks for the following conditions and qualities in candidates:

- married and aged between 25 and 45;
- able to speak, read, and write in the Hausa language;
- able to tell stories well;
- having a mature personality;
- willing to learn and accept new ideas;
- able to communicate well with people;
- having a thorough understanding of the customs, beliefs, and traditional practices of the local people;
- living permanently in the village, with ties of family and property;
- being respected by the various clans, tribes, and religious groups represented in the village;
- being in good health;
- for women candidates, not being more than four months pregnant when starting the training course; if the Committee chooses a woman with a baby on the breast, a nurse-maid should be sponsored to accompany the mother on the course.

At the training centre in Garkida, a staff of four teachers — two male dispensary assistants and two women with primary school education — conduct a three-month course twice a year. A maximum of 20 students may enter each course. The major purpose of the course is to provide VHWs with a knowledge of health education and the basis of disease prevention. This emphasis is maintained so that the VHWs may return to their villages and teach on a regular and daily basis how a person gets sick and what can be done to prevent this. Curative care is taught on a more limited scale: only 10 per cent of teaching time is spent on diagnosis and treatment. The course concentrates on the most common serious health problems in their order of prevalence. Although diseases are named and brief scientific explanations given, the main emphasis is not to prepare health workers for a life of curative care, but one devoted to health promotion.

Clinical teaching is limited to the most common symptoms, the disease causing them and the way it is contracted, with heavy emphasis on prevention through changing health practices. The use of simple medicines is taught in practice clinics with real patients.

Female VHWs are especially trained in the health needs of women and children. They assist in the care of expectant mothers and do monthly examinations in the antenatal clinic. Here they give malaria and anaemia prophylaxis and screen for high-risk pregnancies referring these to maternity centres. They also conduct home deliveries and share their knowledge with traditional birth attendants.

Trainees graduating from the course become VHWs and receive an official certificate. Follow-up and supervision in the field are carried out by a local dispensary attendant, who visits at least once per month. VHWs also return to the training centre twice a year to review and improve their knowledge and skills.

TEACHING METHODS

The distinctive feature of the training programme is its extensive use of stories, drama, and songs – the traditional methods of learning among people still heavily dependent on oral traditions. These methods are used not only in the training course, but also by the VHWs themselves when they start working in their own communities. Experience has shown that non-literate people are often confused by pictures and drawings. For this reason flip charts, slides, cartoons, etc., are *not* used. Bored by purely didactic lectures, most people are very receptive to narrative, dramatic, and musical forms of communication. Since VHWs tend to teach others in the same way they themselves acquired their knowledge and skills, the teaching methods used in the course have a heavy emphasis on traditional oral means of communication. Stories, dramas, and songs are constructed by local people. They include traditional knowledge and beliefs and move towards an action which will help solve a particular health problem.

The course for VHWs is built around 23 lessons of approximately two hours duration each, with additional time allowed for revision, homework, preparation, and practice clinics. A typical lesson runs along the following lines:

1. The teacher tells the story to the class, and asks questions to check what information the students have retained.
2. One student repeats the story and the teacher and students comment.
3. The class divides into groups of four or five persons, each of whom tells the story to the others.
4. Each group creates a drama with each student acting a part.
5. The class reassembles and each group presents its drama.
6. The class evaluates each group's performance and, if desired, chooses the best.

The group chosen as best may collect props such as hoes, water pots, and eating and drinking utensils, and present the drama to a nearby school, a women's club, a village meeting, wedding, or baby-naming ceremony. These occasions provide students with practice and experience which stand them in good stead when they return home and start working in their communities.

Stories are told in simple direct language, building up to one or more health 'messages'. The following story concentrates on how to prevent diarrhoea.

Habu and his wife were farm people who lived in the town of Gardama. The people of the town fetched their drinking water from the nearby river, and they were accustomed to defecating anywhere behind the house or in the bush. Nobody had a latrine.

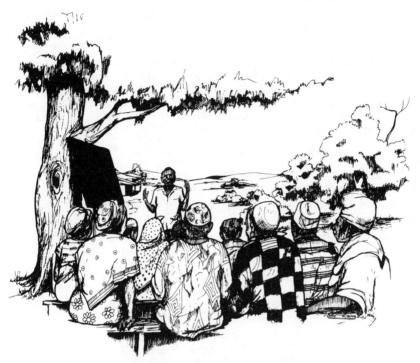

Fig. 10.1. Bored by purely didactic lectures, people are more receptive to narrative, dramatic, and musical forms of communication.

Like many other people, Habu and his wife developed abdominal pain and swollen bellies from time to time. They began seeing blood and mucus in their stools, which they had four to seven times a day. They often felt weak and were losing weight.

One day Habu's wife went to the river to fetch water. When she tried to lift the pot to her head she was too weak. A young man passing by happened to notice her and asked what was the matter. She replied that she needed someone to help her to lift the water pot for she was too weak. Both she and her husband had felt weak since they had started having bloody diarrhoea.

The young man asked if they used a latrine for defecating and she said no, they didn't have one. He asked where they fetched drinking water and she replied 'from the river'. The man suggested they should go to the health post to get medicine for their illness. When they were well again they should dig a latrine for defecating instead of going just anywhere. Diarrhoea is spread by defecating on the open ground. Flies come and sit on the faeces, then fly to someone's house and sit on any uncovered food. Someone eats the food, the germs from the faeces left by the fly enter his body and he gets diarrhoea. He also suggested she and her husband should dig a well. The river water is full of germs causing diarrhoea and other diseases. Then he helped her lift the water pot onto her head and she walked home.

Habu was interested when his wife told him what the young man at the river had suggested. They decided to go to the village health post. The village health worker gave them medicine for their diarrhoea and also repeated what the young man had said about using a latrine and digging a well. He added that it was important to wash their hands before eating and after defecating. Food should be kept covered and fruits and vegetables washed before eating.

When Habu and his wife had recovered, they dug a well and put up a latrine. They soon found that they were enjoying better health. Their neighbours copied them and found that they also could avoid diarrhoea through having safe drinking water from their own wells and disposing of their faeces in latrines. Other people in the town joined in, and the village health worker found that very few people were coming for medicine to cure diarrhoea.

A gram of prevention is better than a kilo of cure!

A popular variation on story-telling and drama is for one or more students to compose a song on a health theme and teach it to the class. The song leader tells the story in verses, while the others join in the chorus after each verse. The following song, for example, tells about the symptoms, cause, prevention, and treatment of malaria:

Chorus: Good health we want
Let's all be healthy

Verses: Fever is bothering me,
Mosquitos bring it.

Standing water around our house
Causes mosquitos to breed.

Let us take the children to the clinic
That they may stay well.

We take them to the clinic for Daraprim
That they may stay well.

Broken pots and tin pans
Let us bury them.

During their three-month course a group of 20 students composes and learns many such songs. They can be practised whenever the group gathers, such as before a drama presentation. When students go home for short breaks, they teach their songs to family members, friends and neighbours, mothers clubs, and school classes. After finishing their training course, VHWs increase their repertoire of songs when they return twice yearly to the training centre for one week.

THE VILLAGE HEALTH WORKER IN THE COMMUNITY

On returning home, the newly trained VHWs start work in a health post constructed and furnished by the community. The building is constructed in local style, has one large room with two or three windows, a table, chairs, and two lockable wooden boxes for carrying medicines. A latrine and water supply also must be provided.

To officially open the new health post and programme, an inaugural ceremony and day of feasting are held. In addition to the usual formalities, Lardin Gabas Rural Health Programme gives a loan to cover the cost of drugs and equipment. This is repaid within about one year.

Daily clinic work begins with a VHW telling an educative story for the people – many of them mothers and children – who have gathered at the health post. The stories include teaching about the value of latrines, hand-washing, well water, home cleanliness, proper diet, family planning, immunization, and antenatal care. This group teaching is followed by individual consultations and treatment. Providing on-the-spot curative care not only helps people overcome the most common diseases, but also gives credibility to the health 'messages' which the VHW tries to convey. It also provides some income for the Village Health Committee to replenish medical supplies, keep the health post in good repair and contribute towards the VHW's salary. Patients whose symptoms are outside the scope of the VHW's training or whose condition does not improve after a few days are referred to the nearest dispensary.

Mother-and-child care is organized around monthly clinics for pregnant women and mothers with under-five children. These are lively occasions, with mothers contributing to the stories, dramas, songs, and word games which introduce, repeat, and reinforce health messages.

Making up stories, dramas and songs is fairly simple for anyone with imagination and some basic health knowledge. The essential ingredients are some specific health teaching messages and a scenario lifted from the local culture. For example, the five infant feeding messages are:

1. breast-feed as long as possible;
2. start feeding ground nut porridge at four months;
3. start giving bean cakes and other soft foods at one year;
4. give at least five feedings a day;
5. delay the next pregnancy at least two years.

This becomes the story of a woman whose nine-month-old baby begins losing weight and becomes weak. When the VHW learns she is pregnant, she explains the feeding plan and how, when this pregnancy is completed, she can delay the next. The story ends happily for mother and child.

Outside clinic hours the VHWs visit local social gatherings such as baby-naming ceremonies and church meetings, as well as school groups and men's and women's clubs. Because VHWs are well-known in their own villages and can communicate health messages in a lively way in the local idiom, their suggestions tend to be accepted more readily.

Experience to date suggests that this form of community-based, disease-preventive health education is much more effective than the previous institutional approach, with its heavy emphasis on curative care. For example, one popular educative story tells of a woman who lost two babies from neonatal tetanus, due to the harmful local practice of cutting the umbilical cord with a corn stalk and applying dirt to stop the bleeding. Her third child, however, survived because the local midwife had been retrained — she washed her hands, used a clean cloth on the floor, severed the umbilical cord with a razor blade and piece of string previously sterilized by boiling. Neonatal tetanus has been virtually eliminated in villages where VHWs have used this story to motivate and educate women.

Immunization coverage of children has been increased by using a story which incorporates a traditional belief which, although medically ineffective, is harmless to children's health. It is common practice for mothers to tie amulets to children's extremities to ward-off disease. The story tells of a child who dies of measles despite the supposedly disease-preventive amulet. The VHW encourages the mother, not to dispense with the amulet, but simply to add vaccinations and malarial prophylaxis to make it more effective. When she does this with her later children, none suffer any serious disease.

Another story tells of a woman who lost three babies with fever. But after taking her fourth child to the health post to receive Daraprim regularly, she saw him grow strong and healthy. Most of the 47 villages where this story has been used report a high percentage of children attending under-fives clinics, and village elders report that women no longer spend many hours walking to distant dispensaries for fever treatment.

In one village a visiting team from the base hospital was greeted by the local VHW who reported that 35 families had dug their own wells in the year since his return from training. At every opportunity he had been telling the story of a village where most of the people had chronic abdominal pain and distention along with bloody urine. Then enough wells were dug to provide sufficient drinking and washing water to eliminate the need for use of a nearby swamp. Following treatment for schistosomiasis at the nearest dispensary, the villagers of the story found little recurrence of this health problem.

Throughout the project area there is an increased awareness of practices which lead to better health, and this has brought a number of positive changes. A marked decrease in the incidence of fever, conjunctivities, neonatal tetanus, leg ulcers, and skin infections also has been observed where health education and health care have been made available by VHWs. The project area continues to expand at the rate of 20 new villages per year, and there is no lack of suitable candidates for the VHW training course. The federal government has also selected Lardin Gabas as a model to demonstrate what it aims to achieve through its own Basic Health Services Scheme.

CONCLUSION

The traditional communication methods of stories, drama, and song have proven to be effective learning methods of VHWs trained by the Lardin Gabas Rural Health Programme. Trained VHWs, on returning to their communities, have used these methods effectively to motivate and teach local people to take greater responsibility for preventing disease and promoting good health. We believe this approach to health teaching and learning could have a wider application in other countries, especially in West Africa, where non-literate peoples use traditional oral methods as the main form of mass communication.

REFERENCES

Hilton, David, Rural basic health services: the Lardin Gabas way. *Contact* **41**, 1–8 (1977).
Hilton, David, *Health teaching for West Africa*, MAP International (1980).
Tarfa, Yautama Fulani, Basic health services for rural areas in Nigeria, In *The Changing roles and education of health care personnel worldwide in view of the increase of basic health services* (ed. R.W. McNeur) pp. 69–79. Society for Health and Human Values, Philadelphia (1978).

11 We are for the people: reflections of a community health worker in the Philippines

Jaime Z. Galvez-Tan explains how working in a remote rural area of the Philippines made him totally rethink his own attitudes, values, and approach to the practice of medicine.

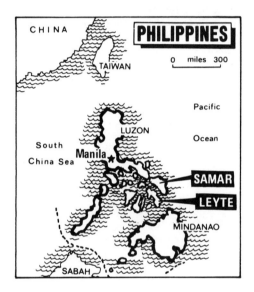

Jaime Z. Galvez-Tan, a Filipino doctor, worked in community health on the islands of Leyte and Samar from 1975 until 1978. He is now director of a health and development programme on the island of Mindanao.

> We are for the people
> We shall remain steadfast
> Strong and firm as the mountains
> We shall remain steadfast.
> Filipino folk song

'We are for the people' — easier said or sung than done. While working among the rural poor of the Philippines I have often recalled those words. I would like to share with you some of my struggles as a physician and community health worker on the islands of Leyte and Samar. In the course of my work I — along

with my fellow health workers — have had to struggle with various contradictions, some arising from our own attitudes and values, others related to the
knowledge and skills acquired through our education and training.

ATTITUDES AND VALUES

One of the most difficult struggles is in dealing with values and attitudes. We ask
ourselves:

- Will we impose our ideas and decisions on the people or will we encourage
  their participation?
- Will goal-achievement be emphasized or will the process be given more
  importance?
- Will we encourage individual freedom more than the discipline of collective
  life with the staff and the people?
- Will we maintain a middle class or a simple lifestyle?
- Will our services be limited to our families and those who can afford to
  pay, or will our services be for all the community?

Our tendency is always to take the easier road — the path of least resistance:
to impose decisions, to use methods more familiar to us than to the people, and
to be individualistic. But serving the people is not an easy road. It is a path
full of difficulties.

Imposition versus democratic process

We always declare that we are for people's participation in decision-making. But
how much do we really involve them in the planning, implementation, and
evaluation of programmes intended for them? How much do we consult them
in an open and honest manner? How much feedback and ideas do we receive
from them? Too often, people's participation is practised only in the implementation stage and very rarely in the planning and evaluation phases.

Planning with the people is a painstaking task, as we have found out. It means
being creative, being flexible, and effectively communicating with them. Our
project staff used to meet people in big village assemblies, but we soon discovered
that only a few people talk in these large assemblies and they are usually the rich
peasants, the store-owners, and the moneylenders. These people wield power in
their villages. They are not the poorest of the poor, the most oppressed. So now
we meet people in groups of 10–15 families, following the village pattern of
houses in clusters. In these small group meetings, the villagers are more expressive
and open. The discussions are more lively. Everybody gets a chance to voice
their opinions and sentiments.

Planning with the people demands perserverance in facilitating the small
group meeting, carefully explaining the issues and encouraging responses, which
are not usually spontaneous. After a question is thrown into a meeting, there is a

long period of silence. The silence can be discouraging if one is not patient and hopeful enough to wait, to give time for the people to think and formulate their ideas. The silence of a few minutes can seem like hours to us – but we manage to take a deep breath, say to ourselves 'relax, don't hurry' – and soon enough the responses come in.

The small group meetings are teaching us to listen, to wait, and to be patient. By listening, we discover the wisdom of the peasants; by waiting, we get their true feelings; by being patient and supportive, we stimulate their participation in matters that will affect their lives.

To impose on these people, long accustomed to domination, is the easy way out. But it is not necessarily the most effective way. As a concrete example of this, consider what happened in one of the villages in Leyte where we were working. The sanitary inspector of the town's health centre had scheduled an immunization for typhoid and cholera. Upon his arrival in the village, only a few people showed up for vaccination. The sanitary inspector cursed the people for being uncooperative and not being interested in taking care of their health. What he did not know was that it was the rice harvest season in the village. The villagers had to choose between food for the stomachs and a cholera-typhoid vaccination. Had the sanitary inspector consulted the people and involved them in the planning of the vaccinations, they would have advised him to come after the harvest. Had he done this, health services would have been more effective and the people would not have been blamed for being uncooperative (Fig. 11.1).

Achievement-orientation versus process-orientation

Numbers and statistics are important in health records. But when we start viewing people and patients in terms of the number of capsules taken, the number of injections given or the number of laboratory examinations done, these numbers and statistics become dehumanizing tools. Yet doctors are easy prey to this. In medical school what was important was the highest grade, the cut-off point for passing, who is first and who is last. In the hospital, the concern was the case number, this bed number, that disease. The patient's name and feelings were not the main focus, but only incidental. In public health, we became entangled with morbidity and mortality rates, the incidence of such and such diseases. We never asked why the people were still dying from pneumonia and gastroenteritis; why there had been no change in the patterns of tuberculosis and schistosomiasis despite so many control programmes. In professional practice, what was pertinent was how much you earned, how many cars and houses you had, how many patients you had treated. Our achievements were measured in numbers, figures, and statistics. It was so ingrained in us that it was nearly impossible to escape this system of numbers. Such a system insidiously educates us to relate in a cold, detached, mechanical, and unemotional way to our patients and their families.

Working in the community and being touched by the varied facets of the people's simple lives helped change our attitudes. In the community, at times, we shared the people's feelings by sharing their experiences: the long hike under the sun, fetching water a kilometre away, washing clothes in the river, planting and harvesting, joining in social life and festivities. We were moved when we saw Violeta, a malnourished child, hungry and crying while her mother, Clara, searched desperately for food for the next meal. We sympathized with Manuel, a farmer who, exhausted by the harvest work, felt cheated every time half his harvest went to the landlord. We were angered when we talked with Jose, bitter because he was dispossessed of his land by a moneylender. The 'community' was no longer something to be quantified, but consisted of individual people whose feelings and emotions we shared. They could never be mere numbers to us.

Thus we realized that there was something much more than merely quantifiable results. We had to be concerned more with the changes in attitudes of the people, the cultural and sociological impact of our work on the community, the degree of people's participation we encouraged and the upliftment of their

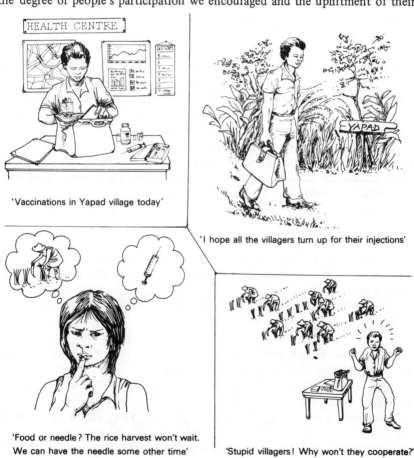

'Vaccinations in Yapad village today'

'I hope all the villagers turn up for their injections'

'Food or needle? The rice harvest won't wait. We can have the needle some other time'

'Stupid villagers! Why won't they cooperate?'

Fig. 11.1. The sanitary inspector's visit.

quality of life. Such endeavours could not be expressed in numbers.

The poverty, helplessness, illiteracy, oppression, and exploitation of the masses in our country have made us re-examine our values. We constantly have to ask the question – why? Why are the people poor? Why are the people hungry despite the wealth of resources around them? Why is the gap between the rich and the poor getting wider? To answer these questions, we have to look into the relationships among the different classes existing in society. We have to go back into the historical background of our people and our country. We have to examine the processes of economic production. We have to dig deep into the people's beliefs, values, and attitudes. In short, we have to be more human.

Individualism versus collectivity

Fighting individualism is difficult, especially as the free enterprise society in which we live supports and nurtures it. This is further reinforced by the training of health professionals where the world of dog-eat-dog competition pressures students to elbow out each other instead of fostering cooperation and camaraderie.

How do we combat individualism? In our staff development, we give time to developing attitudes, as well as to the usual business and evaluation meetings. Importance is given to criticism and self-criticism among the staff members and a spirit of team work is emphasized. Doctors, nurses, community organizers, parish priests, peasants, and fishermen all work as equals.

This collective living and sharing is also transmitted to the community health workers and the small family groups in the villages. Community spirit is reinforced among the people through activities such as labour-exchange in farm work, planning and implementation of activities like community petitions to government and other agencies for services, and social activities like fund-raising for a village project.

Decision-making in vital matters is likewise shared. One of our mottos in community work is 'Never decide on anything alone'. This encourages consultation not only among programme staff members but also the people, thus reinforcing unity among us.

Adjustment in lifestyle

Urban-bred and having stayed in the cities most of our lives, the shift to the rural areas brings feelings of fear and inadequacy among us.

'There is no electricity. The people go to bed early. What will I do in the evenings?'

'There are no movies, disco houses, or theatres. What will be my form of leisure?'

'There are no soft beds. Will I be able to sleep on the floor and manage with just one room for my family?'

'There is no regular transportation. Can I make it hiking along trails over hills, mountains, and rivers?'

'There are no toilets, taps, showers, newspapers, televisions, or telephones. How am I going to cope without all these?'

Threats, anxieties, and insecurities again! However, we are realizing that adjustment in lifestyle is really more of an adjustment in outlook which entails a great deal of psychological preparation and practice.

When I was about to start my work in the community, I was asked how long I intended to stay in the rural areas. I said I would give it a year. That was how insecure I was. Could I tackle life in the boondocks? What kind of life awaited me there? It was generally a fear of the unknown. At the same time there was the threat of separation from my family, my friends, and the comforts of city life that I had grown used to.

Sooner or later, I found out that there were a lot more things to take the place of movies, disco houses, showers, television, electricity, and other luxuries. The hospitality and warmth of the rural people were more than a match for the impersonal behaviour of city dwellers. The seas, rivers, waterfalls, and springs could rival any shower in the bathroom. The sunrise, sunsets, native music and dances, village festivities offered a totally different recreation. The cool breeze, clean fresh air, colourful butterflies, the chirping birds, majestic scenery along the trails and tracks made the hikes not just bearable but even pleasurable. Life in the rural areas was not as bad and lonely as I had feared.

Food adjustments

We learned many lessons in adjusting to the food and meal schedules in rural areas. City lifestyle offers three meals and two or three snacks a day. In rural areas, there are seasons of plenty and seasons of hunger. During seasons of hunger the people eat only one or two meals a day, a 'meal' consisting of rice or root crops and dried fish or salt. It was shocking to me to discover that the majority of our people had not enough food to eat.

This brings to my mind an experience in one of the Samar villages. A meal of wood potatoes and salt was served at the breakfast table. I thought it was just an appetizer. After finishing the food, I asked whether there was more to come. How I regretted the question! It was the hunger season and there was no other food except wood potatoes and salt. Tears of embarrassment and sadness were in my eyes as I nibbled the precious pieces of salt left.

It is easy to say we want to adjust to the lifestyle of the people, but actually it is often the people who feel obliged to adjust to our chosen 'simple' lifestyle. Out of their inherent hospitality and as victims of advertising, the people tend to serve us special foods which are actually a big drain on their meagre incomes. I told the people I would eat whatever they ate, like sweet potato leaves, watercress, and edible ferns. I noticed, however, that these were never served to me. People would rationalize: 'Doctor, these vegetables are food for the pigs only'.

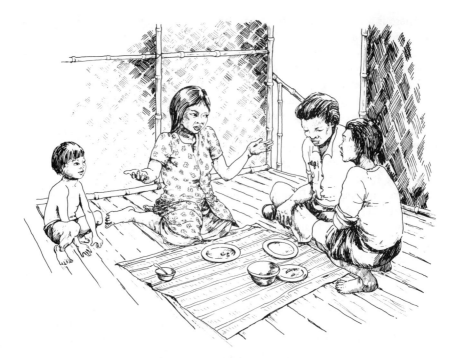

Fig. 11.2. 'The food's finished.'

Every time a doctor enters a village, there always seems to be an 'epidemic' affecting the chickens. The doctor finds he is being served chicken for breakfast, lunch and dinner. One would think doctors carried a virus that killed the chickens every time they visited the villages! And when the doctor leaves, the people go back to eating rice, root crops, and salt.

One morning in a Leyte village I was served instant coffee from a bottle. When I removed the cap, I found out that the contents were still sealed by a foil wrapper. The coffee had not yet been used. I learned that it had just been bought from the store. The villagers did not regularly drink instant coffee, which is expensive, but prepare cheap 'coffee' made of corn or rice, or ginger tea.

So we had to explain painstakingly to the people that they need not serve us anything special. We said if such practices went on, the village would go bankrupt buying special food for us. Instead of helping the village, we would become a burden.

Family pressures

Our families have great expectations of us, having sent us to medical school. They expect us to comply with the conventional roles of doctors and health professionals. Being a community physician does not fall within their expectations or their idea of one who has 'made it'.

My parents were initially disappointed with my decision to go to the rural areas. Their vision was for me to work in a big city hospital, specialize abroad, and become a big-time doctor like most of the others. I had to keep on communicating and relating to them about the joys and wonders of my activities in the community. It took quite some time before they accepted the work I was doing. Now what is important to them is that I am happy and fulfilled in my work. They have since become very supportive of my work.

A few of my colleagues have not been as fortunate as I am with regard to their families. The greatest pressure is economic – the need to augment the family income, to support brothers and sisters who are studying. Their parents often remind them that they have spent so much money on their education so they are expected to return the goodwill. Emotional appeals are also frequent. Families usually say 'You are the only doctor in the family. We need you to take care of us'. One of our doctors was even 'blackmailed' by her mother to go to the United States. Her mother, who was in the United States, said that her presence was needed for a serious heart operation and the family sent several cables urging her immediate presence. So she accepted her pre-paid plane ticket and off she went, only to find that her mother was not very sick. Unfortunately, she could not come back home since she only had a one-way ticket.

The community worker is faced with the dilemma of choosing between the family good or the greater good of the rural community. The pressure not to go against convention is very great.

Something positive

Imposition, achievement-orientation, individualism, and elitism – these are the residual attitudes from our feudal and colonial history. The Philippines, like various other Asian countries, has been under the colonial rule of the Spanish, Americans, and Japanese over four centuries. Such attitudes hamper our growth and work with the people. The positive thing about it is that we are now becoming aware of this attitudinal struggle going on internally in us and we are doing something about it.

KNOWLEDGE AND SKILLS

Another area of the struggle emerges when we consider our knowledge and skills. Will we use only Western ideas and techniques or be open to traditional practices and beliefs? Shall we concentrate on curative means or give emphasis also to prevention? What about the new roles demanded of us; and with these roles, our fears of professional and intellectual stagnation and isolation?

Western system versus indigenous practice

Our educational system is highly westernized, mainly patterned after the system of the United States. I remember the time when we were even fined for speaking in our own language in school.

We always had to talk in English. Just as westernized too is the Philippine medical educational system. We were taught more about North American diseases and how to pass the United States board examinations than about diseases afflicting our own people. The hidden goal of most Filipino medical and nursing students is to go abroad and serve in another country and make a comfortable living abroad. The current trend is to specialize in cardiovascular and degenerative diseases. Communicable diseases are neglected. We were taught to rely so much on laboratory aids and sophisticated instruments for diagnosis that we have failed to develop our five senses. We became dependent on the hospital setting and on expensive curative techniques and interventions. We learned to belittle our traditional healers and dismissed them as quacks.

With this type of educational background, working in the rural areas initially causes a cultural shock. There are no laboratory aids, sophisticated instruments or hospitals. People die of pneumonia, tuberculosis, and gastroenteritis, not of coronary heart diseases and diabetes. Disease prevention, rather than curative skills, is crucial. The rural people regard their traditional healers highly. It was only after spending some time in the rural areas that we realized how inappropriate our training had been. How irrelevant we were to most of our people!

Many pains and frustrations accompany our de-schooling and re-schooling process. We literally have to undo practically everything we have learned. We have to admit that we are not at all prepared to answer the health needs of our people. We have to review and study more about tuberculosis, schistosomiasis, malaria and other communicable diseases. Our work must emphasize health education, sanitation and hygiene, maternal and child health care, the use of medicinal plants, and traditional massage. We have to research and document our indigenous forms of medicine. To make our communication and training methods effective, we have to translate scientific, medical jargon into a language more understandable to the people. We have to learn from the people, especially from the traditional healers. We have to be humble. Indeed, we are continually humbled by the people.

Curative versus preventive measures

The temptation to remain locked into curative work can be very great, since the majority of our training time has been on clinical medicine. Aside from this, curative measures give immediate, tangible results, while disease-preventive measures take a longer time before their effects are felt. Concentration on curing is ego-boosting. This not only gives personal satisfaction but reinforces our god-like status and role.

Rural health needs, however, centre on primary health care. Prevention therefore should take precedence over curative care. Good water supply, sanitary disposal of waste, health education, immunization, and control of communicable diseases should receive priority over big hospitals, sophisticated instruments, and expensive medicines (Fig. 11.3).

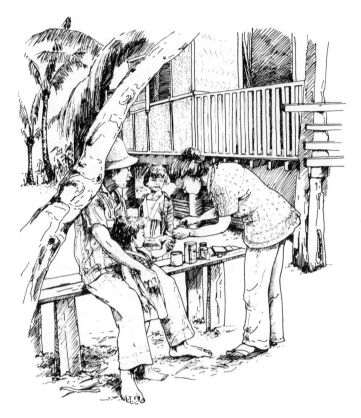

Fig. 11.3. A community health worker takes a blood sample: malaria control is an important priority in primary health care.

Fear of intellectual stagnation

Intellectual stagnation is again a matter of outlook. The rural areas offer a wide range of intellectual pursuits and activities. Although most of us do not initially have the academic skills for research in rural areas, we can learn by observation and participation how to document the patterns and determinants of certain diseases in the villages, the scientific practices of our traditional healers, the people's concepts and responses to health and diseases. All these have become useful guides in improving our service to the people.

In relation to community health, I have learned more from the people than I did at medical school. The field is open for community-based research on relevant subjects. More documentation has to be done on the pharmacology of medicinal plants, the systematization of indigenous theories on health and healing, the development of appropriate medical technology, the production of teaching aids for illiterate groups, and analysis of prevalent health problems in the rural areas.

New roles

We did not envisage that working among the masses would require new roles for us. We were trained in medical practice. The situation is demanding that we take on the role of a change agent with special skills in health care.

To be a change agent, we have to be a community organizer, catalyst, teacher, learner, researcher, conscientizer, coordinator, supervisor, and health worker all at the same time. We have to learn how to motivate and organize the people, systematize their experiences, their feelings, their skills and actions as well as their dreams so that they can mobilize themselves to move out of their dehumanized conditions. These multifaceted roles often evoke strong feelings of insecurity and inadequacy in us at first. With the realization, however, that these roles are necessary to be of total service to the people, initial feelings are superseded by hope, enthusiasm, and optimism.

Our miseducation has isolated us from the majority of our people who need us. We have to adapt our knowledge and skills so that they can be more appropriate to the masses. More importantly, we should use our knowledge and skills for the benefit of the many rather than the few. We should be trying to transform the present unjust situation rather than to reinforce it.

SOCIETY'S VALUE SYSTEM

Handout mentality

We are for self-reliance and self-determination of the people. Obstacles in the prevailing value system of society, however, create great challenges in our work with the poor.

An obstacle to the achievement of self-reliance is the handout mentality that has been and is still being propagated by many government, private and Church organizations. It is frustrating to see the effects of these so-called humanitarian programmes. They have reduced the people to begging. They have stifled the people's creativity to utilize resources within their midst. They have distorted their values and ideas and have concealed the structural determinants of the health-disease process. Their only satisfaction is in pacifying the social pressures of hunger, injustice, and exploitation.

In a community where dole-out programmes have been previously introduced, we have to double our efforts in explaining to the people that our programme is not just another health programme, but one that carries with it a liberating alternative to dependency and helplessness.

In working for people's self-determination, we are confronted with values of leader-centredness, fatalism, superstition, tribal feuding, and submissiveness. Through immersion with the people, constant dialogue with them, through home visits and small group meetings, conscientization and leadership seminars, mobilization on community issues, village creative dramatics and core-group building, the people show us that they are capable of forming their own collective political will.

External contradictions

External contradictions are the forces in the environment that affect our work with the people. The most prominent of these are society's value system, militarization, feudalism, and imperialism.

In several Asian countries today, military rule is a matter of fact. The Philippines has been no exception to this for the past eight years. This has created great challenges for us to work with the people for human rights, justice, peace, and freedom. The present situation has generated tensions and fear. Such feelings are evident in the villages where we work. We try to overcome this by showing our sincerity in helping the people, by being conscious that the people should be able to express their problems themselves, analyse them and propose and work for their solutions together. It will not be the staff who will solve the problems for them but the people themselves.

Some 90 per cent of the farmers in our communities are still semi-feudal tenants. They are plagued by unjust sharing of harvest products with the landlord, high interest on loans (20–30 per cent) from moneylenders, unfair pricing of their goods on the market, high costs of fertilizers, seeds and insecticides, and low wages for agricultural workers. In the mountain villages, the farmers have not been given land title rights to their farms even though they have been tilling the land for more than 20 years.

Given this situation, how do you campaign for food production when the people do not own the land? How can we preach eating the correct diet when half of their harvest goes to the landlord? As to credit unions and cooperatives, all their savings go to repay the moneylenders.

The farmers in one town in Samar met together and discussed their common problems. They decided that it was time to assert their rights as farmers. Land reform and the emancipation of farmers was declared in 1972 but the effect of these measures is still to be felt, especially in Samar. They agreed to hold a Farmers' Day Celebration to reflect on whether farmers have indeed been emancipated already. They were able to get support from the other neighbouring villages. They invited representatives from the different government agencies concerned so that they could present their grievances. Around 600 farmers attended the rally. They were able to get written pledges from the government officials that their seven demands would be answered. The demands were basic indeed:

1. stop the unjust practices of the landlords regarding harvest shares;

2. declare the town a land reform area;
3. stop high interest rates on loans;
4. investigate unfair pricing of goods by middlemen;
5. look into anomalous activities by the administrators of landholdings;
6. implement the minimum wage for agricultural workers; and
7. give land titles to smallholders.

Peasants who have become aware of their situation have realized that it is indeed they who must and can truly solve their problems. With the concerted and organized action of the farmers, the answer to the problems of feudalism may not be long in coming.

Foreign domination of every aspect of our lives has been with us because of the centuries of colonization. Political independence was announced as given to our country in 1946 but in reality we are a neo-colony of the United States. In the health system alone, we can see evidence of this new form of colonialism: 70 per cent of our drug companies are controlled by foreign transnational corporations; 95 per cent of our drug requirements, hospital, and medical supplies are imported. Government health programmes are funded and policies dictated by international and foreign agencies and foundations. Medical education and training is so Americanized that most of our doctors and nurses still prefer to go to the United States to work.

At the village level, this foreign domination is operative indirectly with very direct consequences of poverty and control over people's lives. Most of the products of the rural areas — copra, abaca, sugar, lumber, and minerals are exported. These raw materials come back to us in the form of finished products — soft drinks, cosmetics, soap, cooking oil, cigarettes, canned products, etc. These the rural people can hardly afford, but through widespread and enticing mass media propaganda, they are bought. Encroachment on rural property is becoming more evident since the transnational companies are now going aggressively into agri-business and corporate farming, expanding their mining claims and fruit plantations and setting up their factories and industries in agricultural land through blatant land-grabbing.

The fight against imperialism is becoming a widespread national effort, but it is a long and arduous struggle. At the village level, we have created awareness among the people that their economic underdevelopment has historical and structural roots traceable to monopoly capitalism. Broader perspectives are given so that they can see their problems in the context of the national situation. Once the peasants have been organized, they will want to join forces with other sectors of society. These steps will be necessary initially in finding solutions to the problem of imperialism.

Beyond medicine and health

My work with the peasants has led me to a rude awakening that the health problems of our country are inter-related with the problems of economics, politics, and culture of our country and our people; and that the health situation will remain basically the same unless fundamental structural changes are made to effect solutions to the problems of imperialism, feudalism, and militarization.

Resolving these problems will not be easy. How should a Filipino doctor answer this challenge? It is not enough to attend to health needs. If being a Filipino is foremost, then it certainly means going beyond medicine and health. It is vitally important to enable people to understand the sociological and structural basis of why they suffer from poverty, disease, exploitation, and oppression.

Doctors who consider themselves Filipinos first and doctors second cannot remain apolitical. We have to be aware of what is happening around us. We have to be organized to be of greater service to the masses. We have to unite with the peasants, workers, fishermen, tribal communities, urban poor, students, and other professionals in their struggle for nationalism and democracy. We need to utilize our expertise in health for the majority of our people who are poor, deprived, and oppressed.

Postcript, January 1983

The programme in Leyte Province continues in four urban and five rural areas, with a fulltime staff of one doctor, one nurse, one midwife, and four community organizers. Community health workers run clinics for under-five children. The main form of organization consists of family groupings of 5–15 families.

The programme in the Gandara-San Jorge area of Samar Province has suffered from the increased militarization of the region. The doctor in charge was murdered by the military in April 1982. The parish priest, on whom an arrest warrant was served in December 1982, has gone into hiding. The people are subjected to harrassment, arrest, torture, and summary execution by the military. Community health workers trained between 1977 and 1979 still function in their own villages, but without medical supervision.

12 The ant and the elephant: voluntary agencies and government health programmes in Indonesia *

Mary Johnston describes and analyses how voluntary agencies have made decisive contributions to the development of two government primary health care programmes in Indonesia.

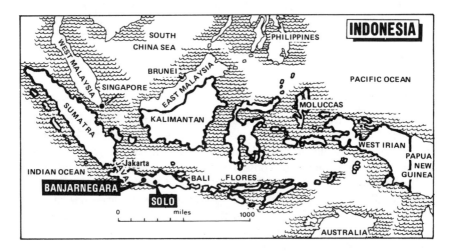

Mary Johnston works as a trainer and a producer of educational materials with the Indonesia Sejahtera Foundation in Solo, Indonesia.

Although voluntary agencies have devised successful primary health care projects in a number of countries, few of these have been transformed into large programmes. The populations covered by such projects usually range from 10 000 to 50 000. Some observers conclude that government agencies – by their very nature – cannot replicate the 'success stories' of voluntary agencies, whose projects are typically small-scale and isolated and enjoy charismatic leadership, highly effective management and generous outside funding – factors which the government can seldom reproduce (Golladay and Koch-Weser 1977).

The experience of some PHC projects in Indonesia, however, appears to

*The author acknowledges the invaluable assistance of Soetrisno Kh., Dr Yoshimiko Kobayashi, C. Sri Sumiwi, Wursito Larso, Purwono, and Dr Arif Haliman in the preparation of this article.

contradict this conclusion. During the Third Five Year Development Plan (1979–1984), the Ministry of Health aims to cover one-third of Indonesia's 60 000 villages with its Village Community Health Development Programme (Ministry of Health R.I. 1978). The design of this programme owes much to the experience of PHC projects pioneered during the 1970s by voluntary agencies in two areas of Central Java Province: the city of Solo and the rural regency of Banjarnegara. In both these cases the local government adopted and expanded a small-scale PHC project initiated by a voluntary agency.

SOLO: 'SLOWLY DOES IT'

The city of Solo[1] lies on the banks of the Solo river in southern Central Java. The population of 451 000 lives in crowded conditions typical of Javanese cities. Markets sprawl over footpaths and hawkers, peddling their wares, patter along the busy streets. Batik and textile factories employing landless labourers from nearby villages are dotted around the fringes of the city.

Until the early 1940s, social life revolved around the two royal houses, whose palaces are now museums. This feudal heritage still marks the city's administration: paternalistic, intricately hierarchical work styles predominate and change is immensely slow. (A popular Solonese proverb says: 'Slowly does it, as long as it goes'.) Community development has also been retarded by poverty and lack of education. Health facilities are inadequate, living conditions are cramped and environmental sanitation is poor. Health status is generally low, with high incidence of infectious diseases and low nutritional status, especially among children under five years.

SEARCH FOR A STRATEGY

During the late 1960s Dr Gunawan Nugroho and his team from the Solo-based voluntary agency YAKKUM took the first steps towards developing a community health strategy. Working from a 20-bed maternity hospital with a small out-patients' clinic in the ward of Kerten, on the western fringe of the city, Gunawan and his team worked towards a programme which ideally would be simple, inexpensive, comprehensible to the community and appropriate to its needs, and also within the scope of the small hospital's limited financial means, staff, and equipment. Their method involved much trial and error. First they approached the leaders of Kerten with a proposal for a community health insurance fund called *Dana Sakit* ('sickness fund'), but this was rejected. Two years later, however, the team offered to help the community clean up their drains which were a breeding site for mosquitos causing malaria. This practical gesture was greatly appreciated, and a process of dialogue between the clinic staff and the community began. One sub-hamlet agreed to try out the idea of a health insurance fund, renamed *Dana Sehat* ('health fund'). This scheme entitled members to a doctor's examination and two days medication in exchange for monthly contributions of 25 Rupiah (equivalent to 0.5 per cent of average household income). The idea caught on quickly, and after three years more than 75 per cent of households in Kerten were paying their monthly contributions. But the Dana Sehat programme did not stop with a mere health insurance scheme. Several groups of households, with technical guidance from Gunawan's team, started curative-surveillance and health-promotive activities. TB detection and treatment, vaccination services, construction of latrines, weighing posts for under-fives, and courses for volunteer health workers on child health, nutrition improvement, and family planning were held in several parts of the ward. In a few cases, credit cooperatives for income-generating activities such as goat raising also started up. Though the programme still retained the original name of *Dana Sehat*, it now covered a wide range of preventive, promotive and curative health care activities, including small-scale economic development schemes. What had begun as a small health insurance scheme had grown rapidly into a multi-faceted community development programme of modestly impressive size.[2]

By 1974 the YAKKUM team was convinced that the Kerten model of *Dana Sehat* could be replicated on a much wider scale within the city of Solo by following the five basic stages of programme development pioneered in Kerten:

1. Preparation of the community health team, involving motivation, team building, and training.
2. Getting to know the people and their problems through observation, informal discussions, and attendance at meetings.
3. Motivating the community leaders and people through informal discussion, and talks at meetings using audiovisual aids.
4. Preparing the community to assume major responsibility for the programme through training of committee members and volunteer health workers, discussions, and meetings.
5. Programme implementation.

The main obstacle to expansion was administrative: government regulations restricted YAKKUM's operations to Kerten ward only. Up until 1974 the programme had run virtually independently of the local municipal government. It had become clear, however, that this state of affairs could not continue if the model was to be tested outside the boundaries of Kerten.

High hopes, breakdown, and deadlock

The imminent prospect of a new mayor assuming office in Solo provided YAKKUM with a chance to legitimize their work throughout the city. The mayor-designate was invited to Kerten where community leaders and YAKKUM staff gave him a full explanation of the health and community development programme. Evidently the mayor was impressed. Soon after assuming office, he declared *Dana Sehat* an official government programme for the whole city. Senior officials were designated as promoters and organizers of the programme, with Dr Gunawan and his staff as their partners. The stage seemed set for the rapid expansion of Dana Sehat throughout the normally slow-moving city of almost half-a-million people.

But with hopes riding high, disaster struck the YAKKUM team. Dr Gunawan, whose dynamic, demanding work style caused frictions within the organization, suddenly was ousted from his position. Some of the community health team followed him and shortly afterwards set up the Solo office of a newly formed agency called the Indonesia Sejahtera Foundation (YIS) established by colleagues in Jakarta earlier that year. Dr Gunawan, however, left Indonesia for an overseas post in 1975.

Despite this serious setback, YIS, in cooperation with a Catholic hospital and a government clinic, successfully introduced the Dana Sehat programme to four wards outside Kerten during 1975. Yet the YIS team felt uneasy about the government's apparent lack of commitment to the programme. Granted, government officials attended community meetings and helped train volunteer health workers in the four new wards. But not a single initiative had been taken by the government itself to introduce the programme to new areas. Even the government doctors in charge of community health centres throughout the city knew little or nothing about the Dana Sehat programme. What had gone wrong?

After a series of introspective discussions, YIS staff arrived reluctantly at the conclusion that their alliance with the municipal administration was little more than a marriage of convenience, which legitimized YIS's work throughout Solo but did not commit the government to any specific steps within a certain time period. A further problem was that many government and private doctors believed that Dana Sehat threatened to reduce their own private practices, overload paramedical clinic and hospital staff, and place too much responsibility in the hands of 'incompetent', ordinary people.

Meanwhile, however, the Kerten programme was attracting interest from health professionals, government planners and community leaders from other areas in Indonesia and overseas. By 1977 a curious paradox had been reached: while Dana Sehat in Solo had virtually stagnated, the programme was receiving national and international acclaim, and the approach was being applied in other parts of Indonesia.

'MAKE OR BREAK'

In mid-1977 YIS took a bold initiative to try to get Dana Sehat on the move once more in Solo. They proposed to the municipal authorities that, in view of the slow implementation of Dana Sehat, the Health Service should organize a three-day workshop for government officials, health workers and community leaders throughout the whole city. The bureaucratic wheels turned slowly but finally, in December 1977, the workshop took place. A major effort was made to enthuse the participants about the advantages of Dana Sehat: lively talks were followed by discussions, a film strip shown and a visit made to Kerten. Finally, the participants drew up plans for action programmes.

Results were not long in coming. Almost immediately a two-pronged process began: on the one hand community leaders approached the government health service and YIS for help in starting Dana Sehat activities, and on the other hand the government health service itself became much more active in informing communities about the advantages of the programme. By the end of 1981 some 27 of Solo's 53 wards had started Dana Sehat activities, about 75 per cent of these during the period 1977–81 (see Fig. 12.1).

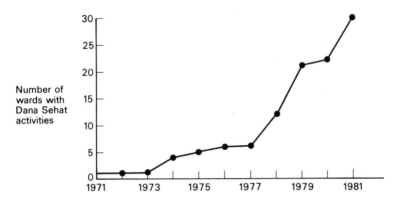

Fig. 12.1. Spread of Dana Sehat in Solo, 1971-81.

FOR EXAMPLE: PURWOSARI

A closer examination of Purwosari ward, where community health activities began in 1974, illustrates some of the dynamics and details of the programme. The ward is divided into four hamlets and 44 sub-hamlets, and has a total population of 11 250. By 1980, around 70 per cent of the sub-hamlets were running two or more health-related activities (see Table 12.1).

The Dana Sehat programme in Purwosari — as elsewhere in Solo — has evolved in fits and starts. Some groups ceased certain activities for a year or more, resuming them later on. The main factors influencing the fluctuating development of activities were:

Leadership

Activities multiplied rapidly during the first two years, when the *lurah* (ward leader) actively supported the programme. During the next two years, when a caretaker lurah was in control, health activities tended to stagnate, reviving only in 1979, when a young, enthusiastic lurah was elected.

Community participation

Initially, the YIS health team played an active role in setting programme priorities

Table 12.1. Cumulative development of Dana Sehat activities in
Purwosari Ward, 1974–80

Activity	Number of active sub-hamlets, by year						
	1974	1975	1976	1977	1978	1979	1980
1. Health insurance scheme	2	13	13	11	16	15	21
2. Weighing of under-fives	2	13	12	12	12	25	27
3. Nutrition rehabilitation centres	–	2	3	5	5	7	30
4. Credit cooperative	2	12	14	16	18	23	27
5. Volunteer health workers	3	11	16	16	16	16	30
6. Vaccinations	–	3	3	3	3	3	20
7. Tuberculosis control	–	11	20	24	26	26	26
8. Environmental sanitation	2	6	20	22	26	30	37
9. First-aid post	–	14	18	11	17	17	21

and carrying out tasks such as weighing under-fives and encouraging leaders to
hold meetings. But after two years the team began to question whether their
highly active role might be hampering community participation and prolonging
dependency. They decided to make a conscious effort to reduce their own involvement and encourage community members to become more active. As a
result, community meetings actually increased, more people volunteered to be
trained as health workers, and greater responsibility for expanding the programme was assumed by women's organizations and community leaders.

Choice of starting point

During the first few years most sub-hamlets began health-care activities with
the health insurance scheme, Dana Sehat, which first gave the programme its
name. But this scheme involves the collection of money on a regular basis – a
delicate and potentially divisive matter. Several sub-hamlet health insurance
schemes went defunct because of financial squabbles and other sub-hamlets were
resistant to the idea of even starting such a scheme. As a result, both YIS and
government staff decided not to stress health insurance as the most appropriate
starting point for health-care activities. In recent years many sub-hamlets have
begun their health programmes with preventive and promotive activities such
as environmental sanitation, nutrition clubs, and weighing of under-five-year-old
children. This greater flexibility in choosing an initial activity related to community needs results in a quicker and more enthusiastic response from the
people.

Role of women

Initially, Dana Sehat activities were administered by the sub-hamlet committees, which have a predominantly male membership and are burdened with many local government duties. Gradually, however, two women's organizations – the Family Welfare Movement and the Family Planning Acceptors Group – assumed greater responsibility in the management and organization of the programme. The active involvement of women has given the programme much greater momentum in recent years.

Personal and political rivalries

From time to time serious disruptions, for example in the weighing programme and collecting health insurance contributions, have been caused by personal or political rivalries between community leaders and volunteer health workers. In such cases the activity could be revived only after one or other of the feuding parties had withdrawn from the stage. Religious issues also posed a serious threat in one or two sub-hamlets, but these were neutralized in the course of time.

PROGRAMME RESULTS

Some of the most important results defy quantification. For example, the physical improvements resulting in a cleaner, more attractive and healthier environment, which are immediately apparent to a visitor. Likewise with human development, such as the new skills and confidence gained through active participation as a volunteer health worker, or a member of one of the numerous committees organizing the activities. Each weighing post, for example, involves at least 10 mothers in making decisions and participating actively in a community activity. Through this and other Dana Sehat activities people have gained greater control over factors influencing their health.

The quantification of programme results in Purwosari is fairly rudimentary – as is common with many primary health care programmes. Perhaps this is not surprising, since the data base is compiled largely by volunteer health workers with little or no training in the collection and use of health statistics, and handicapped by inadequate tools and financial restrictions.

In Purwosari ten sub-hamlets have reliable data about changes in nutritional status (indicated by weight for age) of under-fives over a five-year period; seven others have data over a three-year period (see Figs. 12.2 and 12.3).

In both sub-hamlets there was a marked improvement in nutritional status, with substantial increases in the proportion of children in the 'well-nourished' category. These changes cannot be attributed to any single activity of the Dana Sehat programme, but to a combination of several factors. One important factor may be a sharp reduction in the number of mothers believing in food taboos (see Table 12.2). Taboos forbade the consumption of certain nutritious foods by infants, children under five, and pregnant and lactating mothers – precisely the groups whose nutritional status is most at risk. The sharp drop in the prevalence of food taboos, indicating a receptive response by mothers to nutrition education,

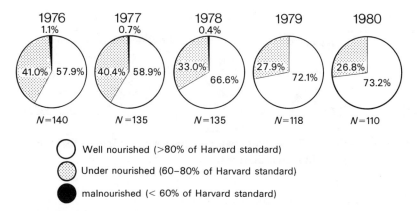

Fig. 12.2. Nutritional status of under-fives in ten sub-hamlets of Purwosari Ward, 1976-80.

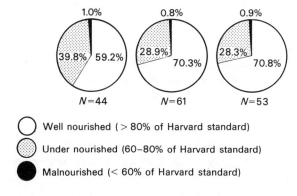

Fig. 12.3. Nutritional status of under-fives in seven sub-hamlets of Purwosari Ward, 1978-80.

is paralleled by an improvement in the nutritional status of these vulnerable groups.

FUTURE PROSPECTS

The development of Dana Sehat in Purwosari is typical of the way it has spread throughout other wards of the city. The programme continues to gain greater acceptance from community leaders, government administrators, doctors, paramedics, and the media. No longer is it forging a new approach to the delivery of health services, but it is providing content to the increasingly community health-oriented health programme of the national government.

Therefore the future development of the programme through the government system is guaranteed. Voluntary agencies, however, still have a role to play in

Table 12.2. Mothers in Purwosari ward believing in food taboos

	Proportion of mothers believing in food taboos, according to group affected			
Year	Infants (12 months)	Children (1–5 years)	Pregnant women	Lactating mothers
1975	37.4%	22.2%	33.3%	52.6%
1981	4.9%	1.2%	3.7%	5.8%

ensuring that the social impact of the programme is maximized so that the people participate meaningfully in achieving healthier lives.

BANJARNEGARA: A SNOWBALL EFFECT

The regency of Banjarnegara, situated in a mountainous area in the middle of Central Java Province, has a population of 678 000 living in 279 villages. Most people work as small farmers or agricultural labourers. Average per capita income is among the lowest in the province, and illiteracy exceeds 50 per cent in most villages. In 1971 the local government faced a typical syndrome of health problems: high infant mortality (150–180 per 1000), low nutritional levels, high incidence of infectious and communicable diseases, and low utilization rates (15–20 per cent) of government health services.

Tentative beginnings

The modest beginnings of Banjarnegara's primary health care programme owe much to the pioneering work of Dr Gunawan and his team in Solo. In 1971 Yahya Wardoyo, a young energetic doctor, spent a few weeks working with the Solo health team before moving to Banjarnegara and taking over the YAKKUM clinic in the small town of Klampok. Yahya began community health work by taking a mobile clinic once a week to the nearby village of Sirkandi. The people's response was lukewarm: a few utilized the curative service, but they showed no interest whatever in paying for it through a health insurance scheme. Yahya and his team went back to square one, and conducted a community survey. This indicated that the people of Sirkandi were much more concerned about agricultural problems than health. So the YAKKUM team changed their approach, firstly by providing funds and technical guidance to help the villagers build a dam which would increase rice production. Other schemes followed: the planting of fruit and clove trees, a revolving loan fund for purchasing goats and finally health activities starting with training of volunteer health workers, who began a nutrition improvement programme for under-five children. Meanwhile, in a neighbouring village, a government doctor was reaching similar conclusions. Dr Elias Winoto, head of the district government health service clinic in Klampok, tried to set up a health post in Karang Salam village staffed by volunteer health workers. The people complained, however, that they were too busy to help run it. Elias then decided to take more interest in the people's daily problems, and found they were spending very long periods of time collecting fuel used in boiling up palm sugar. After some experiments, Elias devised a method of boiling palm sugar using less fuel, and this won him genuine appreciation from the villagers. From this point onwards the people started to organize their own health-care activities, with technical guidance from the government clinic staff.

The community leaders of Klampok now began to take an interest in the latest developments in Sirkandi and Karang Salam. The innovative village head and several other community leaders made visits to Sirkandi, Karang Salam, and Solo to learn from the experiences of those who had pioneered community health in these places. On returning to Klampok, they drew up a plan to develop health care in their own community. Although Yahya provided some technical guidance, this plan was basically the achievement of the village leaders. Their first priority was not to start an income-generating scheme, but to train volunteers (called *kader*) as village community development workers, with special

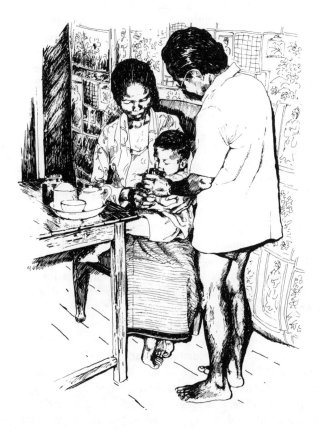

Fig. 12.4. A volunteer health kader shows a mother how to use oral rehydration therapy to treat diarrhoea.

emphasis on health and nutrition. This strategy of investing first in developing human resources before moving into programme implementation was totally successful in Klampok, where community health care activities developed much faster than in Sirkandi or Karang Salam.

Government recognition and expansion

In 1974 the newly appointed Regent of Banjarnegara suggested that the local health service should consider ways of spreading the Klampok approach to other villages throughout the whole regency. The head of the Health Service, Dr Arif Haliman, faced a daunting task. Trained medical manpower was critically scarce: there was only one doctor for every 160 000 people, one midwife and one nurse for every 105 000 people, and one dentist for the whole regency. Communications were poor, with all-weather roads confined to the valley of the Serayu river. (In any case the Health Service had only one vehicle.) Moreover, relations between Dr Yahya's YAKKUM team and the local government were strained.

The Regent therefore established a committee called the PPSE (Committee for Socio-Economic Development). The Committee was given the functions of promoting cooperation between government and voluntary agencies, and co-ordinating the inputs of these agencies into the community health programme. The PPSE also acted as a clearing house and channel for funding from foreign donor agencies. The Regent himself acted as Chairman of the PPSE, with Dr Arif Haliman as Executive Director in charge of day-to-day activities. Other members included the heads of the Planning Board, Agriculture, Animal Husbandry, Fisheries, Education, and Rural Development Services, as well as representatives from YIS and YAKKUM.

Though the PPSE suffered from managerial weaknesses, it eliminated some bureaucratic problems and provided the minimal operational structure needed for the Health Service to promote community health activities on a systematic basis throughout the regency. (In this respect Banjarnegara avoided the pitfall into which the Solo community health programme had fallen.) The PPSE met at regular intervals to set priorities, make detailed plans and review progress and difficulties encountered along the way. The general operational pattern was to invest first in human resources, as in Klampok, before moving into programme planning and implementation. The first step was thus to train government staff, including Health Service personnel, in the basic principles of community health management. Then followed the process of outreach to communities. At the start of each year the PPSE decided how many new villages could be covered by the programme, and kader training sessions were organized in the villages.

Training a group of health and nutrition kaders is not simply a matter of imparting certain technical and managerial skills. It also provides trainees with a theoretical framework within which they and their communities can establish PHC activities according to local needs and capacities. No village is expected to implement simultaneously, across-the-board, all the activities which could form part of a PHC programme, such as first-aid posts, nutrition surveillance and education, installation of safe water supplies, construction of latrines, road and housing improvements, home garden intensification, animal husbandry, agricultural schemes, school health programmes, and credit unions. Each community works out the 'mix' of activities most appropriate to get the programme on the move, and new activities are added as the people feel more confident of their organizational capacity.

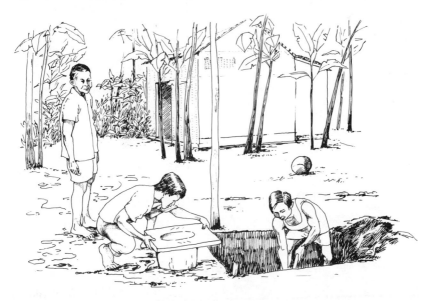

Fig. 12.5. Communities decide the most appropriate activities: building latrines helps reduce infection.

During the nine years from 1972 until 1980 a total of 4000 health and nutrition kaders were trained and the number of villages running PHC activities grew from two to 210 (see Fig. 12.6).

Human development and training strategies

All personnel involved in the programme – government staff with health and other technical and administrative backgrounds, community leaders, and kaders – have taken part in activities designed to familiarize them with PHC and to support its establishment and consolidation in the community. Workshops, refresher and 'upgrading' courses, and group visits to other PHC programmes are a high priority at all levels of the programme. YIS, YAKKUM, and other Indonesian voluntary agencies have played important roles in all types of training and human development efforts, but their roles have eventually been taken over to a large extent by government personnel and village kaders.

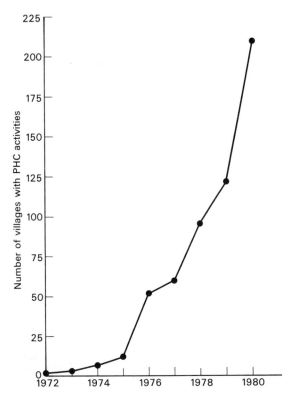

Fig. 12.6. Extension of PHC activities in Banjarnegara, 1972–80 (total villages: 279).

One particularly innovative form of motivation and maintenance of pro-grammes is the *kring* ('circle') – a grouping of about ten villages, of which two are relatively advanced in their development and the others less so. Village leaders and key kaders from each village meet every three months on a rotating basis in order to see and discuss one another's development and plan village development activities for the next quarter. Government and voluntary agency personnel are on hand to give technical or managerial guidance. In this way the psychology of peer group pressure is brought into play to stimulate communities to take new initiatives and to 'reward' those which have made progress.

Measuring results

The medical effectiveness of the programme is indicated by changes in patterns of morbidity, mortality, birth rate, and nutritional status of children. Monitoring of several key health indicators in ten sample villages from 1972 until 1980 showed some important changes.

The infant mortality rate (IMR), which reached 176 per 1000 in 1972, was reduced to 80 during this period (see Fig. 12.7).

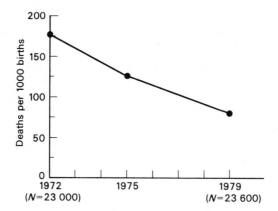

Fig. 12.7. Infant mortality rate in ten villages in Banjarnegara, 1972–79.

This sharp decline in infant mortality perhaps can be attributed in part to improved food production and availability. The main reasons, however, almost certainly are to be found in the PHC programme. Neonatal tetanus has been cut by vaccination of pregnant women, improved water supplies have reduced the incidence of diarrhoea and many deaths avoided by the spread of oral rehydration therapy administered by mothers, nutritional status of mothers and under-five children has improved, and progress made in controlling tuberculosis and malaria.

The maternal mortality rate (MMR) was also halved between 1972 and 1980 (see Fig. 12.8).

This improvement can be attributed largely to better ante-natal and delivery

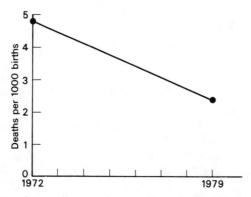

Fig. 12.8. Maternal mortality rate in ten villages in Banjarnegara, 1972–79.

care. In 1972 less than 10 per cent of mothers received maternal care, other than that provided by untrained, traditional midwives. During the past decade over 700 traditional midwives have been trained and given safe delivery kits. By 1980 almost half the mothers giving birth had received ante-natal care from a government or private clinic, largely because of the motivational and educational work carried out by the midwives. Wider coverage by maternal services during the next few years will reduce the maternal mortality rate still further.

The crude birth rate, another factor influencing the health of mothers and children, remained a constant 26 per 1000 during the whole eight-year period, even though family planning is widely in use. This apparent anomaly may be due to under-reporting of births during the early 1970s, resulting in an unrealistically low crude birth rate estimate for that period.

The nutritional status of under-fives is measured by the proportion of the total number of children whose weight rose or fell during a particular month, rather than by the more static measure of weight for age. As the programme has expanded, there has been a steady increase in the proportion of under-fives who gain weight each month (see Fig. 12.9).

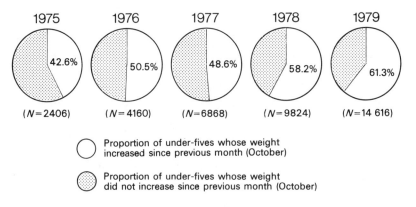

Fig. 12.9. Nutritional status of under-fives in villages covered by Banjarnegara PHC programme 1975-79.

The steady improvement in the nutritional status of under-fives is due to a combination of factors, including nutritional surveillance of children, nutrition education for mothers, increased food availability (in some cases only), and wider coverage by disease-preventive activities such as environmental sanitation, water supplies, and housing.

Although these achievements indicate very substantial gains for the state of the people's health, the PHC programme in Banjarnegara still faces a number of difficulties.

Constraints and problems

Supervision and follow-up

The rapid expansion of coverage has increased the need for suitably trained and motivated health professionals to consolidate PHC activities already under way. Devolving more responsibilities on to village heads, volunteer health and nutrition kaders, the non-health sector, and staff of Indonesian voluntary agencies has overcome this constraint to a considerable extent. Yet there are still problems in trying to maintain a high level of community participation and motivation on the one hand, and staff performance and morale on the other.

National and international recognition of individuals because of their role in the Banjarnegara programme has helped to maintain enthusiasm and commitment in a number of cases. But those who are 'left out' of this reward system sometimes feel disappointed and experience at least a temporary lack of interest in their work.

At community level, initial enthusiasm may suddenly evaporate if the original motivation to start the programme was simply a desire to follow the current mode or to accept the suggestions of a prestigious, external or supra-village agency. Hence regular visits by PPSE staff and government workers are organized to help kaders and community leaders understand the rationale behind activities and accruing benefits. Simple monitoring tools have also been designed to enable health personnel, kaders, and village leaders to follow progress and check health changes on a quarterly basis. One of these monitoring tools is an illustrated card which is punched to indicate the participation of a family in community activities (see Fig. 12.10). Such tools help reinforce the motivation and enthusiasm of the kaders, leaders and people.

Government bureaucracy

The effectiveness of present staff is hampered by bureaucratic procedures, restricted individual authority, minimal hopes of promotion, frequent transfers, and limited material or other incentives for staff to work in primary health care. The regency doctor maintains that 'a far more organized and regular system of staff upgrading and career development would go a long way to solving the problem of health centre staff motivation' (Haliman and Rohde 1980, p. 12). In addition, the training of health professionals still emphasizes curative care above prevention and promotive work. With only a fragmentary knowledge of PHC, some paramedics and doctors continue to regard village health and nutrition kaders as competitors rather than partners.

Involvement of low-income groups

The programme does not involve all socioeconomic groups equally in decision-making and programme implementation. For example, a survey in Klampok subdistrict in 1978 found that programme planning, implementation, and evaluation were dominated by individuals from the upper 60 per cent of the community.

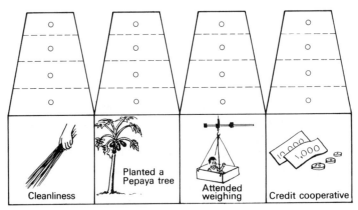

Fig. 12.10. Family participation in community activities

Another 30 per cent tended simply to utilize the services (weighing posts, curative care, etc.) and the bottom 10 per cent were completely untouched by the programme. The strategy of the programme generally favours projects which develop the whole village rather than the poorest groups in particular. Special efforts have been made to overcome this problem, such as forming functional literacy groups and small credit clubs, but they have met with limited success to date. The regency doctor admits frankly: 'We have not effectively solved the problem of the poor. We have found, for instance, that even when they are approached directly to provide manpower and other forms of participation, they are suspicious of groups and prefer not to participate. A few villages have attempted to set up PHC activities exclusively for the poor and this has fared no better.'[4] One of the challenges facing the programme now is whether there is sufficient enthusiasm, knowhow, skills, and funds to reach this group.

Multisectoral cooperation

This has been hampered by inter-departmental rivalries, vertical planning (especially budgeting), frequent transfer of government officials to other areas and a lack of financial and personnel resources for re-orienting and re-training officials in ways of cooperating across bureaucratic dividing lines.

Funding

Shortages of funds for training materials, transport, and fuel still continue to restrict the capacity of the programme to cover the whole regency. Funding of projects at village level is also a problem. For example: an enormous capital investment would be required to provide safe drinking water in every village within the next decade. Even when funds are available for such village projects, they must be handled with great sensitivity so that the participatory nature of the programme is not compromised.

Relations between voluntary agencies and government

Both the government and voluntary agencies — more so the latter — have had to make adjustments to avoid friction in a relationship loaded with sensitivities. The very strengths of the voluntary agencies — staff commitment, flexibility, innovativeness — are at times perceived by some officials as threats to their own prestige and authority. The voluntary agency may find itself accused — quite unjustly — of promoting certain religious or political causes, or simply with trying to undermine government development efforts. (Community leaders sometimes contribute unwittingly to souring of government–voluntary agency relations by expressing a strong preference for the work style of the latter in discussions with government officials!)

Another source of tension may be reporting on the use of funds. Voluntary agencies, with access to only limited funding, tend to be more exact and meticulous in this respect than government departments.

A further problem also arises if voluntary agency staff ignore normal bureaucratic channels. In their enthusiasm to achieve results, they may simply fail to communicate sufficiently with government officials. The existence of the PPSE, though it minimizes this problem, does not eliminate it entirely.

CONDITIONS FOR SUCCESS

The Solo and Banjarnegara PHC programmes have developed at varying tempos and used different organisational structures, yet both programmes have important elements in common, namely:

- a supportive political climate;
- decentralized, multisectoral planning;
- material support from the community and flexible supplementary financing;
- regular follow-up;
- provision of incentives;
- indicators of results and success;
- willingness by government to use voluntary agency resources;
- readiness of voluntary agencies to cooperate with government.

Examining each element in turn:

1. *Political climate*

Official espousal of PHC by international agencies and governments throughout the world since the late 1970s undoubtedly has been useful to both programmes. Yet the crucial political support in both cases was at the *local* level. The Mayor of Solo and the Regent of Banjarnegara endorsed the programmes well before PHC was elevated to its present official status at international level. The Solo experience, however, demonstrates that generalized expressions of support by top government officials are not enough. Detailed operational procedures must be worked out so that all levels of the government hierarchy understand the aims and methods of the programme and their role in its implementation. Great care also must be taken to neutralize problems caused by power struggles at all levels from village head upwards. Village leaders and government officials must be persuaded to see voluntary health workers not as threats to their own authority but as partners in a common struggle for better community health.

2. *Decentralized, multisectoral planning*

In both programmes the government has delegated authority to committees responsible for designing strategies for training, expansion, and consolidation. Decisions on programme activities and methods of implementation have been delegated to community organizations and groups. This approach means trusting the community to make responsible decisions and to implement them effectively. It also requires government staff to maintain a flexible approach including their time schedules, since they are participating in the community's programme, not the reverse.

Government planning for a wide spectrum of community needs demands a multisectoral approach – a difficult and usually lengthy process. Experience in Banjarnegara shows that multisectoral cooperation is feasible, at least to the regency level. Integration takes place when all the 'actors' know each other and belong to the same community. Hence integration is automatic in the village, likely at the sub-district and less likely at the regency level without imaginative, and possibly unorthodox, approaches (in Banjarnegara the creation of a non-government agency within the government itself).

3. *Material support from the community and flexible supplementary funding*

The core activities of both programmes were financed almost entirely by the communities themselves. This high degree of self-reliance strengthened the people's sense of identity with the programme and gave them a real sense of achievement and pride. It also encouraged greater thrift and responsibility in handling money, while still allowing sufficient flexibility.

In Banjarnegara, financial support from foreign donor agencies enabled the semi-autonomous development committee PPSE to develop flexible medium-term budgets covering items such as training, transport, financial incentives for fieldworkers, equipment, and communications material (written and audio-visual). The PPSE also channelled outside funds into capital investment projects such as water supplies, small-scale irrigation, and animal husbandry. The key factor in the usefulness of this outside support was not the (relatively small) absolute amount, but its timeliness and flexibility of usage.

4. *Follow-up*

Follow-up and maintenance consist of managerial and technical guidance as well as a portrayal of real interest in developments. Because of the multisectoral nature of programme planning and implementation, each sector should possess the managerial skills needed to maintain a programme, as well as providing its own specific technical and educational inputs. An agricultural extension worker, for example, should be able to motivate and guide a mother's club running a nutrition surveillance and education programme. By the same token, an auxilliary nurse should be able to help motivate a group of farmers to form a revolving loan fund to buy goats or cows. This multisectoral approach enables problems to be handled with greater speed and flexibility.

5. *Provision of incentives*

The Solo and Banjarnegara programmes have demonstrated that while incentives are needed to give voluntary health workers a sense of achievement and sustain interest and enthusiasm, they should *not* be financial. In both programme areas a sense of community spirit and mutual responsibility has motivated ordinary people by emphasizing the *human* element of health care. Even in urban Solo, voluntary health workers have remarked: 'Why should we be paid for helping ourselves?' Increased knowledge and skills, greater social status, and wider contacts and a desire to fulfill religious obligations have been sufficient justification for thousands of volunteer health workers to spend hours each week working for better health and living standards within their communities.

For government staff, however, highly desirable rewards are career development opportunities and wage adjustments. Other incentives include T-shirts, visitors, courses, visits to projects in othe parts of the country, articles on their work in the press, and interviews.

6. *Indicators of results and success*

Feedback of results is important to maintain the interest and enthusiasm of both the community and the professional health workers. Government planners and administrators also need reliable indicators of what is being achieved with public funds invested in health care. The Solo and Banjarnegara programmes highlight three main problems in this field.

— What are the most appropriate indicators of a successful PHC programme (e.g. number of on-going activities, the extent and quality of community participation, or changes in quantitative indicators such as nutritional status and infant mortality rate)?
— Which indicators are most meaningful to policymakers, programme planners, and the community?
— In what form should these indicators be presented to all parties so that interest is retained, and critical, creative responses generated?

From the Banjarnegara experience the conclusion has been reached that indicators must reflect action, i.e. largely process indicators such as current users in the family planning programme, total number of kader, vital events, attendance at weighing posts, and weight increases for nutrition surveillance. All are comprehensible, and easy to measure and compare, in contrast to infant mortality and morbidity rates, which are technically more sophisticated measures.

However, it is admitted that further efforts need to be put into determining the most sensitive indicators, and to methods of communicating results so that the enthusiastic, creative participation of implementors can be sustained, and policy makers can be convinced of the relevance of PHC.

7. Willingness by government to use voluntary agency resources

In both programmes the local government has consistently tried to make maximum use of the resources — both human and financial — of voluntary agencies. The minimal bureaucracy of voluntary agencies, the commitment of their staff, the flexibility of their budgeting and accounting processes and their readiness to experiment with new approaches to solving old problems enable them to assume innovative roles for which the government is poorly equipped.

8. Readiness of voluntary agencies to cooperate with government

Close cooperation with the government in expanding PHC in Solo and Banjarnegara has placed rigorous demands on the voluntary agencies concerned. The voluntary agencies have accepted their role as junior members in the partnership with government, even though they initiated the programmes in the first place. The following lessons have emerged for the voluntary agencies:

— They must keep a low profile and avoid taking credit for achievements of the programme;
— They must thoroughly understand the intricacies of the government administrative machinery and adjust their own work styles and procedures to fit in;
— They must accept the role of 'gap filler', taking on tasks for which the government is not yet equipped;
— They must be prepared to change their function as the government takes on new responsibilities and as new needs arise.

CONCLUSIONS

The experiences of PHC programmes in the city of Solo and the rural regency of Banjarnegara suggest that, under certain conditions, the creativity and enthusiasm of voluntary agencies can be combined successfully with the authority of government structures to develop health services covering large populations.

The most crucial elements in forging this combination are the will to create a political climate supportive of community initiative on the part of the government, and the readiness of voluntary agencies to make adjustments enabling them to work within the government system. This demands openness and tolerance to criticism from the government and a realistic, sensitive attitude on the part of voluntary agencies.

Despite their potentially valuable role in developing PHC services, voluntary agencies remain vulnerable. On the one hand they must retain their political independence, clearly articulated objectives and flexible operational procedures. But on the other hand their financial viability may depend on the decisions of committees in the national capital or in countries thousands of miles away from their work. Their very existence may depend on retaining the favour of governments whose policies reflect a bias towards the rich and powerful rather than the low-income groups. Yet the experiences of PHC programmes in Solo and Banjarnegara suggest that in Indonesia – a country whose development policies during the past decade still leave much to be desired in terms of equity – voluntary agencies can cooperate with certain levels of government in developing PHC services through which low-income communities can participate in determining the direction and momentum of their development.

NOTES

1. Also called 'Surakarta'.
2. For an account of this programme from 1967 until 1974 see Newell (1975) pp. 102–11.
3. Data taken from a baseline survey of a random sample of 171 married women in 1975 and a follow-up survey of 162 women in similar socioeconomic conditions in 1981.
4. Personal communication to author.

REFERENCES

Golloday, F.L. and Koch-Weser, C.K., The new policies for rural health: institutional, social and financial challenges to large scale implementation. *Proceedings of the Royal Society of London* **B199**, 169–78 (1977).
Haliman, Arif, and Rohde, Jon E., Case study of primary health care in Banjarnegara (1980). (Unpublished.)
Ministry of Health, Republic of Indonesia, *Primary health care (village community health development) in Indonesia,* Jakarta (1978).
Newell, Kenneth W. (ed.), *Health by the people.* World Health Organization, Geneva (1975).
Nugroho, Gunawan, A community development approach to raising health standards in Central Java, Indonesia. In *Health by the people* (ed. K.W. Newell). World Health Organization, Geneva (1975).

13 Contrasts in community participation: case studies from Peru

Frits Muller argues that 'community participation', now generally accepted as essential to primary health care, should not be interpreted as merely the *mobilization* of human and material resources. Rather, it should be understood as the community increasing its *control* over the social, political, economic, and environmental factors affecting the health status of all its members.

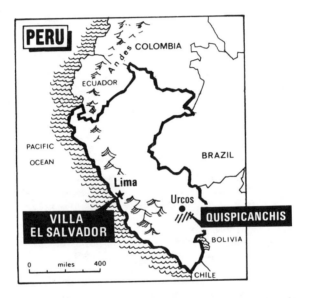

Frits Muller, Ph.D., M.D., worked from 1972 until 1977 in the two health programmes described in this chapter. He now works as a primary health care consultant, based in Holland.

Community participation is generally considered a fundamental element in primary health care (PHC) strategy. Yet there is considerable confusion about the meaning of this term. Most commonly it is conceived of as the *mobilization* of community resources – such as manpower, money, materials, and 'creative capacities' – in order to carry out health programmes. This view is based on the assumption that the community has certain capacities which have been hidden under apparent passivity or resistance to change.

An opposing view is that community participation consists of increasing people's *control* over the social, political, economic, and environmental factors determining their health. Many communities do not control the main factors determining their health at present. Peasants who do not own enough land to feed their families, who have to walk long distances every day for drinking water, and who do not have access to decent health services can hardly be blamed for being in poor health. According to this view, poor communities already are using their creative capacity to the maximum in trying to alleviate their health problems through traditional medicine. What these communities lack, however, is the opportunity to participate, not only in health, but also in education, housing, and many other benefits of society.

These two opposing views of participation reflect a different analysis of society, especially of the distribution of wealth and power among different social groups. For the sake of clarity, the view that community participation consists of the mobilization of community resources will be referred to as *direct participation*. Increasing community control of the factors determining health status on the other hand, will be called *social participation*. Ideally direct participation is merely a strategy for attaining greater social participation, but in practice it is often regarded as an end in itself.

To add to the difficulties of defining community participation, communities are rarely the homogeneous units which many health workers expect them to be. They tend to be divided into groups with different — even opposing — interests and varying degrees of power. Moreover, there may be enormous differences in the structure and composition of communities in different parts of the same country.

This study describes and analyses the reactions to PHC programmes of communities in one rural and one urban area of Peru. It is argued that different socioeconomic, political, and historical characteristics account for the major part of the communities' different reactions.

QUISPICANCHIS — A RURAL PROGRAMME

Background

The Andean province of Quispicanchis is situated in the department of Cusco, in the southern region of Peru. The province is about 250 kilometres long and 60 kilometres wide, and consists of two main regions: the Valley of the Vilcanote river, dissecting the province from north to south, at about 3100 metres altitude; and the uplands averaging about 4000 metres but including peaks of over 6000 metres. The capital city of Urcos, with a population of 4000, is situated in the river valley.

The province has a population of about 80 000 mostly Quescha-speaking Indian peasants (*campesinos*) living in widely dispersed hamlets. They grow crops of corn, barley, vegetables, beans, and fruits in the fertile river valley, while the poorer soils of the uplands support mainly potatoes, beans, and barley. Higher up, where there is only grass, sheep and llamas are grazed. Trade, transport, and administration are dominated by the *mestizo* (mixed Spanish and Indian descent) population, living in the eleven district capitals. Social and health indicators for the region are extremely unfavourable. Illiteracy, for example, stood at 85 per cent (including *all* women) in 1975, and infant mortality at 251 per 1000.

Quispicanchis is situated near Cusco, centre of the former Inca civilization. Under the Incas the state owned all the means of production, but peasants were allowed to till the soil in exchange for sharing the crop with the dominant classes and the non-productive population. The arrival of the Spanish conquerers in the sixteenth century destroyed this system and led to the establishment of large, privately owned farms (*haciendas*). A large proportion of the Indian population was assigned to a landlord, on whose land they worked in return for a small plot to work themselves. The rest were allowed to continue to live and work in their own communities on communally owned land. In the following centuries little changed in this system, not even after Independence in 1820, when a national bourgeoisie took over from the Spanish crown and its representatives. Gradually the *haciendas* grew at the expense of the land of the Indian communities. The Agrarian Reform Law, decreed by a military junta in 1969, aimed to eliminate this exploitation through selling off *haciendas* to workers' cooperatives. In Quispicanchis, however, the reform brought little change, as the landlord was simply replaced by government officials, and no investments were made to increase agricultural production.

Development of primary health care

Western medicine was introduced into the area through traders selling analgesics and antibiotics at high prices. A missionary organization also opened a clinic, concentrating on curative work, in Urcos. The government clinic, built in 1965, was not staffed by a permanent doctor until 1974. The government also established dispensaries, staffed by attendants (*sanitarios*) in each district capital.

The PHC programme started in October 1974 when the population, assisted by a local group of Jesuit priests, successfully demanded that the Health Ministry assign a doctor to the clinic in Urcos. The health team consisted of one doctor, one dentist, one nurse, two auxiliary nurses, and eight dispensary attendants. The team was assisted from the start by the Jesuit-run adult education school, later by the communities themsleves, and finally by the Ministry of Health. Funds for the programme came from foreign donor agencies and the Ministry of Health. Over the three years 1974–76 capital expenditure amounted to US $0.70 per person annually, and running costs at US $0.80 annually.

The programme aimed to extend coverage, which was nil in 1974. Implementation took place in three phases. Phase One aimed to improve the performance of the dispensary attendants through better supervision and support. This had limited success, because most of the attendants had long settled into the routine of exploiting the local population with their knowledge of medicine. The second phase was to teach schoolteachers the principles of PHC. This failed because the *mestizo* teachers lacked the necessary commitment to help the local population. Only in Phase Three was the training of health promoters selected by the community for work within the community begun. This approach eventually was modified to include health training for groups of volunteers within the communities themselves.

The programme was developed through visits of the health team to 40 communities in five districts. The areas of programme concentration were selected by the team on the basis of marginality: the poorest and most isolated had highest priority. Curative services were provided during these visits — not only were they badly needed, but they also demonstrated the value of western medicine, of which few people had any experience. As the trips were long and arduous (by foot or on horseback), the team stayed overnight with the *campesinos*. In discussions by lamplight during the long, cold evenings, the team pieced together a better understanding of the campesinos' interpretation of health and disease; at the same time, the campesinos moved towards a greater understanding of the biological and social causes of ill-health and disease.

The team encouraged each community to select a candidate for the health promotor course to be held in Urcos. The only requirement was that the candidate could read and write, which virtually excluded women. Some 34 communities finally selected and sent a trainee health promotor to the course. Training, which lasted two weeks full-time, covered the most common health problems in the region, starting with the trainee's own perceptions of the problems. Curative training was limited to elementary diagnostic and therapeutic skills. Administration procedures and an examination of the social origins of ill-health and disease were also part of this initial training course. To assist their work, the promotors were given a manual which they had helped compile during their training, as well as a stock of 12 basic drugs purchased by the community. In addition, they were entrusted with medical equipment (valued at US $100) from the project, for which the community as a whole was responsible.

The health promotors began their work by concentrating on curative care, for which there was a great need and which was more acceptable to the people than preventive measures. According to a project survey, the average consultation rate in 1976 was about 20 per month, with a minimum of seven and a maximum of 37 per promotor. Around 70 per cent of diagnoses were correct, but only about 50 per cent of the therapies prescribed. (Since the drugs had been carefully selected, however, there were no negative side-effects.)

The communities maintained strict control of drug supply, pricing, and replenishment. Not a single case of overcharging by a promotor was reported during the three year period from 1974 until 1977. The communities also decided whether the promotor could charge patients, apart from the actual cost of drugs. A nominal charge was usually fixed, but in some cases the promotor was exempted from communal work (*faena*) in return for providing patients with a free service.

Field supervision of the promotors' work was carried out by a member of the project team visiting the community every month. Supervision was closely linked to the training course and aimed at *supporting* the promotor, not merely assessing his performance. The team member would meet with the promotor and discuss his work on the basis of a review of his records of patient visits and drugs prescribed. Every six weeks the promotors met as a group with the health staff to share experiences, improve their knowledge and strengthen friendships. The team also encouraged community supervision of the promotors through village assemblies to discuss topics such as the promotors' performance, the effectiveness of treatment, and the pricing and control of drug supplies.

At the time of the evaluation in 1977, the programme was delivering health services through a clinic in Urcos, dispensaries in seven of the 11 district capitals and a network of health promotors in rural communities. Of the 25 promotors originally selected in 1974, 15 were still active in 1977. The evaluation noted a marked improvement in the delivery of curative care. Medical records had been introduced at the clinic and dispensaries, a drug supply system established, regular supervision of promotors was taking place and a referral system had been set up. These simple measures resulted in a rapid rise in consultation rates, from 80 to 600 per month within the first half year. But this meant that health clinic staff were spending insufficient time in the field. Consultation times therefore were reduced to four hours a day. This enabled the nurse to concentrate on fieldwork and for the doctor to spend about 30 per cent of his working time outside the clinic. Preventive and promotive measures concentrated on vaccination of mothers and children, protection of water supplies, and nutrition improvement through production and consumption of vegetables.

Relations with the government were complicated. Most participants in the programme were opposed to complete integration with the Ministry of Health because they felt the Ministry did not share the interests of the campesinos. On the other hand, everyone agreed that the Ministry was obliged to ensure everyone's right to adequate health care, and thus should pay for the programme's activities. The Ministry began taking an interest in the programme at the time preparations for the WHO–UNICEF conference in Alma Ata were under way, and provided the programme with drugs, vaccines and the salary for one staff member. Yet it also threatened the programme leader at various times with replacement.

Results

It is useful to distinguish between the *medical effectiveness* and the *social impact* of the programme. Medical effectiveness is evaluated in terms of the changes in morbidity and mortality patterns brought about by the programmes. Social impact, on the other hand, is indicated by the community's increased awareness of health problems and capacity to organize itself to solve these problems.

The medical effectiveness of the PHC programme in Quispicanchis between September 1974 and September 1977 could not be quantified because no reliable base-line data on morbidity and mortality were available. Some reduction in these indicators, however, can be assumed, given the increase in health service coverage. Curative coverage[1] rose from virtually nil in 1974 to 19 per cent in 1977, when 18 000 consultations were made, 60 per cent of which were first consultations. The referral system, however, was greatly under-utilized, because the campesinos distrusted state hospitals. 'You only go to hospital to die', they said, so they refused to go. Preventive and promotive activities had modest success: 2000 children below the age of five (about two-thirds of the total) were vaccinated in 1976 and 1977; wells providing safe drinking water were constructed in five communities in 1977; and in one community 17 families started home gardens growing vegetables for their own consumption. The main weaknesses of the programme were limited coverage, insufficient concentration on high-risk groups, and lack of maternal services.

The social impact of the programme was also unevenly spread. Health became a subject of interest and discussion in many community meetings, and in many cases people's interpretation of health moved from traditional to biological or even social.[2]

Some structural aspects of the programme were weak: staff members were not able to transfer medical knowledge and technical skills to community members other than the health promotors. For their part, the promotors also were generally unable to share their knowledge within the community, so no 'ripple effect' developed. Overall control of the programme was too firmly in the hands of the doctor in charge of the provincial health service. This centralized leadership caused dissatisfaction among some other workers and created

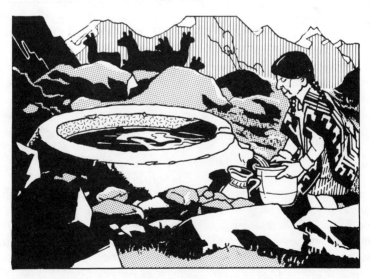

Fig. 13.1. Five communities built wells providing safe drinking water.

an exaggerated sense of dependency on the doctor among the campesinos. The central position of the doctor also restricted the programme's possibilities for continuity after he left at the end of 1977. At this time the programme was re-organized under the leadership of the Jesuit school for adult education.

Involvement of local communities in the programme was generally limited to direct participation in implementation. The functions of planning and management control were completely in the hands of the health staff. Social participation also occurred to a limited extent, but only where local conditions were especially favourable.

Three case studies

Of the 34 communities involved in the Quispicanchis programme, three were chosen for detailed study because each reacted differently to the programme: Occoran rejected it; Pinchimuru collaborated with it; and Pampaccamara — to whom the programme was not offered originally — demanded assistance from it. Let us firstly examine the socioeconomic, political, and historical background of these three communities during the mid 1970s.

Occoran lies about three hours on horseback from the provincial capital of Urcos, at a height of 3800 metres. The population of about 200 lives in 36 houses, scattered far apart. The soil is very poor, the best parts yielding only a meagre crop of potatoes and barley. Each family keeps a few animals such as sheep and llamas. To help their families survive, men are forced to migrate to seek work in the lowlands for up to four months of the year.

Until 1972 the land belonged to an absentee landlord, whose administrator nominated a local man to organize the labour force. He controlled the community to such a degree that there were no autonomous institutions, and the only other local person of any influence was the traditional healer. The land is now held collectively in a 'pre-cooperative' but is worked individually by each household. The agrarian reforms of 1969 also made it necessary to hold regular meetings, for which the people were totally unprepared. The local school teacher keeps records of these meetings.

Health problems were interpreted in a traditional way. The local traditional healer, an old, blind woman, had the complete confidence of the population. Apart from her healing function, she also carried out religious duties such as making offerings to the gods in the hope of a good harvest.

The second community, Pinchimuru, is only half an hour by foot from a dirt road, about 80 kilometres east of Urcos. The 38 hectares of land belonging to the community consist of poor soil supporting only grass for animal fodder and potatoes. The 76 families of the community live around the former hacienda house, which now serves as a school. Pinchimuru was formerly a small hacienda. Relations between the workers and the landowner were good, even to the point where the workers defended the land against incursions by a powerful neighbour. This history of shared struggle with the landowner against the neighbour's attacks favoured community organization. In 1965 the workers bought the hacienda from the owner and formed an 'Indian community' — a legally recognized organization within which the land was distributed evenly among the members. But the conflict with the powerful neighbour — now in the shape of a cooperative — still continues.

Health problems in Pinchimuru were interpreted in the same traditional way as in Occoran. The traditional healer is the person with most authority. The most notable difference in comparison with Occoran is the much stronger community organization expressed through regular meetings of all community members (including women) to discuss common problems.

The third community, *Pampaccamara*, lies next to the main road in the Cctaca Valley, at an altitude of about 3500 metres, about 40 kilometres from Urcos. The relatively fertile soil produces crops of potatoes, beans, barley, and corn. Production exceeds local needs, and the surplus is sold in nearby towns. The 306 families own 10 000 hectares among them, and live in two-storey houses with tile rooves. The land officially belongs to the community as a whole, but in practice each family works its own plot, although some land is set aside and worked collectively. The crop is sold and the money used to finance community needs.

Pampaccamara has a long history of common struggle, mostly about land ownership, with the nearby hacienda, the greater part of which (originally usurped from the community more than two centuries earlier) was allocated to the community in 1974. Because of this long experience of common struggle, community organization is strong. General meetings are held regularly and are of great importance.

In addition, frequent contact with urban life through trade has created urban-type expectations among the farmers. They want the same services as cities. During the past 20 years the community has used its own resources for communal activities such as the construction of a school, a centre for community activities, a post office, a medical post, and even a police station.

Although health still tended to be interpreted in a traditional way, frequent contact with western medicine was leading to a biological interpretation.

Reactions to PHC programme

In *Occoran*, the community rejected the programme out of sheer inertia. When visited six times in 12 months by health team staff, the people came together for consultations, but only after much persuasion by the local school teacher. Then they asked, 'What use are those drugs? What will happen to our money?' At first nobody was willing to serve as a health promotor. When, finally, a young man was chosen and trained, he went off to a big city and did not return. Even then, the community did not demand his replacement. The community was simply unable to organize itself sufficiently to utilize the services offered by the health team, let alone demand better services or take any initiative to start their own programme. Crushed by poverty and repression, and lacking any history of shared resistance to outside control and the process of marginalization, the community remained indifferent to the failure of the programme. The people's interpretation of health remained traditional, and the health team was unable to help start a process of direct or social participation in health care.

In *Pinchimuru* the programme attracted considerable direct participation and even a certain amount of social participation. The son of the local traditional healer was chosen as the health promotor and his services were well used after he returned from training. He used both traditional and western medicine in providing curative care, and the community collected money for the purchase of medical supplies. His work was twice evaluated positively at general meetings of the community, yet only two friends helped him build the village well, and only his own family helped him construct his small medical post. In 1977, some 17 out of the 76 families started their own vegetable gardens, after a two-week course given on the spot by staff of the Jesuit adult education school from Urcos, and following the example of the health promotor, who had begun his garden the previous year.

Pinchimuru was just as poor economically as Occoran. But, unlike Occoran, the community had a history of common struggle against the neighbouring hacienda. Consequently, they already had built up some effective leadership and organization when the health programme started. The programme had the effect of strengthening community organization. Moreover, many people's interpretations of health problems shifted from purely traditional towards biological and social. Health was seen, for the first time, as something which an organized community could influence, rather than simply a gift of the gods.

In *Pampaccamara* the programme attracted by far the greatest amount of direct participation and also some social participation. Initially this community was given low priority by the health team and so was not invited to send a trainee to the health promotor course. But the community had already constructed their own health post at a cost of US $10 000 and had been struggling for years to obtain their own health worker. (They had even sent representatives to far-away Lima, the national capital, and submitted their request to the Minister of Health himself.) When they heard about the health promotor course in nearby Urcos, they simply chose a trainee at a general meeting and sent him to the course, where he was accepted. On returning to Pampaccamara the promotor worked effectively for four months in the health post until the government health worker finally arrived and displaced him. The government health worker discouraged the local health promotor from playing an active part in community health work, so he returned to farming and his health skills were lost to the community.

Pampaccamara had an even stronger base of community organization due to surplus agricultural production and an even longer history of common struggle than Pinchimuru. The people did not merely collaborate in the implementation of the programme, but actually demanded its services and contributed a substantial sum of money to construct a health post. But in making this large financial commitment – an impressive act of direct participation – the people relieved the Ministry of Health of an obligation, so endorsing the system which had deprived them of health services in the first place. Thus, paradoxically, direct participation by the community weakened the people's critical awareness of health problems and tended to reduce their social participation in health!

These three rural communities, each with different economic, political, and historical backgrounds, reacted differently to the same PHC programme: Occoran rejected it completely; Pinchimuru showed considerable direct and some social participation; Pampaccamara showed by far the greatest participation – but direct participation tended to undermine their social participation, and the community became even more dependent on the formal health care system.

VILLA EL SALVADOR, AN URBAN COMMUNITY

The experience of community participation in a PHC programme in the urban environment of Villa el Salvador provides some interesting contrasts with the rural situation of Quispicanchis.

Background

Villa el Salvador is one of about 350 slum areas in Lima, capital of Peru. The phenomenon of rapid urban growth is fairly recent in Peru, originating from the growing imbalance in economic development between urban and rural areas. The shacks of Villa el Salvador, inhabited by 125 000 people, sprawl across a barren stretch of land ('the sandbin' to the locals) about 12 kilometres from the centre of Lima. The settlement's history began during the night of 28 April 1971, when about 2000 homeless people invaded and occupied a privately owned, sandy area called Pamplona Alta, on the outskirts of Lima. Within three weeks, the population of illegal occupants had swollen to 50 000. But after heavy government pressure, backed by police and Army troops, the people agreed to move further out to an officially approved site called Pampa de Lurin, 8 kilometres long and 4 kilometres wide, where two main roads had been laid out but no other preparations made. Each household was entitled to a tiny plot of land, just sufficient for a shack. Here, in overcrowded, unsanitary conditions, the slum now known as Villa el Salvador grew up.

The people faced innumerable hardships. Their flimsy straw and cardboard shacks were in constant danger of going up in flames. Thieves invaded to steal the people's few precious possessions. Drinking water was an acute problem. Men, women, and children had to trudge for hours through the burning sand to reach the main road to buy drinking water from a tanker which called every day. No trained medical care was available because the slum could not be reached by road. These shared hardships helped motivate the people to organize themselves for survival. Among the first community organizations were 'common pot' committees providing food to groups of people during the initial stages of the illegal occupancy. Committees for schools and health care soon followed. Most important however, was the community's own organization based on blocks of houses, which provided local government. This political organization 'from below' had to compete from the beginning with the government organization SINAMOS.[3]

The community's organization aimed at the greatest possible independence from national society, as the people blamed the government and 'free enterprise' for their own problems. SINAMOS, on the other hand, wanted to fully integrate community organization and projects (in the form of cooperatives) into national society. Efforts to resolve the differences failed, and in November 1973 the community formed its own organization known as CUAVES (Urban Community of Self-Sufficiency, Villa el Salvador). CUAVES enjoyed considerable success, at least during the first few years of its existence. A community bank was formed, acting as a savings bank and a source of credit for communally-owned enterprises such as a bakery, a hardware store, a kerosene pump, and a pharmacy. CUAVES also arranged for a loan from the Banco de la Vivienda, enabling each block of houses to have access to a public water tap and for most houses to have electricity.

Living conditions, however, remained precarious. In a community health survey carried out in 1976, the health promotors concluded that half the population was under 15 years; that only one in 20 houses was solidly built and fewer than half had a latrine; that in every fifth household three people had to share one bed; and that an average of 75 households had to share one water tap. The same study also found that only 15 per cent of adults had a stable job. As a result of these conditions, health conditions were highly unsatisfactory: infant diarrhoea, dehydration, tuberculosis, typhoid fever, and scabies were frequent diseases. Infant mortality was at least 60 per 1000, and probably higher.[4] The survey also showed, perhaps ironically, that families who had adhered strictly to a traditional interpretation of health while still living in rural areas soon started spending more money than they could afford on western medicine after settling in Villa el Salvador.

The primary health care project

Health services in the form of privately owned pharmacies and doctors' surgeries began operating soon after the people were moved to Pampa de Lurin. At the same time, however, the people themselves began organizing their own health care. In regular meetings of blocks of houses, health problems were discussed and solutions suggested. Many such meetings chose one person to be responsible for health care, starting with simple tasks such as collecting drugs to form a basic pharmaceutical kit and organizing the burning of waste. Funds were collected through Sunday dances and lotteries. The first health committees were elected in 1971. These made a census in each block of houses and collaborated in the government's mass immunization campaign. The people's own initiatives in health care later received help from doctors of the National University of San Marcos, who not only provided curative care but also participated in meetings at which the root causes of ill-health and poverty were discussed. Ten health committees were formed and 20 health promotors trained. But as the promotors had little technical and organizational support or supervision, they soon began using their knowledge of medicine as a way of making extra income. Signs appeared above their doors announcing 'Injections for Sale'.

In November 1973 a new health plan for the whole of Villa el Salvador was submitted to a general meeting of delegates from the whole community. The plan, drawn up by community leaders in dialogue with University doctors, proposed the establishment of a Health Committee consisting of elected representatives from the 67 blocks (around 300 families each). Each block also would have an elected health promotor, who would be trained to carry out primary health care. The organizational centre of the programme would be a community pharmacy, to be built at a cost of US $20 000 and financed by the community bank. The plan was opposed by people who argued that it was the government's responsibility to establish effective health services, but finally it was approved and went into operation.

The community pharmacy was soon constructed. A concrete, one-storey building without water, electricity, or other 'luxuries', it still serves as a meeting place, training centre, and a place for doctors' surgeries and dispensing basic drugs. In 1978 the pharmacy staff consisted of one permanent doctor assisted by various voluntary doctors and nurses, and four health promotors receiving a small remuneration for their work. The programme was carried out within the community by 60 health promotors, virtually all of them women. About half the promotors were politically motivated to do the job, while others were just interested in medicine and in helping their neighbours. All were aware of the fundamental problems of inequality and injustice. One promotor commented: 'In our block of houses we have succeeded in having everyone pay for communal services according to their capacity. But this is much more difficult at the level of a whole neighbourhood. As for establishing a fair and just community for all of Villa el Salvador, that is even more difficult still.' Her motivation for doing this modestly paid work was clear: 'I became a health promotor to help bring about a just community'.

The training of health promotors is continuous and rather informal. There are weekly training sessions in the community pharmacy, linked to the promotors' work in their own blocks. The results are analysed and a plan of action drawn up. The promotors then begin carrying out their tasks: registering under-fives and arranging their vaccinations; registration and referral of chronic cough patients; first aid and the organization of waste burning. Discussion of the promotors' activities at the start of the weekly lessons is an effective form of on-going supervision.

Nine traditional midwives have been trained in the community pharmacy since 1976 in courses of three months duration.

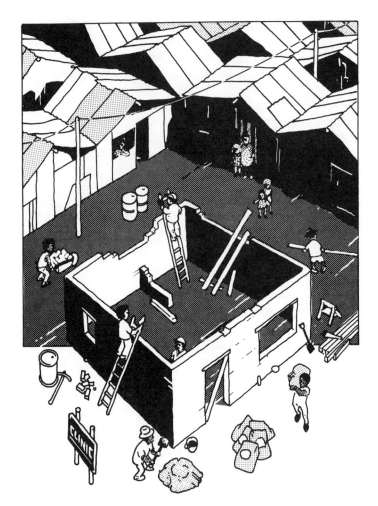

Fig. 13.2. The people construct a community pharmacy.

Relations with other health projects

Apart from the CUAVES-sponsored PHC programme, three other organizations have taken initiatives in the field of health in Villa el Salvador: SINAMOS, Jospice International, and the Ministry of Health.

SINAMOS introduced female health promotors in 1972, but they had little success. This probably was due in part to their not living in Villa el Salvador, which limited their acceptability to local people. In addition, many people might have viewed SINAMOS as more interested in their political allegiance than their health.

Jospice International, an international aid organization, started a maternity clinic in 1973, at the instigation of the local Catholic Bishop. It was staffed however, by expatriate nurses, and was felt by the community to be something of a 'foreign body' with little sensitivity to local needs. In 1975 CUAVES organized a massive public demonstration outside the clinic, demanding its transferral to the Ministry of Health. As a result, the clinic now serves as one of the two health centres run by the Ministry in Villa el Salvador.

The Health Ministry, for its part, has not provided the CUAVES-sponsored health project with adequate support, and has opposed it in various ways. For example, when the health promotors identified 140 sputum-positive tuberculosis cases in 1976, the Ministry did not send the free drugs to which the patients were entitled. A more subtle form of official opposition was the installation of a much better equipped health centre two blocks away from the community pharmacy. In contrast to the people's pharmacy, however, the health centre was under tight government control. A similar event occurred in 1976, when CUAVES submitted a comprehensive, community-based health programme to the authorities. This was ignored. Yet shortly afterwards the Ministry produced its own, much more expensive plan, financed by an international agency.

Although the Ministry has never officially denounced the CUAVES-sponsored health project in Villa el Salvador, it still seems uneasy about the existence of a health programme outside its own direct control, and therefore withholds the support which is in its power to provide. The Ministry of Health has thus attempted to undermine the project by a strategy of withholding logistic support and offering alternative, technically more sophisticated, health services under tight government control.

Results

The medical effectiveness of the programme is probably limited but impossible to quantify, given the availability of other health services to the population – two clinics, 24 doctors, and a number of pharmacies. Curative coverage in 1976 was 7 per cent with 12 000 clinic consultations. The other main elements of the programme – health education, mother-and-child health, promotion of sanitation, and health monitoring – have achieved about 10 per cent coverage of the potential target groups in the total population of 125 000.

The programme's main importance, however, is as an expression of popular concern about community health. It resulted originally from the people's efforts to overcome certain health problems. But, once created, it developed its own dynamic and helped the people towards a critical analysis of the reasons for their health problems. Health became one of the main themes of popular demands *vis-à-vis* the government authorities and other 'outside' bodies. The programme thus had a much wider social impact than its limited medical effectiveness might suggest. Its replicability, however, is probably limited because few – if any – other slums in Lima have such strong, well-organized leadership. External support (in this case, from the University Medical Faculty) may also not be available elsewhere.

CONCLUSIONS

The main reasons for the limited *medical effectiveness* of both the Quispicanchis and Villa el Salvador programmes are as follows:

— *Limited health resources*: Despite severe problems in both areas, only limited financial and health manpower resources are available. The average per capita expenditure on health by the government in 1977 was only US $0.25 in Quispicanchis and US $0.30 in Villa el Salvador. — compared with the national average of US $8.00. In other words, primary health care in these cases meant cheap health care for the poor, with inadequate coverage to be effective.

— *Curative bias*: Both programmes were heavily oriented towards cure rather than prevention of disease, with consequent loss of effectiveness.

— *Lack of government support*: Government support was needed (as is the people's right) to provide drugs, personnel, and specialist referral services. But very little such support was provided, and on several occasions the government authorities were obstructive, seeming to distrust a community initiative outside their own direct control.

— *Lack of monitoring*: Though both programmes started with a community health analysis, no on-going monitoring of health levels was carried out. It was thus impossible to correct the courses of the programmes and match them to the people's needs.

— *Ignoring traditional health systems*: In neither programme was the people's traditional interpretation of their health problems taken into consideration during the planning stage. This led — especially in Quispicanchis — to a lower utilization of health services than otherwise would have been possible.

— *Poverty*: Neither programme did much to reduce poverty, the basic cause of the people's low health status.

— *Duration of the programme*: At the time of the evaluation both programmes had been running for around three years. It could reasonably be expected that both programmes would be more effective after a longer period of operation.

The *social impact* of the programmes differed greatly — from nil in Occoran to considerable in Villa el Salvador. The structure of the communities themselves, rather than the nature of the programmes, was the main determinant of the ways in which the communities participated. Within the community structures the main factors were as follows:

— *Type and degree of economic marginalization*: Communities producing an economic surplus — such as Pampaccamara and Villa el Salvador — had greater freedom to decide whether or not to participate than did Occoran and Pinchimuru, which were much more constrained by economic marginalization.

— *Shared experiences of struggle*: With the exception of Occoran, all three communities had experience of collective struggle, which formed a viable basis for direct participation in the programmes. In Pinchimuru, which was just as poor as Occoran, the community's experience of shared struggle against a neighbouring hacienda was an important factor in their much more positive response to the health programme.

— *Local organization and leadership*: Pampaccamara and Villa el Salvador had particularly strong leadership and well-developed community organizations: Pinchimuru was fairly well organized and led; Occoran was very weak in both respects.

— *Interpretation of health problems*: If people blame their health problems on individual failure to make suitable offerings to the gods, there is little motivation to organize a collective struggle against disease. This traditional interpretation of health applied in Occoran and to some extent in Pinchimuru. A purely biological interpretation of health, which leaves the struggle against disease to the health 'experts', is also inadequate — as was seen above all in Pampaccamara. A social interpretation of health, recognizing poverty as the main cause of disease, was found mostly in Villa el Salvador — the only community which challenged the government's system of health services.

Although in general the community structure was more important than the health programme, the latter did have an important influence in Villa el Salvador, where doctors from the University helped the people towards a social interpretation of health by offering alternative directions and ideae. This sort of external agent was lacking in Quispicanchis. For totally marginalized communities like Occoran only an external agent promoting land reform and radically different community organization offers any hope of overcoming the present inertia. In Pampaccamara an external agent could have offered the people alternative ways of viewing the government health system. They might thus have avoided their present position, in which their direct participation relieves an unjust system of some of its responsibility to provide adequate health care for the whole population.

WIDER RELEVANCE

Community participation in health care will continue to be a theme of lively debate and discussion. There are no simple recipes for success, as conditions vary enormously between countries and, indeed, between communities and regions within the same country. A number of general principles, however, emerge from these case-studies of two programmes in Peru. Community health workers elsewhere may find them of some relevance.

In promoting *direct participation*, the following principles are important:

— Believe in the people, and accept the relativity of western medicine.
— Place your knowledge and technical skills at the disposal of the population and serve as a critical partner in discussions of health problems.
— Base the programme on a community health diagnosis, made by the community with your help. Discuss the results and conclusions with the

people; keep monitoring and analysing health in a constant dialogue with the community.
- Preserve the people's control over their own health services by introducing only those programmes which they can understand and control. Do not create new organizations to run the programme where viable ones already exist.
- Be democratic in the running of your own programme.

In the much more difficult task of promoting *social participation*, three general principles should be borne in mind:

- Encourage and participate wholeheartedly in critical discussions of the perceived causes of health problems: traditional, biological, and especially social.
- Promote critical assessment of the existing health services in all their aspects: traditional, scientific, and managerial.
- Do not isolate the health sector but let it be part of a more general discussion of the community's place in society.

Health workers and community organizations do not control all the factors causing disease and poor health. A well-conceived primary health care programme, however, can start a *process* of social participation leading to a greater degree of community control over the complex network of political, social, economic, and environmental factors which determine whether 'Health for All' becomes a reality or remains an illusion.

NOTES

1. The concept of 'curative coverage' was developed by the author in order to have an indicator of health service utilization in PHC programmes where little data is available. It is based on the assumption that a normal population needs about 700 first consultations a year per 1000 inhabitants (Kohn and White 1976, pp. 148–9). An indication of the utilization rate of services offered compared with existing needs is obtained by comparing the number of first consultations with the estimated needs. Thus for the Quispicanchis programme the figure is arrived at as follows:

Number of first consultations made: $\frac{700}{1000}$ × 80 000 (total population) = 56 000

Number of first consultations carried out   = 10 800

Curative coverage: $\frac{10\ 800}{56\ 000}$ × 100   = 19 per cent

2. Three interpretations of health are referred to in this article:
- *Traditional interpretation*: health seen as a state of equilibrium between different forces such as hot and cold, present-day man and his ancestors. It is part of the people's vision of the cosmos.

— *Biological interpretation*: based on knowledge of the biological origins of disease. It is part of a belief in western science.

— *Social interpretation*: analyses the origins of health and disease in terms of social, political, and production relationships.

3. SINAMOS stands for *Sistema Nacional de Movilizacion Social*, a once-powerful organization established by General Velasco's military regime to generate popular support for the military-led revolution. It was dissolved in 1978.

4. Infant deaths were almost certainly under-reported in the survey.

REFERENCES

Kohn, R. and White, K.L., *Health care: an international study*. Oxford University Press (1976).

Muller, Frits, *Participation in primary health care programs in Latin America*. National School of Public Health, University of Antioquia, Medellin, Colombia (1981).

14 Sociopolitical constraints on primary health care: a case study from Indonesia*

Glen Williams and **Satoto** describe how the rigid, hierarchical power structures of a community in rural Java brought a popular health project to a virtual standstill.

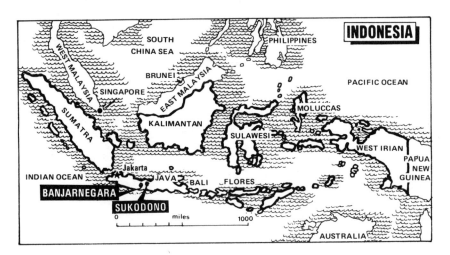

Glen Williams is a writer on Third World development issues, based in Oxford, England.
Satoto, M.D., is a lecturer in Nutrition in the Medical Faculty of Diponegoro University, Semarang, Indonesia.

In Indonesia, under the Third Five Year Development Plan which started in 1979, the Ministry of Health (1978, p. 41) aims to expand its primary health care (PHC) programme to reach 20 140 villages by 1984.

The success of this programme, however, depends largely on factors outside the field of health *per se*. The PHC concept has important sociopolitical and institutional implications, in particular:

- *Sharing of responsibilities* across socioeconomic, sexual, and political divisions within communities.
- *Decentralization* of administrative authority within government structures.

In other words, PHC implies the sharing of power both within communities

*An earlier version of this article appeared in *Development Dialogue* Vol. 1 (1980).

and the government apparatus itself. Indeed, Banerji (1978, p.25) argues that 'a "people-oriented" health service' can serve as 'a lever to bring about social, economic, and political changes so that the exploited find a rightful place for themselves in society'.

Since PHC is closely related to power structures, it may be useful to examine briefly the dominant tradition of power in Java, where nearly two-thirds of Indonesia's population of 150 million people live.[1] According to Anderson, Javanese culture is based on the concept of power as being constant: 'For political theory, this has the important corollary that concentration of power in one place or in one person requires a proportional diminution elsewhere' (Anderson 1972, pp.7-8). In other words, since the absolute amount of power in any given situation is constant and cannot be increased, any new holder of power is assumed to have taken it from its source at the centre. The newcomer on the periphery is thus seen as a usurper of power which rightly belongs to the original authority at the centre, who will try to wrest it back at the first opportunity.

In practical terms, this means that power must be invested — and more importantly be *seen* to be invested — in the hands of one individual: at village level the *lurah* (village head), at provincial level the Governor, at national level the President. PHC, on the other hand, is based on *power sharing* — a concept running counter to the dominant tradition of centralized power.

The Indonesian government's PHC programme may thus be set on a collision course with its own centralized policies in fields such as regional autonomy, public finance, security, rural development, and local government. Either there will be collisions, in which PHC will be the victim, or there will be a series of compromises.

The experience of a PHC project in the village of Sukodono[2] may serve as an illustration of some of the institutional and sociopolitical constraints facing the Indonesian government in implementing a nationwide PHC programme.

THE SUKODONO VILLAGE HEALTH ORGANIZATION

Sukodono is situated on the northern coastal plain of Central Java, separated from the Java Sea by a few kilometres of ricefields and brackish water fishponds. Most of the population of 2150 people live in houses of wood or bamboo thatch with tiled roofs, shielded from the harsh tropical sun by a canopy of coconut palms. Irrigation facilities are good and most of the arable land is planted with rice for the greater part of the year. Tobacco and sugarcane are also grown, while fish and prawns are caught in the ponds. Socioeconomic divisions are sharply defined: a mere 8.1 per cent of Sukodono households own 51.1 per cent of the ricefields, while 48.8 per cent own no rice fields at all (Hart 1978, p.91). (Figures of this kind are not unusual for rice-growing areas in Java.) The people are devout Moslems and are strict in their observance of religious duties.

Although religiously homogeneous, Sukodono society is divided by political affiliations and family ties. The two main political groups are the government-backed GOLKAR organization and the Moslem party PPP. The leading family is that of the lurah, whose political affiliation (as a matter of course) is with GOLKAR. The other main family is that of the *carik* (village secretary), most of whose members support the Moslem party.

The lurah is a tall, thin man aged about 60. By nature reticent and socially rather awkward, he has presided over village affairs in a firm, paternalistic way for the past 35 years. Perhaps his most notable achievement has been the enforcement of a total ban on the sale of land in the village to outsiders, a measure which undoubtedly has been of considerable benefit to the village as a whole.

The Sukodono PHC project began as an indirect, unintended offshot from a nutrition research project carried out by the Medical Faculty of Diponegoro University (UNDIP), Semarang, in 1975. Concerned about the nutritional and health status of the people of Sukodono, the research team cast about for ideas to start an action programme which the people would be able to manage themselves after UNDIP's withdrawal. One of the UNDIP doctors had read about an apparently successful PHC programme in Banjarnegara regency (see Chapter 12), so it was decided to invite a group of villagers from Sukodono to visit Banjarnegara in the hope that they might learn something which could prove useful in trying to solve Sukodono's health/nutrition problems.

The leader of the UNDIP team took this idea to the lurah of Sukodono, who expressed interest and gave his blessing to the enterprise. However, for reasons unspecified, he declined to join the expedition himself and appointed the carik as group leader.

The expedition to Banjarnegara consisted of four UNDIP doctors, 13 village elders (*pamong desa*)[3], and the carik's third son, Ali. Having studied for three years at the Islamic University in Semarang, Ali was highly articulate and was therefore invited to be official spokesman for the group. Ali also happened to be an enthusiastic supporter of the government-sponsored political organization GOLKAR, which probably enhanced his acceptability as the group's spokesman.

The PHC programme in Banjarnegara regency began in the village of Klampok in 1973. When visited by the Sukodono group, in September 1975, it had reached about 35 other villages. The approach is based on the participation of village people in planning, establishing, and maintaining simple, low-cost, curative, preventive and promotive health services. Training of community health workers, known as *kader*, who work without remuneration of any kind, is carried out mainly by sub-district health centre staff, under the guidance and supervision of an intersectoral team led by the regency doctor. Two non-government agencies have also played an important role in establishing and developing the programme.

Although the Banjarnegara programme suffers from managerial and other deficiencies, it has achieved encouraging results.[4] The relative success of this programme is due to the persistent efforts of the local government — especially the Regent himself — to create a sociopolitical climate in which:

- At village level, ordinary people, including many women, play an important role in planning, implementing, and evaluating PHC activities. (Landless villages, on the other hand, still have only a very limited role in decision-making processes.)
- Between the regency and sub-district levels of government on the one hand and village level government on the other, two-way communication is carried out with greater frankness and mutual respect than is usually the case elsewhere.

During their two days in Banjarnegara, the Sukodono group visited four villages, including Klampok, where they saw PHC activities such as health insurance funds, medical posts, *taman gizis* (neighbourhood nutrition clubs), housing and sanitation improvement programmes in action. They talked informally with many health kaders and villagers using the PHC services. In addition, they were warmly received by the Regent himself, whose backing for the programme has been of crucial importance. The regency doctor also gave generously of his time, accompanying the group for two days and explaining the importance of community participation in the programme.

Greatly impressed by what they saw, the Sukodono village leaders were eager to start a PHC scheme in their own village. Lively late-night discussions took place in the guest-house where the group was staying. Ali, the youngest member of the group and the only non-pamong desa, gradually emerged not only as the official spokesman but also as the group's unofficial leader. After returning to Sukodono, the group met with the lurah and Ali took the lead in reporting their impressions of the Banjarnegara PHC programme and their hopes of implementing such a scheme in Sukodono.

FORMATION OF VILLAGE HEALTH ORGANIZATION

A few days after hearing the report on the Banjarnegara trip, the lurah called a meeting to discuss the possibility of starting a health/nutrition project in Sukodono. The meeting was attended by about 35 people, including all 13 pamong desa, several of their wives, and a number of men aged between 25 and 35 who belonged to the larger land-owning group in the village. The lurah invited these younger men in the hope that they would be willing to become health kaders.

The meeting was held along Javanese *musyawarah* lines, with the discussion being introduced and guided by the lurah and decisions made on the basis of consensus (*mupakat*). This traditional practice reflects the paternalistic nature of Javanese village government and social organization, as expressed in the norm *Manunggaling kawulo lan Gusti* ('The people and the leader are one'). According to Sutrisno, 'Those who lead the village meeting or musyawarah should possess the wisdom to perceive what constitutes the common purpose and interest in the matter under discussion' (Sutrisno 1977, p.35). Participants in the musyawarah generally try to avoid open clashes of opinion and Sutrisno comments: 'The decision is taken on the basis of discussion, in which the pamong desa understand

and perceive the interests of the village as a whole, while each villager also understands and perceives the interests of others (including the poor and underprivileged) as well as his own interests' (Sutrisno 1977, p.36).

It should be noted that no landless or near-landless household attended this meeting. Furthermore, the wives present did not participate in the discussions, which at times were quite lively, especially concerning the question of whether better-off households should contribute more than poor households to a health insurance fund.

The meeting finally agreed on two points:

1. To start a health insurance fund based on monthly contributions of Rp 50 (US $0.12) per household to meet the costs of medical supplies and referring patients for treatment at the local hospital.[5]
2. To request assistance from the UNDIP Medical Faculty for training and equipping health kaders, who would all be men, and nutrition kaders, who would all be women.

After discussing this request with Sukodono village leaders UNDIP contacted the local Regent and the regency doctor, both of whom approved the scheme. As part of its programme of research and community service, UNDIP therefore agreed to provide basic PHC and nutrition training, regular supervision, an initial stock of medical supplies and weighing scales. OXFAM, an international development assistance agency, provided UNDIP with financial assistance for these inputs. The running costs of the programme, however, particularly the replenishment of medical supplies, were to be the responsibility of the village.

The Sukodono Village Health Organization (VHO) was formally established at a meeting of about 40 people in Sukodono in February 1976. Ali was appointed chairman and the lurah's son became secretary (a neat reversal of the roles played by their fathers in the village government). The lurah's son-in-law was appointed treasurer.

Health cadre training was held in the village school from February to July 1976, at the rate of two afternoon sessions per week. The opening ceremony was attended by dignitaries such as the Regent, the regency doctor, and the Dean of UNDIP Medical Faculty, who all made speeches congratulating the Sukodono Village Health Organization and wishing it every success.

Training for the health kaders covered the following fields: community health problems; health education; socioreligious aspects of health; mother and child health; first aid; nutrition; and identification and treatment of communicable and high prevalence diseases.

Although it had been agreed that staff from the near-by government hospital would teach some subjects in the course, this plan had to be abandoned after hospital staff failed to appear for training sessions on several occasions.

Of 34 people who began the course, only three – two pamong desa and Ali – had participated in the Banjarnegara trip five months previously. Six schoolteachers also enrolled, but five soon dropped out, complaining that the other trainees (all farmers) made them feel 'uncomfortable'. Apparently, the farmers learned at a slower rate than the school-teachers and therefore felt some resentment towards the latter. The only school-teacher who completed the course also happened to be the only woman trainee. Unfortunately, she was transferred to another village soon after the course ended.

Fifteen health kaders, all married men aged between 25 and 35, passed the final examination and were given a supply of drugs for the treatment of ailments such as respiratory tract infections, diarrhoea, skin infections, and eye diseases, as well as dressings for wounds, burns, and fractures.[6] None of the health kaders were pamong desa but all owned or controlled at least 0.5 hectares of ricefields, which put them in the top 30 per cent of village society. All agreed to work as health kaders without remuneration.

The main tasks of the health kaders were defined as follows:

— To motivate and inform their neighbours about health and health-related subjects.
— To organize their neighbours to work towards a healthier environment, e.g. by improving sanitation facilities.
— To treat minor ailments and give emergency first aid.
— To supervize home care of patients.
— To identify serious illness and diseases, and refer cases to hospital.

An impressive ceremony was held to mark the health cadres' graduation. The regency doctor made a speech and presented the kaders with certificates as recognition of their competence to carry out their duties. The speech of the regency secretary, however, struck a different note altogether. He warned the kaders not to get exaggerated ideas of their own importance, but to bear in mind their subordinate place in the structure of the village and regency governments. This was an ominous sign of the difficulties to be encountered later by the VHO.

A group of 20 village women formed the Nutrition Section of the VHO and UNDIP staff taught a nutrition course from August 1976 until February 1977. Eleven women passed the course and were each given a set of scales to start weighing posts in their homes for children under five.

The tasks of the nutrition kaders were defined as follows:

— To weigh children once a month and record their progress on a weight chart.
— To spot illness early and advise mothers on treatment.
— To teach mothers about nutrition, especially those whose children were suffering from undernutrition.

From its inception, the Nutrition Section was very much under the domination of the male-run VHO. For example, five women school-teachers who wanted to join the training course withdrew after several male health kaders objected that their wives would not be able to learn at the same rate as the teachers. Their wives, on the other hand, had no objection at all to the teachers attending the courses. (It is perhaps noteworthy that in Banjarnegara regency, where many nutrition projects are running successfully, the organizers are often women school-teachers.) The men also insisted on a strict division of tasks: male health kaders on the one hand and female nutrition kaders on the other.

FINANCE

While health kader training was still taking place, monthly contributions of Rp 50 per family to the Health Insurance Fund had been made on an informal *ad hoc* basis. Some families made larger contributions, but most did not contribute at all during this period. The lurah, however, released the handsome sum of Rp 60 000 from village funds.

After receiving their certificates and medical kits in July 1976, the health kadres decided that it was time to start collecting fees regularly. However, bearing in mind the hierarchical structure of the village government and the very sensitive nature of this task, the kaders felt it would be advisable if they were each accompanied by a pamong desa on their initial visits to collect money. The VHO asked the lurah to instruct the pamong desa to this effect, but the lurah failed to issue the instruction. He did not actually refuse to do so, but simply delayed on the matter. As a result, only Rp 8000 (US $19) were collected between July 1976 and March 1977, although it had been expected that at least Rp 200 000 (US $480) would be raised during this period.

At the same time, the VHO's funds were being whittled away steadily by hospital referrals and replenishment of supplies for the kaders' medical kits. By June 1977, the Sukodono VHO had no funds at all and its future looked bleak. However, it was able to obtain medical supplies on credit from a clinic in Semarang, so that the treatment of patients could be continued.

In August 1977, the health kaders hit upon a bold and original way of raising funds for the continuation of the VHO: the rental and cultivation of a ricefield on a communal basis. This field, known as *wakaf* land (that is, land donated to the community for religious purposes, in this case by a well-off villager), has good irrigation and is highly productive. The rent money is used for the maintenance of the village mosque.

The kaders decided to ask the lurah's permission to rent this land and to use half the profits from the rice crops to finance the activities of the VHO. The other half of the profits would be used to pay for the maintenance of the village mosque. The lurah, however, rejected this request, deciding instead to throw the wakaf land open to auction: the highest bidder would obtain the rights to the land for four consecutive seasons.

Ali, representing the VHO, entered the auction. To the great surprise of the lurah and other pamong desa, Ali stayed with the bidding even when it reached a very high level and finally won the land.

Cash was now urgently needed to pay a deposit on the rent and to buy seeds, fertilizers, and insecticides. No wages would be paid to workers for cultivating the field, because it was expected that most villagers would give a few hours of

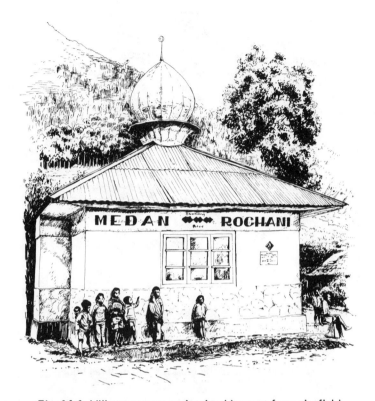

Fig. 14.1. Village mosque maintained by rent from ricefield.

their time for this purpose. An UNDIP doctor came to the rescue with a personal loan of Rp 100 000 (US $240).

The lurah was highly sceptical of the wakaf land operation. He himself had tried and failed on three separate occasions to organize the village people to work voluntarily on village-owned land in order to raise money for the construction of a village office and road. How could a bunch of 'youngsters' possibly hope to succeed where the lurah himself had failed?

Realizing that no help could be expected from the lurah or the pamong desa, the health kaders went directly to the villagers, visiting people in their homes, explaining the purpose of renting the wakaf land and asking them to give a few hours of their time in order to cultivate it. The response was encouraging: 355 households (65 per cent of the total) participated in cultivating the field. Men hoed the heavy mud for two or three hours and women planted rice seedlings, as well as weeding the field twice. Some families supplied cooked food to the workers. One man agreed to regulate the water and to fertilize and spray the field, in return for the use of a small piece of land bordering it, where he planted beans.

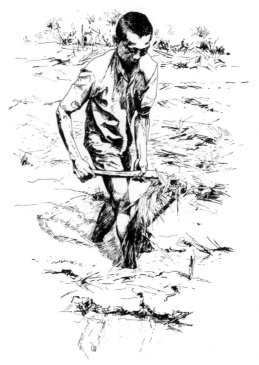

Fig. 14.2. Men hoed the mud for two or three hours

After three months, the health cadres were able to look with satisfaction on a field of golden paddy almost ready to be harvested. Then disaster struck. A rat plague destroyed two-thirds of the crop. The kaders' morale sank to an all-time low. The crop failure meant they were unable to repay their debts (as devout Moslems this was particularly worrying), no financial assistance could be given to patients referred to hospital for treatment, and medical supplies were getting very low.

However, there was no time to be lost brooding about the crop failure. The wakaf field had to be prepared and planted once more. So again the kaders went knocking on people's doors, asking them to give a few hours of their time to help cultivate the field. Once again, the people came out and worked. The field was planted and there was a fair harvest, although about 30 per cent was again lost to rats. The profit from this crop was just enough to pay the next instalment of the rent on the land. The money was not paid to the lurah but directly to a contractor hired to carry out repairs on the mosque. The kaders took this bold step because the lurah had failed to carry out a promise made several months earlier to form a special committee to handle rent money from the wakaf field. However, bypassing the lurah amounted to a serious personal insult and contributed to the process of alienation between the lurah and the VHO.

Meanwhile, there was a dispute among the kaders themselves, one of whom wanted to use part of the wakaf land for his rice seedbed. He and a number of other villagers had been granted this privilege during the interval between the first harvest and preparation of the land for the second planting. Most of the other kaders, however, felt that this practice reduced the yield of the second crop. Finally, after several heated debates, it was decided not to allow the wakaf land to be used a second time for seedbeds.

While the kaders were debating this matter, precious time was slipping away. The wakaf field urgently needed to be hoed and planted, but nobody had yet begun to contact other villagers to ask for their voluntary participation. In addition, utilization of the medical posts had sunk to a low level because many supplies had run out. Those who had already worked twice on the wakaf field had thus received little or no reward for their labours, and the kaders felt it would be difficult to motivate the people to work voluntarily on the field a third time. For this reason, they decided to hire workers to cultivate the wakaf land. They realized that this decision would probably lessen the villagers' sense of belonging to the health insurance scheme, but they felt that there was no alternative.

The third harvest was extremely good. With a great feeling of relief, the health kaders were able to repay the VHO's debts. They also paid for further repairs to the mosque, purchased supplies for the village medical posts, and still had an unspent balance of Rp 160 000 (US $385). This is a considerable sum for a Javanese village, amounting to nearly half the annual *Bantuan Desa* ('Village Assistance') of Rp 350 000 (US $843) from the central government at that time. With the rent of the wakaf land fully paid, the profit from the fourth and final harvest was expected to increase the VHO's funds even further.

The wakaf field was once again prepared and planted, using hired labour for the second time. The harvest, however, was only mediocre, due to another rat infestation. By May 1979, the VHO's funds had dwindled to about Rp 100 000 (US $240).

ORGANIZATION OF VILLAGE HEALTH COMMITTEE

When first formed, in February 1976, the Sukodono VHO had the status of a section of the Village Social Committee (*Lembaga Sosial Desa*),[7] of which the lurah is chairman and Ali deputy chairman. In October 1978, however, after the VHO's successful third rice harvest on the wakaf land, the lurah announced that the VHO had 'too much autonomy' and was 'not running well'. He proposed two steps to remedy the situation.

First, the VHO should be brought directly under control of the LSD by fusion of the role of chairman of both organizations. The old VHO management committee was therefore dissolved and, after considerable behind-the-scenes lobbying, a new management committee was formed with the lurah himself as chairman. Ali's elder brother, Achmad, was appointed executive officer and Ali was relegated to the position of assistant executive officer.

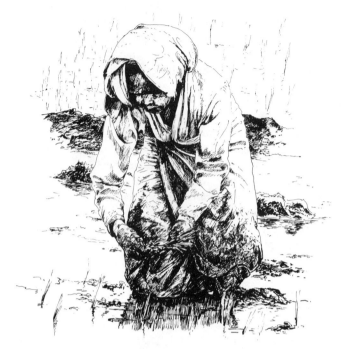

Fig. 14.3. Women planted the ricefield.

Second, health kaders should be given remuneration for their services in the
form of the right to use a small piece of land. To achieve this, the lurah effected
the redistribution of rental rights to a six-hectare strip of unirrigated land
running along the banks of the irrigation canal which passes through Sukodono.
This land, known as *tanah berem*, is actually owned by the Public Works Department of the local Regency government and rental rights are granted on an annual
basis. Some 60 households – about one-third of which have no other farming
land – had been planting tiny plots of berem land (each about the size of a
tennis court) with dryfield rice and vegetables for many years. However, the
lurah convinced the Public Works Department of the need to hand over rental
rights to the 43 members of the Village Home Guard (WANRA)[8] and the 15
health kaders. But there was one condition: the kaders would have to join the
Home Guard. This condition they accepted unanimously.

Angry protests followed from the evicted households. They took their case
to the regency government, but were told that the redistribution of the land
rental rights would stand. At the time of writing, however, almost a year after
the redistribution of rental rights to the berem land, the new tenants have not
yet begun to cultivate their holdings. The berem land has become a sort of 'no
man's land'. The new tenants do not feel sufficiently sure of their rights to start
dividing up and cultivating the land, while the old tenants have not been

sufficiently bold to reoccupy the land from which they were evicted.

The size of the plots – 0.1 hectares on average – is actually very small, much smaller than the ricefields already owned or controlled by the health kaders. They see the lurah's action, however, as a symbolic expression of good will, and they are delighted to have harmonious relations with their leader again. The actual additional income from the berem land means little to them. Although they admit that people who have lost their rental rights may feel wronged, the kaders do not believe that this will have an adverse effect on people's attitudes towards the VHO. However, for the evicted landless households, the loss of income and security is a real hardship.

The health kaders admit that most people in Sukodono have a fairly ambivalent attitude towards the Home Guard. At certain times – for example during General Elections – there is considerable resentment of what many people consider to be heavy-handed actions by the Home Guard in preserving 'law and order'. Some of the kaders actually have optimistic plans for reforming the Home Guard from within. Whether this will be possible remains to be seen.

PREVENTION OF DISEASE AND HEALTH PROMOTION

One of the health kaders' main tasks was to motivate and organize their neighbours towards creating a healthier environment, for example by improving sanitation facilities. Most Sukodono households use open drains and canals for defecation and disposal of household wastes. This practice poses a serious health risk, especially during the dry season.

The VHO decided, therefore, to try to start a sanitation programme, beginning on a small scale by constructing a simple, low-cost squatting plate toilet. This experiment attracted interest from some villagers, but the programme was stopped by the lurah, who informed the VHO that two projects which he had been struggling to finish for some time – the village office and road – demanded a higher priority. This was a great disappointment to the kaders.[9]

The Nutrition Section of the VHO began its activities in February 1977 with 180 children under five (about 60 per cent of the total) attending 11 weighing posts. One nutrition kader was responsible for each post. No particular day was set for weighing sessions. Mothers could bring their children whenever it suited them, as long as the period between each visit was about one month. No supplementary feeding was given to the children, the emphasis being entirely on educating mothers to make better use of foods already available. In addition, no curative service was provided, since the male health cadres – who controlled the medical kits – did not see the need to become involved in the *taman gizis* (neighbourhood nutrition clubs). As far as the health cadres were concerned, these were entirely the women's affair.

It proved difficult to motivate mothers to bring their children to be weighed. The main reason given was lack of time, but it seems that most mothers simply did not believe their children were getting much benefit from the weighing sessions. Attendances steadily declined and all activities stopped in mid-1978.

A CURATIVE SERVICE

The health kaders' record books provide a fairly complete picture of the extent to which patients used the medical post during the period July 1976 to October 1978, shown in Fig. 14.4.

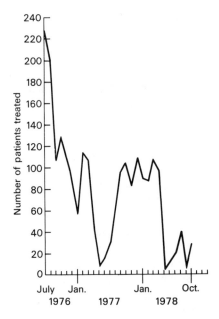

Fig. 14.4. Number of patients using medical posts July 1976 to October 1978.

During July and August 1976, patients treated averaged 212 per month, but many of these visits were probably made out of curiosity. Between September 1976 and March 1977, patients averaged 102 per month. Then followed a five-month period during which, as a result of social tensions before and after the general elections of May 1977, the activities of the VHO were disrupted: between April and August 1977, the average number of patients treated per month fell to only 33.

After the relaxation of social tensions caused by the general elections, normal curative activities resumed: an average of 97 patients per month were treated between September 1977 and April 1978. Utilization of the medical posts then slumped again: from May until October 1978, an average of only 19 patients per month were treated. During this period the VHO was in debt and unable to purchase supplies to restock depleted medical posts. It was hoped that a utilization rate of about 100 per month would be resumed after the purchase of medical supplies in late 1978, but this was not achieved. The kaders' record books are incomplete after October 1978, but according to their verbal reports the utilization rates between November 1978 and October 1979 averaged 30-40 patients per month.

These performances were an encouraging achievement, especially if compared with those of official government health services. During the first six months of 1978, the utilization rate of government health services at sub-district level in Central Java Province was 1050 per month, for a 'target' population of about 50 000 (i.e. an average of approximately 40 patients monthly per village).[10] Which socioeconomic groups used the medical posts? Since landless households were not involved in planning the establishment of the VHO and had no role in its management, it might be supposed that many would be reticent about coming to the health kaders for treatment. However, this was not the case. Table 14.1 shows utilization of the medical posts according to socioeconomic status of patients during the period April 1977 to October 1978.

Table 14.1. Patients using medical posts, according to land-ownership status of households, April 1977–October 1978[11]

Patients' land ownership status	Visits to health posts		Proportion of total village population
	No.	%	(%)
Class I (owning 0.5 ha of ricefields)	210	20	29
Class II (owning 0.0–0.5 ha of ricefields)	305	29	22
Class III (owning no ricefields)	543	51	49
Total	1058	100	100

Source: Health kaders' record books.

The high utilization rate of the medical posts by patients from landless and small landowning households is an impressive achievement. These groups, which previously received little or no regular medical care, were certainly greatly in need of the curative service provided by the health kaders. The relatively low utilization of the medical posts by the larger of the two land-owning groups may be due to a tendency among well-off households to seek medical treatment from itinerant hospital staff working in their off-duty hours, from the hospital itself, or even from doctors in the near-by town.

However, the sharp fluctuations in the utilization of the medical posts reflect the vulnerability of this service to disturbances both from within the village (e.g. conflicts with the village head) and from outside (e.g. elections). Furthermore, the poorest households are the most seriously affected, because they can ill-afford the cost of obtaining medical care elsewhere.

The women of Sukodono were also denied a direct role in establishing and managing the curative work of the VHO. In addition, it might be expected that women in a strict Moslem community such as Sukodono would feel inhibited about visiting fairly young male health cadres who were not close relatives. However, this does not seem to be the case. As Table 14.2 shows, adult women utilized the medical posts at more than twice the rate of adult men.

Table 14.2. Patients using medical posts according to age and sex, April 1977–October 1978

Children (< 12 years)		Adults (> 12 years)				Total	
		Male		Female			
No.	%	No.	%	No.	%	No.	%
456	43	184	17	420	40	1060	100

Source: Health kaders' record books.

The other main aspect of the VHO's curative activities was the referral system, initially to the government hospital in the near-by Regency town. This proved difficult. Staff at the hospital refused to treat Sukodono patients on a credit basis, with payments being made by the VHO at the end of each month. Treatment was given strictly on the basis of immediate cash payment. Since all VHO funds obviously had to be held by a single kader, rather than distributed among all 15, immediate cash payment at the hospital was impractical. Nevertheless, during the period July 1976 to March 1977, 20 referrals were made to the local hospital and ten to the government university hospital in Semarang.

CONSTRAINTS FACED BY THE SUKODONO VILLAGE HEALTH ORGANIZATION

The sociopolitical and institutional constraints faced by the Sukodono VHO can be divided into two main categories: those at village level and those at supra-village level.

Constraints at village level

Relations between the lurah and non-pamong desa

The lurah's strong reluctance to allow meaningful responsibilities to be entrusted to a group outside his immediate and complete control has severely handicapped the programme. As he felt his position of authority threatened, the lurah's initial endorsement of the VHO quickly turned into distrust. He felt humiliated when the VHO was able to organize the villagers on two successive occasions to cultivate the wakaf land without pay, a feat which he had never been able to achieve. To compound the insult, the VHO paid the rent directly to a building contractor for repairs to the mosque, rather than to the lurah. He brought the sanitation programme to an abrupt halt because he did not want the people's attention and energies diverted from his village office and road projects. Furthermore, it was galling for him to see so much power — in terms of popular support and hard cash — in the control of someone who was neither a pamong desa nor even a member of his own family. Finally, three years after the founding of the VHO, the lurah arranged for himself to be appointed chairman of the Management Committee. Power has thus returned to its 'rightful' place, or so it seems.

Women

The village men have not allowed women to participate in decision-making and this has contributed to the failure of the VHO's nutrition programme. From the outset, the male-dominated VHO decided that women's activities would be restricted to the field of nutrition, which the men saw as separate from their own domain of general health. In the eyes of most villagers the male health kaders, equipped with their medical kits, had a much more important role than the women. The 'merely' educative function of the women nutrition kaders seemed far less prestigious than the more obviously active role claimed by the men. Furthermore, the men blocked the participation of women school-teachers — who might well have provided much-needed leadership and organizational skills — in the nutrition programme. Petty rivalries among the women themselves also handicapped the nutrition activities. The main reason for the failure of this programme, however, would seem to be the village women's limited opportunity for taking part in decision-making about the VHO's activities as a whole and taking on meaningful responsibilities in the management of the programme.

Landless households

This group, nearly 50 per cent of village households, had no say at all in planning, establishing, and running the VHO. The composition of the VHO management board was decided by a meeting of land-owning households called by the village head. The young men appointed to the management board, who all became health kaders, also belonged to the larger land-owning group in the village and did not consider it important for landless households to be involved in decision-making concerning the VHO.

The exclusion of the landless group from an active part in VHO affairs probably contributed indirectly to the failure of the sanitation programme, from which landless households had most to gain, since they cannot afford luxuries such as wells and WCs. Yet they were almost totally unaware of this programme, let alone of its potential benefits. Had they been involved in starting the sanitation programme, many landless households might well have joined the health kaders in opposing the lurah's decision to close it down.

The most dramatic demonstration of the consequences of leaving landless households out of decision-making processes affecting their welfare was the case of the berem land. Had the 20 landless households who previously cultivated some of this land been consulted about the lurah's plan to evict them and re-distribute the land to the Home Guard, the evictions almost certainly would never have taken place, and the VHO would not have become embroiled in a totally unnecessary land dispute which may well have done irreparable harm to the health cadres' image as healers of the sick and health promoters.

Constraints at supra-village level

Regency health service and hospital

Hospital staff withdrew from health kader training sessions, were uncooperative over referrals, and did not provide the cadres with any follow-up service. In fact, it seemed as though hospital staff regarded the Sukodono health cadres as rivals in the health 'business'. (Several hospital paramedics augment their incomes during afternoon and evenings by travelling by cycle and motor bike around the villages to treat patients.)

Regency government

The initial goodwill of the regency government disappeared after a few months. The government's change of heart was conveyed in the Regency Secretary's speech at the kaders' graduation ceremony, when the kaders were reminded that they occupied only a lowly rung in the village administration, which itself was subordinate to higher levels of government authority.

However, the regency government only rarely intervened directly in village affairs. Instead, it worked via the lurah, who performed to perfection his role of client to the supra-village authorities.

The lurah and the regency authorities cooperated closely in efforts to bring the VHO to heel. These moves centred on the related issues of rental rights to the berem land and recruitment of the health kaders into the Home Guard. By distributing the berem land to the Home Guard and inducing the health kaders to join this paramilitary organization, the lurah and regency authorities succeeded in strengthening the forces for 'law and order' within the village; weakening the position of the Moslem party; and manoeuvring the VHO into a position of dependence on both the lurah and the regency authorities.

This was achieved at the expense of the former tenants of the berem land, and at the same time transformed the image of the health kaders. Whereas previously they had been seen as healers of the sick and promoters of health, they are now identified with a government organization entrusted with the role of enforcing 'law and order'. Whether this information will have an effect on the people's willingness to approach the health kaders for medical care remains to be seen.

CONCLUSIONS

After three years of friction with authorities at village and supra-village level, the Sukodono VHO has finally settled into a compromise situation: the lurah is in charge of the VHO, while the health kaders have promised to submit to the discipline of the Home Guard. As far as the village and regency authorities are concerned, the VHO is now well in hand. In other words, a source of power which had sprung up on the periphery, thereby threatening the position of authorities at the centre, has been brought under the control of the central authorities – or so it seems at least.

What did the Sukodono VHO achieve during the first three years of its existence? Its most obvious achievements are the following:

1. A curative service, consisting of eight medical posts (out of an original 15) used by all socioeconomic groups at an irregular level of utilization, and a hospital referral system on a limited scale.
2. A self-financing scheme using village resources to provide funds for the running costs of the VHO's activities, especially the curative work. This scheme, however, has ceased to be a community effort in the full sense, because the wakaf ricefield has been cultivated using paid labour for the past two seasons.
3. A certain amount of participation by a group of villagers outside the village government hierarchy in planning and implementing activities in the field of primary health care.

Considering the obstacles placed in its way, these achievements are very creditable. On the other hand, the preventive and promotive services have stopped, with no prospects for their revival in the foreseeable future. In addition, it seems open to question whether the health cadres retain the confidence of most people in the village after adding the task of defending 'law and order' to their healing and health-promotion functions.

On the basis of the Sukodono experience, it may be possible to make some tentative general remarks of relevance to attempts to implement PHC programmes in other parts of Indonesia, or at least in Java. Two important sociopolitical and institutional constraints with which the Indonesian government's PHC programme may have to come to grips can be summarized as follows:

At village level

1. An unwillingness on the part of the ruling elite, especially the village head, to allow authority and responsibility to be exercised by a group (or groups) *outside* the existing village government hierarchy.
2. An aversion on the part of men to allow women to participate in decision-making processes.
3. A reluctance on the part of land-owning farmers to allow participation of landless villagers in decision-making processes.

At supra-village level

1. A tendency by *kabupaten* and *kecamatan* authorities to exercise their 'law and order' functions at the expense of efforts to improve the people's welfare.
2. A general disposition of authorities to enhance and strengthen the position of village elites, rather than focusing on the needs of the poor and underprivileged which are sometimes at variance with those of the elites.
3. A certain distrust by sub-district and regency level health staff of village level initiatives that seem to threaten their positions of authority.

Perhaps the ideal sociopolitical climate for starting a PHC programme would be one in which:

1. At village level, non-pamong desa, women and landless villagers are encouraged to participate in decision-making processes which affect their interests and to take on positions of responsibility in village affairs.
2. A process of frank, two-way communication, marked by mutual respect, occurs between government agencies at regency and sub-district levels on the one hand and village level organizations on the other.
3. Supra-village authorities allow village institutions to develop at their own pace, intervening only when the interests of poor and underprivileged groups are endangered.

There are, of course, very few rural areas in Indonesia today which even approximate to these conditions. In fact, they seem almost Utopian. But should one therefore conclude that PHC programmes should be held back until the right socioeconomic and political conditions have been created? This conclusion would be defeatist and unimaginative. It may well be that a PHC programme, in itself, will have the indirect result of introducing some flexibility into rigid institutions, attitudes, and sociopolitical structures, while also awakening communities to interests and needs that cut across socioeconomic divisions.

The authors believe that the sociopolitical constraints faced by the Sukodono VHO are representative of present conditions in many parts of Indonesia, particularly in Java. Centre-periphery power problems of this kind are not, of course, limited to Indonesia. The WHO Report to the Alma Ata Conference on Primary Health Care stated quite bluntly:

'It has been shown that primary health care has a great variety of implications and consequences that go far beyond technical considerations. National strategies are therefore required that take into account all political, social and economic as well as technical factors, and that help to overcome obstacles of any nature' (WHO 1978, p.45).

As far as Indonesia is concerned, it can simply be stated that efforts to introduce primary health care must be accompanied and supported by fundamental changes in sociopolitical structures, procedures and attitudes at both village and supra-village level.

Postcript, December 1981

By the start of 1981 the PHC project in Sukodono had ground to a complete halt. The last of the Village Health Organization's funds were used to buy medical supplies in December 1979. Curative services stopped after these supplies were used up the following year. In 1980 the remaining three cadres made only five referrals to the University hospital in Semarang. None were made in 1981.

Cultivation of the tanah berem was begun by members of the Home Guard, several pamong desa, and the lurah himself in late 1979, a year after the eviction of the previous tenants. As for the health kaders, only six of the ten joined the Home Guard, and two of these soon dropped out. Most kaders simply decided to become 'ordinary people' again. Ali, their leader, left to seek work in the national capital, Jakarta. Another found a job in Semarang. The lurah, speaking in mid-1981 about Sukodono's former health kaders, said: 'They weren't really wrong. At the time, the regency people approved of what they were doing. But you know what young people are like – give them an inch and they take a mile!'

NOTES

1. Generalizations about Java are not necessarily true for all parts of Indonesia. The Javanese, however, exert a strong influence on government policy, both by occupying key administrative posts and through sheer weight of numbers.
2. Fictional name for a village in Central Java.
3. The village elders, of whom there are 13 in Sukodono, make up the official village government. They almost invariably are drawn from the relatively well-off, land-owning section of the village population and usually are appointed by the lurah himself. In lieu of a cash salary, they are granted free utilization rights to a piece of village-owned land.
4. By late 1980, PHC activities had been established in 210 villages (out of a total of 279) in Banjarnegara Regency.
5. Since Sukodono is situated in the same sub-district as the Regency town, it is served by the Regency hospital rather than by a sub-district health centre.
6. Nineteen people actually passed the course, but four – including the woman school-teacher and a pamong desa – were not given medical kits.
7. The *Lembaga Sosial Desa* was a village development committee composed of community leaders (and the lurah), to promote general welfare in the village. All Indonesian villages were supposed to have such a committee. In 1980 its name was changed to *Lembaga Ketahanan Masyarakat Desa* ('Village Community Defence Committee'). Although the new name has strong political overtones, there have not yet been any fundamental changes in the committees' activities.
8. This paramilitary organization has the function of maintaining general 'law and order'. Members of the Home Guard are issued with uniforms and are empowered to deliver suspects over to the authorities. However, they are not issued with weapons, except for unloaded rifles on certain ceremonial occasions.
9. Three years after this incident, the village office and road were still unfinished.
10. Personal communication from Dr S. Gunawan, office of Central Java Provincial Health Service, Semarang.

11. Land-ownership was taken as the criterion for socioeconomic status because virtually all households in Sukodono make their living from agriculture; either by cultivating riceland or fishponds, or by working for wages as agricultural labourers.

REFERENCES

Anderson, Benedict R. O'G., The idea of power in Javanese culture. In *Politics and culture in Indonesia* (ed. C. Holt). Cornell University Press, Ithaca (1972).

Banerji, D., Health as a lever for another development. In *Development dialogue*, Vol. 1. Dag Hammarskjold Foundation, Uppsala (1978).

Hart, Gillian, Labour allocation strategies in rural Javanese households. Unpublished Ph.D. thesis, Cornell University, Ithaca (1978).

Ministry of Health, Republic of Indonesia, *Primary health care (village community health development) in Indonesia.* Jakarta (1978).

Sutrisno, P.H., *Filsafah Hidup Pancasila Sebagaimana Tercermin dalam Filsafah Hidup Orang Jawa*, Penerbit Pendawa, Yogyakarta (1977).

World Health Organization, *Primary health care*. Geneva (1978).

15 Community participation for health: the case of Latin America*

Emanuel de Kadt discusses approaches to community participation in solving health problems in Latin America, and concludes that participation will really thrive only under governments with a strong commitment to overcoming poverty and social inequality.

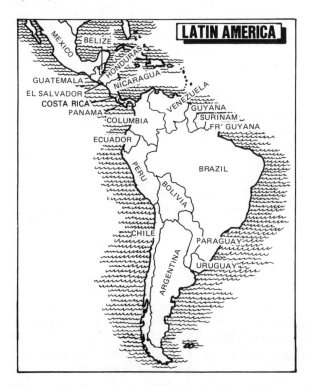

Emanuel de Kadt, Ph.D., is a Professional Fellow of the Institute of Development Studies at the University of Sussex in Brighton, England, where he has worked since 1969.

*A longer version of this article appeared in *World Development* **10**, 573–84 (1982).

Community participation has become a central preoccupation in the health field during the past decade. This upsurge of interest in the community's role in defining and solving health problems may be relatively new among health planners,[1] but the concept of community participation itself has been discussed and promoted as an element of development for more than 30 years. Two main strands can be distinguished: first, the community development movement, with its heyday mainly in India and West Africa during the 1950s and early 1960s; and secondly, the concern with community involvement through *conscientisación*, a mainly Latin American phenomenon of the 1960s and 1970s.

The exponents of community development recognized the shortcomings of promoting economic growth through large-scale capital-intensive projects. Yet they achieved little because they disregarded fundamental issues of inequality, conflict, and power relationships within communities.[2] Those who promoted the *conscientisación* of the masses in Latin America did not make the same mistake. Their analysis began with the existence of socioeconomic inequalities, their origins in the economic system, and their underpinning by the state. The name of Paulo Freire (1967) is strongly associated with this approach. Subsequent events in the continent showed that they had over-optimistic – some would say naive – views of the political reactions which their activities were likely to provoke, and of the people's power to overcome them.

They were, however, well in advance of then current thinking on health promotion. Only recently have international organizations such as UNICEF and WHO recognized the importance of wider socioeconomic factors. Yet this recognition is still expressed largely in terms of the need for 'inter-sectoral collaboration'. Emphasis is placed on the desirability for those concerned with health to work with government agencies with responsibility for public works and water supplies, rural development and agriculture, or education. As yet much less clearly perceived is the backdrop which colours all health promotion: the existence of economic relationships which create inequalities in wealth, political power, income, education, and *consequently* in health. Unequal 'health chances' derive from unequal 'life chances' (de Kadt 1974, p.129). The *conscientisadores*, whatever their precise political ideology, did realize that community involvement in health could be meaningful only if it took account of the basic issues of the political economy of health.

The growing interest in community participation has resulted in a number of recent studies which try to bring some order into what is now an increasingly confused field. Cohen and Uphoff (1980, p.213) survey the literature on participation in rural development and find that the concept has popularity without clarity, and is subject to growing faddishness and a lot of lip service.

Based partly on Cohen and Uphoff's analysis, this review of community participation for health in Latin America will focus on three main issues:

— What *kind* of participation is being discussed?
— Who is *sponsoring* participation?

— How is the community *socioeconomically structured?*

THE NATURE OF PARTICIPATION

Participation in implementation

The argument for community involvement in health in developing countries most widely used today is that public resources are insufficient to extend the basic health services to those at present without access to them. There is a long history in many parts of the world, including Latin America, of government and voluntary agency schemes in which communities share the burden of providing health improvements through contributions in labour, materials, or even money. Muller (1980) gives recent examples of Latin American experiences, notably the people's pharmacy building erected for US $20 000 in Lima's Villa el Salvador. In some of the communities studied by Algara (1981) this kind of activity also was the predominant one — notably in the field of health. Local health insurance schemes, by which communities contribute to the costs of drugs or even to the remuneration of local health workers, are relevant in this context too.

Beyond community contributions in money, kind or labour, community involvement in the implementation of health-related activities frequently involves the incorporation of community health workers in voluntary agency health projects or into the periphery of the health-care system. They are often seen as the simplest means of extending some aspects of the basic health services beyond the health units. This kind of *enlistment* of community members is extremely widespread throughout the Third World. Many examples of community health worker schemes can be found in Latin America, where they are often called *promotores de salud*. All the eight case studies reported by Muller (1980) made use of some type of community health workers, though there were considerable differences in the balance between curative, preventive, and promotive activities, and in the amount of training given.

In Africa and much of Asia physicians have always been in such short supply that the use of paramedical personnel for curative tasks has been widely accepted. African medical assistants or health centre superintendents have effected diagnoses and prescribed drugs in the manner of physicians. Lower level auxiliary personnel have also (perforce) had a considerable degree of latitude in these areas. When community members were enlisted to help extend health care to the rural areas, it was often taken for granted that they, too, would be trained to recognize the most common ailments and then be allowed to prescribe the appropriate medicines. Poor (rural) communities, after all, most want and need curative care; moreover, they know that it is available in the towns. In addition to curative tasks, community health workers in Africa and Asia are often expected to carry out preventive and promotive activities: to help their fellow villagers maintain and improve their families' health, and to mobilize them for collective actions in sanitation, water supply, and communicable disease control.

In Latin America, by contrast, physicians have been relatively plentiful (even

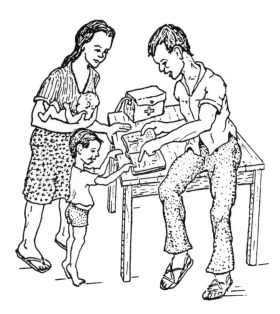

Fig. 15.1. The community health worker: many different interpretations of his role and responsibilities.

though largely concentrated in the major towns), and certainly very powerful. Almost everywhere the medical profession has been able to institutionalize — by law — a strong monopoly over medical knowledge and activity. Even delegation of tasks to fully trained and salaried auxiliaries is very limited. The account by Dr Gonzalez of the Venezuelan 'Simplified Medicine Programme' makes interesting reading in this context (Newell 1975, pp. 169ff). The Venezuelan programme is advanced in comparison with most of the continent, and has clearly made a difference to the previously neglected distant rural areas. But in Africa or Asia a rural auxiliary, operating on his (or her) own for most of the time, is not hedged in by the same formalistic and limiting regulations. For example:

'Of course it is vital to limit the auxiliary to this well-defined set of tasks. To this end, the manual that has served for training is used as the 'bible' for the day-to-day work. The auxiliary is expected to consult the manual at every instance, to follow it exactly and not to take any step beyond the instructions and never to perform anything from memory' (Newell 1975, p. 184).[3]

In this light it is hardly surprising that in Latin America the main concern with the role of community health workers often seems to be that of *excluding* tasks and activities. The most prevalent situation is for them to be given mainly promotive and preventive tasks, though some first aid is usually included in their training, as is the recognition of the most common diseases. However, they are not taught the use or dosage of modern drugs such as simple antibiotics, which they are expressly not allowed to prescribe. They are expected to refer the patient to the nearest doctor for anything that requires, let us say, more than an aspirin or a cough mixture (and full-time auxiliaries, even nurses, do not fare much better in this respect). Werner (1980, p.95) remarks that the community health workers' 'trivial knowledge of medicine, in a community where many medicines are widely used, reduces the people's respect for them and makes them less effective, even in preventive measures'.

This situation produces a number of other possible negative consequences. The community health workers may be discouraged from continuing with their tasks, and so the tenuous link of health service to community is broken. Alternatively, they acquire over the counter, in the nearest pharmacy or even in the village store, the drugs which are officially barred to them (especially, of course, antibiotic injections), and then use these untutored and unsupervised (Muller 1980, p.V.4.8). They thus assimilate themselves *de facto* with the 'practical' healers, many of whom nowadays use a mixture of traditional and modern procedures and remedies (Werner 1980, p.91).

In general, much benefit could be derived from making ordinary people more truly able to cope with health problems without constant and immediate recourse to full-time health workers, especially professionals. In this respect, participation means in the first place *learning* – the broadening of skills and widening of understanding (Dore 1981, p.31). The result would be to break down the self-interested mystique which the medical profession has built around its work, and reducing the domain legitimately considered exclusive to physicians (de Kadt 1981). Even though some of his points were exaggerated, in this respect Illich (1976) was surely right: people have to be given a much greater opportunity to be self-reliant as regards the health problems that afflict them. The role of community health workers must be formulated accordingly.

Relevant in this connection are also the traditional ways of coping with health and disease which (rural) populations derive from their own indigenous cultures. When the health-care system comes to concern itself with the rural masses, little thought tends to be given to the fact that there exist elaborate and deeply rooted responses to health needs in rural communities: the recent survey of 'pre-scientific' medicine by Antonio Scarpa (1981) documents this extensively. Even the Declaration of Alma Ata, and the Joint Report of the Director-General of WHO and the Executive Director of UNICEF to the Alma Ata Conference, do little more than mention traditional practitioners and birth attendants (in passing) as potentially valuable allies in the spread of modern health science (WHO 1978, pp.5 and 63). In practice, it may be recognized that some traditional procedures can be beneficial (parts of herbal medicine, especially), but on the whole little respect is shown for traditional culture, and there is almost no humility when it comes to attempting to convince the 'ignorant' of the 'benefits' of modern health science. If communities are to participate successfully in implementing health activities, their beliefs and behaviour patterns relating to health (often entwined with deep-seated religious beliefs and practices) must be taken seriously, and not just brushed aside as obstacles to health improvement — which they may, or may not, be. This will require above all a capacity to *learn* about, and from, traditional culture. Unless in this respect the people are met on their own ground, past failures will simply be repeated. Of course, such an open-minded attitude need not prevent critical assessment of health practices, behaviour, and wider inter-personal and social relations. This is particularly relevant as regards the position of women, who are often profoundly disadvantaged in health and other respects by traditional (and modern) patterns of the division of labour, and of social subordination.

Finally, it must be emphasized that if resource (mis-)allocation within the health sector remains basically unchanged, then promoting community involvement in the implementation of health programmes may occur side by side with the continued expansion of sophisticated facilities available largely to the better-off in the urban areas. In these circumstances the (rural) poor would be 'taxed' to pay for a second-class service, and community participation would do little more than underpin mechanisms that perpetuate inequality and injustice.[4]

Participation in decision-making

Participation in decision-making for health has, so far, been much less widespread (or genuine) than participation in the implementation of health activities. In part, this results from the class structure of most societies, in part from the problem of medical predominance discussed in the previous section. Medical professionals, especially in Latin America, have found it exceptionally difficult to see why their authority in matters of health should be shared with anyone, least of all with 'ignorant peasants'.

It has thus been left largely to the personal initiatives of rather exceptional individuals to involve community members in the organization and running of health projects,[5] although in certain (for Latin America, unusual) political circumstances government initiatives were taken in this respect. In post-revolutionary Cuba, popular organizations, notably the Committees for the Defence of the Revolution, have played a significant role in health promotion and decision-making about health activities at the local level. At certain times other countries (e.g. Chile between 1970 and 1973; Nicaragua today) have attempted to copy some of these mechanisms.[6] Statutory participation bodies were set up in the early 1970s in Peru and in Chile, and somewhat later in Colombia; however, the real power of decision-making seems to have been left largely in the hands of the medical staff (Muller 1980; de Kadt 1974). The practices of health workers, or the routines of health centres, have been influenced significantly by community members only in exceptional cases.[7] In fact, participation in decision-making may mean little more than that community members choose the persons who will be trained as community health workers, or decide on the place where they themselves will build a health facility. Although community members are often said to have a task in supervising (and hence deciding on) the work of the community health workers, in many places this is insignificant compared to the role played by technical supervisers from the health-care system.

In some small-scale, non-government-sponsored projects, however, there has been a certain amount of sustained involvement of communities in decision-making. At times this appears to have led to the reorientation of originally exclusively medical activities to a much wider concern with other factors that influence health: agriculture, food production, education, feeder roads. This has happened to some extent with the 'Hospital without Walls' programme in San Ramón, Costa Rica (which is attached to a government district hospital but has considerable independence within the government health care structure). It started as a community-centred health care system, based around health posts, using paid auxiliaries and unpaid community health workers who act as liaison between the health post and their neighbourhood. The awareness in the programme of the impact of non-medical factors on health has made it focus on the socioeconomically weakest groups, not least because of the existence of active health committees. The programme has helped raise the consciousness of the communities with respect to these wider factors, and has created organizational capacity to tackle problems in areas such as land tenancy, physical infrastructure (e.g. access roads), and production and marketing. The infant mortality rate in the (largely rural) project area is now below 20 per thousand, more than 10 per thousand lower than the national average (UNICEF/WHO 1981).

In certain parts of Latin America, notably in the Andean highland areas and in Guatemala (Muller 1980, pp.V.1 and V.5), traditional social structures still linger on, in spite of centuries of emasculation by the colonial and post-colonial state. People remain socially and culturally attached to such structures and their traditional patterns of leadership and/or cooperation. These can be helpful in involving community members in decision-making about actions to improve their health and general living conditions. In other parts of the world, particularly in Africa and Asia, this is done to a greater extent than is apparently occurring in Latin America.

A survey by Boutmij (1976) of primary care projects in Indonesia is of interest from a comparative point of view. In Indonesia, traditional authority relations in the mid-1970s were still accepted as legitimate by the villagers. As a result, the village head was in a crucial position for any kind of community mobilization, for health or for other development activities. Things could get done if the traditional processes were activated; and to some extent needs recognized by outsiders but not felt by the average villager could be *transmitted* through the traditional leadership and could thus be 'incorporated' into village life.[8] Fairly homogeneous village communities were often given a lead by their traditional authorities to adopt certain innovations that would be of benefit to all. Examples included the selection and training of village health workers, communal cleaning of the village or building of wells or latrines, the adoption of new agricultural practices leading to greater food availability, or the promotion of forms of commercialization more advantageous to the villagers.

In Latin America, by contrast, the use of such traditional structures remains quite unusual. National governments, on the one hand, tend to look down upon traditional institutions. In spite of the *indigenista* rhetoric often espoused in public pronouncements, the usually centralized political systems and administrations make little effort to open themselves up to indigenous ways of doing things. More radically oriented persons and groups, on the other hand, while glad to link up with traditional institutions insofar as they are cooperative or communitarian, are suspicious of the elements of hierarchy and authority often embedded in them. So they, too, may stand off.

As a result, it remains rare in Latin America for community members to be genuinely involved in decision taking on issues that matter greatly to them. In the terms of Cohen and Uphoff (1980, p.225), the *scope* of the decisions in which communities may participate is usually narrow: even within any sector (such as health) the range of issues on which they can expect to have some say is small. Moreover, the *empowerment* is generally low: where they do participate, their power to influence decisions tends to be limited.

THE SPONSORS OF PARTICIPATION AND THEIR ORIENTATION

Most community involvement is, somehow, 'sponsored' — i.e. brought about by agents external to the community. Left to their own resources, communities are not likely to change their behaviour in or understanding of the world around them, though the mass media (especially radio) may have a catalyzing influence.[9] External agents may be closely linked to official organizations, or they may be supported by voluntary agencies (church groups, international development volunteers, etc.). The sponsors of community involvement usually say they want to make the communities more self-reliant, more capable of influencing their own fate. Yet in reality sponsors may differ considerably in their links with the existing sociopolitical structure, and in the extent to which they would be willing to see communities challenge certain aspects of that structure. This is an issue as much in socialist societies as it is in capitalist ones. Four main types of sponsorship can be identified.

Government sponsorship with conservative orientation

Since Alma Ata, all governments have formally accepted the primary health care approach. This implies that sooner or later some form of community participation is likely to be 'policy' everywhere, also in the case of governments whose overall policies have little or no real concern for the disadvantaged. The state, while essentially supporting the existing social structure through its economic policies (and perhaps also by control, or repression, of trade unions or independent political activities) may want to avoid the potentially explosive effects of great poverty and great inequality. Hence community health programmes may be developed, while the health sector remains nevertheless heavily weighted to urban curative care, which absorbs most of the country's health-care resources.

If communities are being 'involved' by official organizations in such circumstances, 'participation' is likely to be largely a matter of following directives that come from above – of *compliance*. The poor themselves will not contribute much to the definition of the problems, and it is unlikely that attention will be drawn to the main causes of their ill-health, their poverty and underdevelopment. David Werner's conclusion, after visiting and studying some 40 rural health projects in Latin America, may be relevant mainly to this type of situation. He found that:

'when it came to the nitty-gritty of what was going on in the field, many of these ambitious 'king-size' programmes actually had a minimum of effective community participation and a maximum of handouts, paternalism and super-imposed, initiative-destroying 'norms'' (1980, p. 94).

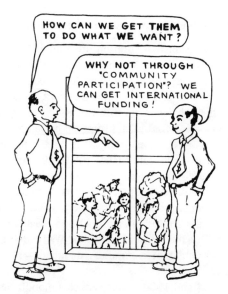

Fig. 15.2. 'Participation' is often a matter of compliance with directives from above.

There is another point. In these situations contributions in time and resources of the rural poor 'let the government off the hook', as the people's activities are accompanied neither by a redistribution of resources within the health sector itself, nor by wider efforts to help the members of such communities improve their socioeconomic well-being.[10]

Non-governmental sponsorship with conservative orientation

Certain health projects sponsored by religious organizations provide examples of this case, particularly in Latin America. Muller cites a number of instances from Guatemala (1980, p.V.6) and Peru (1980, p.V.2). The more 'fundamentalist' or 'messianic' a religious group, the less likely it is to concern itself directly with problems relating to the socioeconomic structure: usually the preoccupation with the Kingdom of God, and with living according to the sect's strict rules, is overwhelming. Of course, by following a demanding code of religious and moral practice the socioeconomic position of the members of the sect may be improved. Nevertheless, this would be the unintended and even unexpected outcome of an orientation that takes the status quo for granted (Pereira de Queiroz 1968).

Outside Latin America the rural health programmes of missionary hospitals are now increasingly imbued with a concern for social justice. Yet many remain conservative in essence, failing to question existing socioeconomic processes. Moreover, they usually need to charge fees for their services, in order to survive: this is another characteristic which may give them a conservative orientation.

Government sponsorship with reformist or radical orientation

Governments with a reformist orientation are found in many countries of the world, the degree of 'reformism' varying considerably from one place to the next. These are intermediate cases, neither clearly conservative nor obviously revolutionary, and there is often wide disagreement in assessing the effects — and intentions — of the policies of governments in this category.

Community participation for health promoted by reformist governments may easily be dismissed as 'integrative', that is as 'strengthening the system [i.e. capitalism] that marginalizes' (Muller 1980, p.VII. 19). And yet, they could also be seen as enabling the disadvantaged groups to relate their health problems to the broader causes of under-development and its perpetuation, and potentially setting in motion dynamic processes of change beyond the health care system. That kind of effect is the aim of the national rural health programme of Costa Rica (partly inspired by the 'Hospital Without Walls' discussed above), which seeks the active involvement of community members — also to some extent in local decision-making.[11]

Chile, between 1964 and 1970, also saw such a mobilizing use of community participation. The years of the Christian Democratic Government witnessed the widespread stimulation of community organizations among 'marginal' groups in towns and among the peasantry in the countryside. The approach has been much criticized for being based on an inadequate — or even deliberately mystifying — interpretation of the operation of the socioeconomic system. Yet many of those involved saw the mobilization of community members through health committees, neighbourhood organizations, or Mothers' Clubs, as contributing to a radical transformation of Chilean society (de Kadt 1967).

More recently, there has been a large-scale government-sponsored rural health programme in Brazil, in which community participation has been regarded as a tool for *conscientisacion*, and eventually for social change. Maria das Mercês Somarriba (1980) has analysed the Norte de Minas community health programme with much insight. She shows how the team responsible for this project (covering over one million people) developed an orientation at odds with that of the State Secretariat of Health. The latter was basically concerned with the extension of health service coverage and promoted the participation of community members in implementation only. The former, on the other hand, convinced 'that the main causes of ill-health in the region [were] related to the existing social inequalities' (Somarriba 1980, p. 64), came to regard participation in the health programme as a means to press for changes in the economic and political spheres.

Success in these circumstances was limited. The aims pursued by the project team were coherent neither with other government policies predominant in the health field, nor with overall government policy. In the mid- and late 1970s, Brazil's health policy revolved around the extension of *curative* services provided in the urban areas through the National Social Security Institute, and bought directly from the private sector. While development policy was groping for a measure of democratization and some reduction in inequalities, the government continued to be extremely nervous of anything that could be interpreted as subversion.

Similar circumstances are described by Algara in his discussion of the Mexican case in the UNESCO-sponsored comparative study of community development projects (Dore and Mars 1981). Here health-related activities were embedded in a broader integrated programme, financed by an agency of the State of Guanajuato. The programme 'sought to create and develop an authentic class consciousness in the peasants, as a basis for the autonomous development of the communities' (Algara 1981, p.358). All went well for a year or so. There was little to condemn in the rhetoric, which is anyway also widely used in Mexico by members of the central government and the ruling party. No great changes took place in the communities: participation was largely confined to local co-operative activities in the agricultural and infrastructure sectors. When, however, the promoters moved into activities which threatened to challenge the existing distribution of power in the economic and political spheres – specifically the proposed establishment of Regional Peasant Councils – the government first clipped the programme's wings financially, then closed it down completely.

These examples incidentally demonstrate that it is wrong to assume that governments are necessarily monolithic. Within any large state bureaucracy there are always nooks and crannies where an orientation can operate which is more progressive – or conservative! – than the dominant government line. But there are obviously limits to the divergence that is tolerated, though these limits can only be known when tested. Moreover, they do change over time, and the 'testing' itself may help to promote change.

Governments may also attempt to mobilize the masses in support of a *radical* change in social and productive relations. Community participation then is part of a strategy for change; it is a weapon used by government or ruling political party to challenge the influence of powerful groups and classes, and to shift power and resources to those hitherto disadvantaged. This happens after a socialist revolution, and in the early years of elected governments committed to a transition to socialism.

During the years 1970-73, when the government of President Allende intended to effect a transition to socialism, community organizations in Chile were given a major support role. They were stimulated in all areas of life, often 'steered' by militants of the various parties which made up the governing coalition of Unidad Popular. In specific sectors such as health, representatives of these community organizations were brought together in formal committees, which were given legal status (de Kadt 1974). Two types of health committees existed at the local level, one rather larger and more diffuse, the other smaller and with somewhat less vaguely defined functions. Even so, whether the latter really had decision-making functions was left unclear in the legislation. At the time, their efficacy varied, and much depended on the relationship between community leaders and health centre personnel, which was partly at least a matter of politics: the different parties constituting Unidad Popular attempted to use such committees to promote their own (divergent) policies. What was lacking, however, were mechanisms to link these committees to those in other sectors, and their attention tended to focus rather narrowly on 'medical' issues.

In Cuba it is a central tenet of ideology that development should benefit the masses, and the inequalities in health-care provision (as in education or housing) which characterize capitalist countries have been greatly reduced. Neighbourhood health committees play an important role in ensuring that preventive and promotive measures are effective for the entire population; with the disappearance of gross socioeconomic inequality, health chances have also been largely equalized (Djukanovic and Mach 1975).

Community participation in health, as in many other activities, is widespread in Cuba and fully integrated with party and government. Using various mobilization structures, such as Committees for the Defence of the Revolution, mass organizations of women or youth, or residents' committees, it serves essentially the function of mobilizing the population behind official policies, and defending the achievements of the revolution as defined by the party, which is the sole legitimate channel of political expression. How far such mobilization provides a channel for, manipulates, or stifles the views and demands of people in the communities, is an issue on which views diverge — even in socialist countries.

Non-governmental sponsorship with reformist or radical orientation

Probably the bulk of voluntary agency projects in Latin America and elsewhere, today, are reformist. Werner (1980, p.94) has defined community-supportive programmes as those 'which favourably influence the long-range welfare of the community, that help it stand on its own feet, that genuinely encourage responsibility, initiative, decision-making, and self-reliance at the community level, and that build upon human dignity'. He found that in Latin America it was small, non-governmental programmes that could be characterized as community supportive.

Because of their smaller scale and more direct human involvement with the communities, the promoters of such projects are likely to listen attentively to the views of community members, sharing a concern for their 'felt needs'. However, when asked about their needs, many poor people do not place health, as such, very high up on their list of priorities. More urgent are food, work and income, job security, or even some important consumer durables.[12] Sponsors of non-governmental health projects with a reformist orientation usually realize that poor people are not 'wrong' to put the emphasis where they do. 'Wrong' are the circumstances in which health improvements are isolated from the wider social and economic context, promoted on their own without thought for the way in which living conditions and social relations may impede their implementation or nullify their effect.

This type of project, then, appears to be particularly prone to move away from isolated health activities (Rifkin 1980, p.3). It can engage in wider development activities rather more easily than government-sponsored community health programmes: the latter are enmeshed in the web of specialized government agencies, each of which has its own bureaucratically separated and maintained sectoral tasks in 'health', 'agriculture', 'education', 'public works', and so on. This division of labour easily obscures the interconnections between different problems; non-governmental organizations are less hampered by this particular constraint.

The success of such projects in achieving improvement for the disadvantaged groups, and in using health as a 'lever' in the wider socioeconomic arena, depends to a large extent on the political context in which they operate.

Non-governmental projects may also see themselves as presenting a radical challenge to the status quo, but this may not always be obvious to outsiders. This ambiguity results mainly from the relationship between projects and the government, or the 'forces of order'. The more repressive the state, the more easily will the authorities define projects as subversive; in the final analysis, any radical project will at some point face the decision whether or not to defy government authority outright (Hollnsteiner 1980). Before that occurs, however, the project's activities may remain within limits acceptable to the authorities, even if its orientation, and hence the nature of what happens in the name of *conscientisación*, point in the direction of basic change.[13] Project leaders will require a capacity for predicting the reactions of potential allies and adversaries, in order to weigh up the chances for success or failure; in Latin America, the latter has, unfortunately, predominated.

Muller's examination of community participation in health projects provides a number of interesting examples of these problems, notably from Peru in the 1970s (see Chapter 13 of this book for Muller's presentation of four case studies from Peru.) In some cases the approach to health problems prevalent among the peasant communities hindered projects in mounting a wider attack on the structural causes of ill-health, in spite of a congenial political climate. Of one Peruvian highland project he writes:

'Neither the community leaders, nor the peasant league, nor the project's staff seem to have [had] a clear social interpretation of health problems, which would have allowed a development of the health programme as social crowbar or as political praxis' (Muller 1980, p. VII.13).

More in general, the authorities appear to have been concerned to keep a fairly strict control of the projects, either through the Ministry of Health or through the popular mobilization agency SINAMOS. However radical the government's orientation at that time, it was not radical enough for certain groups behind some of the projects. In addition to projects in the Andean highlands, the case of Lima's Villa el Salvador is relevant, where political parties of the left and sympathizers from the medical faculty of the National University tried 'to make Villa el Salvador independent of its national environment' (Muller 1980, p.VII.10).

So the effects of projects run by radical non-governmental sponsors are not likely to be all that different from those sponsored by reformists. Both types of project can help to sow the seeds of change. Yet only when their aims and those of the authorities are basically identical can radicals outside the government really stimulate communities to challenge those who remain powerful within the health-care system, in other government departments, or in the local socioeconomic structure.

THE STRUCTURE OF THE COMMUNITY AND ITS SOCIOPOLITICAL CONTEXT

The term 'community' has so far been used without many qualifications. It now needs to be stressed that community involvement for health is likely to present different problems and different opportunities in relatively homogeneous and in relatively unequal or segmented communities.[14]

In rural Latin America, the most significant distinctions in this respect are socioeconomic. In many places the complex of large landowners and small-holders or tenant farmers still predominates. Elsewhere, large-scale modern commercial plantations have taken their place. In both situations rural communities are made up of smallholders or landless workers, while the large land-owners — who may or may not live in the area — monopolize the main productive resource, land, and often also the channels of commercialization. In these circumstances successful community participation depends to a great extent on whether or not formal or informal leadership has developed among the poor majority. Where there is a history of struggle against the local land-owners — Muller (1980, p.V.1) saw this in a number of project areas in the Peruvian highlands — community organization may be strong; then a good basis exists for the development of health activities. If this is not the case — many parts of Brazil have that characteristic (cf. Somarriba 1980) — it is much more difficult to involve community members in health projects, also because of fear of the consequences of undertaking activities without the express permission of the locally powerful (de Kadt 1970, Chapter 13).

Where material resources are more equally distributed, there appears to be a better basis for community activities. Nevertheless, even in such circumstances it may be difficult to involve community members in health promotion if poverty is acute and individualism prevails. This situation may be exacerbated by com-munity segmentation. In Africa this can be the result of tribal or clan divisions; in some parts of Latin America it is more likely to be the result of religious sectarianism, stimulated by missionary activities often promoted from outside the country. Muller describes the negative effects of this kind of community structure on participation in health projects in parts of Guatemala (1980, Section VII). The programmes described in Dore and Mars (1981) also give various examples of such problems.

These structural factors are, however, mediated by the wider sociopolitical context. If the large landowners cannot call upon the state for support when the local peasantry faces them with demands, the outcome of the confrontation is

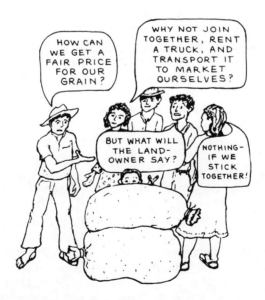

Fig. 15.3. Successful community participation depends to a great extent on whether or not formal or informal leadership has developed among the poor majority.

rather less certain than when they have the police (and judiciary) at their beck and call. Reformist or radical governments can make a difference in this respect, through legislation as well as through the strict control of the local 'forces of order'. In turn, community mobilisation becomes a condition for the successful *implementation* at the local level of such legislation and government-promoted and institutional change, in the face of opposition from the locally powerful. This lesson has been well applied by revolutionary movements in Latin America and elsewhere, but reformist governments have also understood that mobiliza-tion of the disadvantaged groups is a necessary – if, from this point of view, perhaps risky – enterprise.

CONCLUSIONS

Community participation in activities for health is being promoted for a variety of reasons. Perhaps most important is the perceived need of governments to ease resource constraints by sharing the burden with communities themselves. Various modes are reported from Latin America: the use of part-time, unremunerated community health workers; the promotion of local health insurance schemes; and the provision of communal labour for the construction of health care facilities, latrines, water supplies systems, or the cleaning up of villages. There may be no alternative to this if the aim is to improve coverage and access. It can happen, however, that the poor are made to share the burden of providing for their own health needs, while there is little or no change in the biased allocation of government resources to hospitals and (urban) curative care. The politics of most Latin American governments tend to lead to that result.

Community involvement can improve communication between the population and health workers, and thereby enable people to become more aware of their own potential contributions to health, and to engage in health-promoting activi-ties. It may also broaden the range of such activities. Consciousness may develop, among people and health service staff, of the importance for health of wider socioeconomic factors. If sociopolitical circumstances are favourable, this may contribute to the emergence of dynamic processes of change and mobilization, and the health sector can become an entry point to the wider socioeconomic structure.

After his extensive survey of community health projects in Latin America, David Werner (1980, p.95) thought the biggest challenge to rural health care was the adaptation of the 'people-supportive features' of small non-governmental projects to regional or country-wide programmes. The present discussion largely supports that conclusion. It has, moreover, brought out the importance of the political orientation of the sponsors of community-involving health projects, and of the wider political context in which non-governmental projects operate. The seeds of change may (and *need* to) be sown in unfavourable circumstances. Yet community involvement will really thrive only under governments with a sub-stantial measure of genuine commitment to overcoming the poverty and social inequality still so widespread in Latin America.

NOTES

1. Community involvement in health as a phenomenon which has captured the widespread attention of international agencies and national governments dates from the mid-1970s, although it had been promoted for years in China and some other socialist countries, as well as elsewhere; through small-scale projects, often run by voluntary agencies. See Djukanovic and Mach (1975) and UNICEF/WHO (1977).

2. This issue is clearly brought out in Ronald Dore's Introduction to a recent comparative study of community development projects in India, Korea, Mexico, and Tanzania. See Dore and Mars (1981).

3. Another example of the same problem is that of Guatemala's Rural Health Technicians. They have nine years of schooling and three years of specialized training, yet pressure from the medical profession has kept curative medicine almost entirely out of their course (Muller 1980, p.V.5.4).

4. That is, of course, a conclusion that also applies outside the health sector. In general terms, UNECLA (1973) drew attention to the problem with respect to mobilization of voluntary labour for community improvement schemes in some Latin American countries. The theme was recently taken up again in UNICEF/WHO (1981).

5. Muller (1980) mentions the influence of members of Colombia's Escuela Nacional de Salud Publica on a number of projects in Antioquia, as well as the role played by members of the medical faculty in Lima's shanty towns in the early 1970s.

6. Not only in Latin America: Democratic Yemen has also been influenced by the Cuban example (UNICEF/WHO 1981).

7. Muller (1980, p.V.4) relates how in one urban health centre in a Medellin suburb relations between the staff became more democratic as a result of the participation of community members in decision-making.

8. This also is the case in much of Africa, though on the whole health-care projects appear to pay little attention to the relevant mechanisms. On Ghana, see IDS Health Group (1981, Chapters 9 and 10).

9. Even then, the presence in the communities of 'interpreters' of the messages — monitors, teachers, etc. — is usually a condition for action to be taken. For Brazil in the 1960s see de Kadt (1970); interesting also is the description of the Tanzanian health campaign by Budd Hall (1980).

10. The Guatemalan national programme of rural health care described by Muller (1980, p.V.5) would seem to fit this case in general terms — although the rural health technicians appear to be motivated to help communities become conscious of the structural factors that play a major role in the generation of ill-health.

11. Personal interviews with officials and politicians, Costa Rica, January 1980.

12. The surveys carried out in India, Korea, Mexico, and Tanzania, reported in Dore and Mars (1981), attest to this point. There is also much evidence for this from studies among the poor in developed countries, who have been widely subjected to surveys of one kind or another. See Hatch (1970, p.1088); Irelan (1967, p.57); Kosa (1969, p.21).

13. For an analysis of the consequences of a disjunction between the nature (message) of *conscientisación* and the potential for action in Brazil in the mid 1960s, see de Kadt (1970, Chapters 12 and 13).

14. Ronald Dore (1981, p.38) points out that 'natural' differences can also be important: constraints deriving from ecological factors, or from (natural) resource scarcities also differ considerably.

REFERENCES

Algara Cosio, Ignacio, Community development in Mexico. In *Community development* (ed. R. Dore and Z. Mars) Croom Helm/UNESCO, London and Paris (1981).

Batten, T.R., The major issues and future direction of cor munity development. *Community Development Journal* 9, 2 (April 1974).

Boutmij, Hudion L., *Op weg naar nieuwe vormen van gezondheidszorg in Indonesië*. Vrije Universiteit, Amsterdam (mimeo) (1976).

Cohen, John M. and Norman T. Uphoff, Participation's place in rural development: seeking clarity through specifity. *World Development* 8, 3 (1980).

Dore, Ronald, Introduction. Community development in the 1970s. In *Community development* (ed. R. Dore and Z. Mars) Croom Helm/UNESCO, London and Paris (1981).

Dore, Ronald and Zoë Mars (eds.), *Community development*. Croom Helm/ UNESCO, London and Paris (1981).

Djukanovic, V. and E.P. Mach (eds.), *Alternative approaches to meeting basic health needs in developing countries*. A joint UNICEF/WHO study. WHO, Geneva (1975).

Freire, Paulo, *Educação como pratica da liberadade*. Paz e Terra, Rio de Janeiro (1967).

Hall, Budd, Development campaigns in rural Tanzania. In *Health: the human factor: readings in health development and community participation* (ed. S. Rifkin). World Council of Churches, Geneva (1980).

Hatch, John W. Discussion of the 'how' of community participation in delivering health care. *Bulletin of the New York Academy of Medicine,* **46** (December 1970).

Hollnsteiner, Mary Racelis, People power: community participation in the planning of human settlements. In *Health: the human factor: readings in health development and community participation* (ed. S. Rifkin). World Council of Churches, Geneva (1980).

IDS Health Group, *Health needs and health services in rural Ghana,* revised and abridged edn. prepared by Emanuel de Kadt and Malcolm Segall, *Social Science and Medicine* Special Issue, **ISA**, No. 4 (July 1981).

Illich, Ivan, *The limits of medicine. Medical nemesis: the expropriation of health*. Marion Boyars, London (1976).

Irelan, Lola M., Health practices of the poor. In *Low income life styles* (ed. L.M. Irelan). DHEW, Washington, DC. (1967).

de Kadt, Emanuel, Paternalism and populism: catholicism in Latin America. *Journal of Contemporary History* 2, No. 4 (October 1967).

de Kadt, Emanuel, *Catholic radicals in Brazil.* Oxford University Press for RIIA, London (1970).

de Kadt, Emanuel, Aspectos distributivos de la salud en Chile. In CEPLAN, *Bienestar y Pobreza.* Nueva Universidad, Santiago (1974).

de Kadt, Emanuel, Ideology, social policy, health and health services: a field of complex interactions. *Social Science and Medicine* 15A, (1981).

Kosa, John, The nature of poverty. In *Poverty and health* (ed. J. Kosa *et al.*). Harvard University Press, Cambridge, Mass. (1969).

Muller, Frits. *Participation in primary health care programs in Latin America.* National School of Public Health, University of Antioquia, Medellin (mimeo) (1980).

Newell, Kenneth (ed.), *Health by the people.* WHO, Geneva (1975).

Pereira de Queiroz, Maria Isaura, *Réforme et révolution dans les sociétés traditionnelles.* Anthropos, Paris (1968).

Rifkin, Susan B. (ed.), *Health: the human factor: readings in health development and community participation.* CONTACT Special Series, No. 3. CMC, World Council of Churches, Geneva (1980).

Scarpa, Antonio, Pre-scientific medicines: their extent and value. *Social Science and Medicine,* 15A, No. 3 (May 1981).

Somarriba, Maria das Mercês, On the limitations of community health programmes. In *Health: the human factor: readings in health development and community participation* (ed. S.B. Rifkin) World Council of Churches, Geneva (1980).

UNICEF/WHO, *Community involvement in primary health care.* JC 21/UNICEF/WHO/77.2, Geneva (1977).

UNICEF/WHO, *National decision-making for primary health care.* WHO, Geneva (1981).

United Nations Economic Commission for Latin America, Popular participation in development. *Community Development Journal* 8, 2 (April 1973).

Werner, David, Health care and human dignity. In *Health: the human factor: readings in health development and community participation* (ed. S.B. Rifkin) World Council of Churches, Geneva (1980).

WHO, *Primary health care*, Report of the International Conference on Primary Health Care, Alma Ata, USSR, 6–12 September 1978. WHO, Geneva, (1978).

Part III

Programme development

INTRODUCTION

Since the Alma Ata Conference in September 1978 many governments have
attempted to revise their health strategies in the light of their official commitment to 'Health for All by the Year 2000'. The following chapters examine
the process of health programme development in three countries with vastly
different political, social, and geographical characteristics: Indonesia, Ghana,
and South Yemen.

The chapter on Indonesia describes how an effective approach to nutrition
improvement was developed over several years through small, community-
based projects started by voluntary and governmental agencies. These projects
gave rise to a unified strategy consisting of an appropriate technology and an
effective form of decentralized community organization. The strategy was
then adopted by the Indonesian government as the basis for a national family
nutrition programme.

The chapter on Ghana relates how the Health Ministry developed a rational,
quantifiable method of health planning which convinced policy makers at
national level of the urgent need to give priority to primary health care in the
allocation of public funds.

The chapter on South Yemen shows how, even with political commitment at
the highest level, a country may still need several years to develop an appropriate
PHC strategy. Cooperation with international agencies and field visits to other
countries played a constructive part in working out a national health policy em-
bodying all the essential elements of PHC.

These three programmes are all of recent origin. Their effectiveness and impact
will not be fully known for a few years yet. Some issues remain unresolved and
more detailed planning is needed, but in each case an encouraging start towards
'Health for All' has been made.

16 Development from below: transformation from village-based nutrition projects to a national family nutrition programme in Indonesia*

Jon Rohde and **Lukas Hendrata** argue that Indonesia's national family nutrition improvement programme demonstrates how successful pilot projects can be transformed into national programmes.

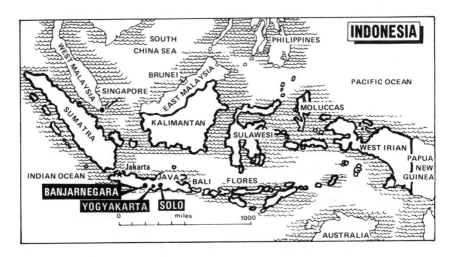

Jon Rohde, M.D., is currently Head of the Management Sciences for Health team working with the Department of Health in Haiti. He was visiting lecturer in the Medical Faculty of Gadjah Mada University in Yogyakarta, Indonesia, from 1973 until 1980.
Lukas Hendrata, M.D., has been General Secretary of the Indonesia Sejahtera Foundation, Jakarta, Indonesia, since 1974. He is also a consultant to UNICEF, World Bank and other international agencies.

During the Five Year Development Plan of 1979–84 (REPELITA III), Indonesia's national family nutrition programme is scheduled to cover 40 000 of the country's 65 000 villages. The evolution toward this programme over the past 10 years provides an opportunity to examine the process of national programme development. While in retrospect there appears to have been a logical sequence of interacting activities, in fact, the many participants in this evolution, both government and private, followed no preconceived plan or pattern to reach the goal of a common programme. Frequent meetings and field visits between government, academic, and private-sector workers, coupled with a genuine

*An earlier version of this chapter is being published by Plenum Press, New York.

commitment to flexibility and innovation, led to a coherent formulation of an affordable and implementable nationwide programme.

In our review of this process, simultaneous development of three crucial areas has become apparent:

— The understanding, acceptance, and articulation by planners and decision makers of the importance of nutrition to national development, resulting in formulation of policy, political will, and resource commitment to specific nutrition goals.
— The development and field perfection of an appropriate technology that not only proved to be effective in terms of nutritional goals, but also proved to be pragmatic and affordable within the means of the country.
— The formation of a comprehensive, intersectoral organizational structure capable of systematically administering and managing a population-wide programme at the village level. The organization had the means to provide training, supervision, information flow, logistical support, and outreach to guarantee coverage of specific targeted groups.

Although in this article we review these three elements separately, we should re-emphasize that the elements evolved simultaneously and synergistically. As in all living structures, the whole exceeds its individual parts.

POLITICAL COMMITMENT

Wide awareness by government decision makers of the extent of malnutrition in Indonesia dates from Sayogyo's evaluation (1975) of the Applied Nutrition Programme (ANP), 1972–73. Physicians and nutritionists alike had long recognized, treated, and researched malnutrition, but their approach, which was reflected in scientific writings, viewed it as a clinical or a biochemical problem of individual patients. Sayogyo's sample survey demonstrated undernutrition on a massive scale; he showed that one-half of Indonesian children were malnourished, that poverty and malnutrition were closely linked, and that existing programmes aimed at increasing protein consumption were largely irrelevant. The report called for specific actions in home food production, nutrition education, and targeted preventive measures.

Of considerable importance, these findings were expressed not in medical-nutrition terminology, but rather in broadly understandable lay terms focusing on poverty, inadequacy of food, and resulting poor child growth and ill-health. The complex web of causation was clearly seen to involve economics, social inequity, traditional behaviour patterns, and agricultural stagnation, as well as ignorance and disease. The nutrition issue began to be seen as an integral part of the development process itself, both as a means to, and an end goal of, the nation's development. Nutrition entered the political arena.

In 1974 President Soeharto called upon 10 ministries to join in a coordinated effort to '. . . improve the nutritional health of the populace . . . as an effort important for national development . . .'. A National Committee on Food was founded, and during the second Five Year Development Plan of 1974-79 (REPELITA II), a large number of approaches were initiated involving agriculture, education, health, information, religion, industries, and internal affairs. While sectoral efforts were limited in extent and impact, momentum was building as more ministries and departments of the government accepted a role in addressing the nutrition problem.

Several groups worked diligently to educate the public and move the nation toward concerted action. UNICEF-Indonesia sponsored a sound-slide show that highlighted both the problems and various programme options. Open dialogue in the press, in seminars, and in other forums kept the issue in the public eye and contributed to the critical re-education of policy makers and top bureaucrats about the issues involved. The importance of these communication strategies in obtaining the needed political commitment cannot be overemphasized. Armed with clear data on the problem and with the increased public interest in nutrition, decision makers could grasp with confidence the issue of nutrition as a major social need with positive political impact.

Following the formulation by Parliament of the development strategy for REPELITA III (1979-84), emphasizing 'equity', the planning board (BAPPE-NAS) has given particular attention to multisectoral approaches to nutrition. With the major plan emphasis on social and economic equity, improved nutrition has become a specific goal of Indonesian development policy, which focuses heavily on the poor. No longer considered as an adjunct programme facilitating national growth through its effect on the economy, good nutrition is accepted as an end in itself, a legitimate and highly desirable outcome to be achieved through multisectoral development efforts. Equitable development means good nutrition.

THE DEVELOPMENT OF A PRAGMATIC FIELD PROGRAMME DEVELOPED IN INDONESIA

In spite of the plethora of small field projects in food raising, nutrition education, and supplementary feeding, a successful and affordable nutrition technology for mass implementation was unknown 10 years ago. The cost of food supplements was too high, the results transient at best, and the dependency engendered was damaging to the family as well as to national self-esteem. World Food Programme milk and fortified cereals provided through mother-and-child (MCH) clinics have served largely as a reward for clinic attendance and have not been highly focused on those who are undernourished and poor. Considerable evidence exists to suggest that those most in need of such supplements do not attend MCH clinics and therefore are excluded from the programme.

The ANP emphasis on production of protein foods was not relevant, given the overall calorie deficit among the poorest groups (roughly 500 calories below the recommended daily average). Sayogyo's finding that protein-energy malnutrition

(PEM) was equally prevalent in 'food-adequate' and 'food-deficit' households gave strong evidence that nutrition education aimed to effect behavioural change within the family should be a central part of action programmes. The ANP failed to select target groups in which a measurable and sustained improvement in nutrition could be expected. The ANP did, however, provide the first experience for many government agencies in an inter-sectoral, community-based development effort and significantly raised awareness of nutritional problems among civil servants in the selected communities where ANP projects were carried out.

During the 1970s, an 'appropriate technology' emerged from the combined field experience and innovative projects of both the private sector and the government. One factor was the development of the hardware for programme implementation on a massive scale – the *dacin* weighing scale and the special weight chart, which have proven simple, practical, economical, and, to a large extent, self-explanatory. But 'technology' is now recognized to include not only scientifically sound equipment and information but also certain organizational elements. Some elements found to be essential to an 'appropriate' nationwide programme are:

– The programme must cover the total population at an affordable cost, with major recurring costs funded by the community itself.
– The community must be involved, not only in a passive way but also in the development of leadership trusted with continued implementation of programme activities.
– Nutrition goals must be understandable to the lay public as well as to the civil leadership to enable mass involvement.
– Activities should be targeted to those most in need, and particularly to those subgroups in which a measurable impact can be expected and obtained.
– A nutrition programme should be framed in terms of multisectoral involvement to insure maximum utilization of existing sectoral manpower and implementation of field activities. It is not, and cannot, be viewed exclusively as a health problem.
– The emphasis should be on the prevention of protein-energy malnutrition rather than rehabilitation of existing undernutrition. This is not only a more efficient use of limited resources but also a more achievable use and, in the long run, more effective on a mass population-wide basis.

While it is not generally considered technological, the inclusion of such social and logistic issues in programme implementation is a vital part of 'appropriate technology' for a national-scale programme. A review of some of the many field experiences leading to these principles highlights the process of the technological transformation from small projects to large-scale programme design.

More than 10 years ago, Dr Gunawan Nugroho, then the Director of the YAKKUM Community Development Foundation in Solo, Central Java, introduced the concept of weighing in the village rather than in the clinic, plus the use of Morley's chart to record growth. In the suburban village of Kerten (see Chapter 12) mothers organized the weighing sessions in each hamlet, but the actual weighing and filling out of the weight chart was done by clinic staff. While it was apparent that mothers were interested in having their children weighed regularly, their lack of involvement in both the measurement and understanding of its implication resulted in a limited impact. The clinic scale, a standard platform Detecto beam balance, was impractical in the village setting and was considered as something alien and peculiar. Lack of specific nutrition messages or activities and passive participation of mothers led to marginal results. However, Kerten showed that higher levels of participation in maternal-child-health-promotive activities could be achieved in the village than in the clinic itself.

In Godean, a subdistrict of Yogyakarta Province (population 40 000 in 17 villages), the community nutrition programme conducted by the Pediatric Department of the Gadjah Mada Medical Faculty in Yogyakarta brought further improvement to this approach.[1] Weighing activities were built into the existing village women's organization, the PKK, becoming a part of the regular *arisan*, a monthly social hamlet meeting. Instead of the clinic scale, the locally made *dacin* market scale was used. This robust bar scale, costing under US $20, was universally available in rural villages, and proved to be accurate and much better understood by the mothers. Sleeping babies could be hung in a sling, while older children were suspended in cloth weighing pants.

Nutrition advice was largely based on the result of each weighing and aimed at achieving gain in weight each month. While surveys demonstrated that roughly 50 per cent were undernourished, those well-nourished were found to be from the same economic and social strata, thereby indicating that the local ecology could sustain good nutrition. The programme focus became positive, emphasizing the 'wisdom of village motherhood' rather than the 'science of nutrition'. Successful village mothers whose children demonstrated persistent normal weight gains were asked to advise their neighbours whose children faltered in growth. This 'pairing method' sought to replace scientific and clinical nutritional advice with practical, affordable action already practised in the same village. While this presents a far more culturally acceptable approach, the lack of specific feeding guidance resulted in a haphazard communication strategy.

Emphasis on weight gain was reinforced by recording, on a large wall chart, the percentage of children who gained weight each month. However, the card on which weights were recorded continued to be seen mainly as a clinical record rather than as a communication tool. The three growth lines, based on the Gomez interpretation of static weight, tended to stratify children as 'good', 'inadequate', or 'bad'. This type of understanding is detrimental, both from the point of view of nutrition and as a communication strategy. It stigmatized about 50 per cent of the target population as failing in their efforts as mothers, and therefore tended to alienate those most in need of the programme benefit. Thus, while the advice attempted to emphasize growth, the weight chart, with its

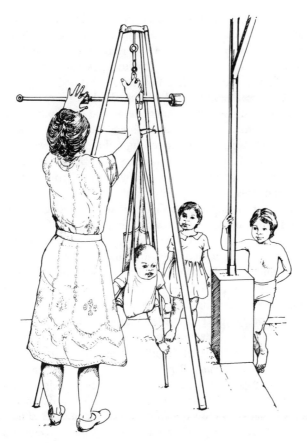

Fig. 16.1. The *dacin* market scale is well understood by mothers.

inherent emphasis on weight category, did not support this concept. The communication strategy was still not consistent.

In Banjarnegara regency (see Chapter 12) the approach in all sectors has emphasized community participation in the design and implementation of development activities. Working within the existing government staff and budget, but through a strong commitment by the regency leadership to decentralize control of village-based activities, Banjarnegara has developed the *kader* system, involving community members as both technical and social motivators for their own neighbours.

The critical elements of this mobilization of community manpower lie in:

- selection of kaders by the community;
- the highly specific nature of their responsibility to the small neighbourhood they serve;
- the totally voluntary nature of the work; and
- regular supervision and continuous in-service guidance from department field workers who provide their initial training.

The small unit of operation is crucial in maintaining the community sense of belonging to any particular action programme, and assures the degree of decentralization and flexibility capable of responding to each community's potential and needs. Kaders chosen for nutrition training are responsible for the monthly weighing programme in their own neighbourhood.

While the *dacin* scale continued to be used, children often cried or fussed about being suspended, relatively immobile, in the cloth pants. Woven baskets or wooden boxes painted to look like an animal, an airplane, or a car suspended under the scale made weighing an interesting and fun game even for shy children and eliminated the tendency of the mothers to avoid the weighing of the children because of the unpleasantness involved. A new weight chart was designed to reinforce the important message of monthly growth.

In adopting the techniques of 'social marketing', a design team was formed that included a communications specialist, an advertising firm, and a group of physician/nutritionists. The marketing goal was set to motivate mothers to seek a monthly increase in the weight of their young children. The goal was understandable, measurable, and attainable. The *weight chart* became the prime communication tool with a market appeal and inherent emphasis on action leading to growth, replacing its usual function as a clinical record of nutritional status. A variety of 'product presentations' was field-tested among potential 'consumers', leading to a 'sales' approach that regularly affected mothers' perceptions of, and attitudes toward, monthly weight gain. A catchy slogan *Anak yang Sehat, Bertambah Umur, Bertambah Berat* ('A healthy child grows in weight as he grows in age') advertised the new, full-colour weight chart on posters.

The care with which the card messages were designed can be seen in the choice of the woman shown on the front, breast-feeding her child. The woman was chosen from a panel of photographs and drawings portraying a wide array of women, poor and wealthy, traditional and modern, each nursing a child. The model chosen represents the image of what the majority of women interviewed stated they would like to be: one cut above their own level economically, modern in appeal, but traditional in dress and reserved in composure. The wide appeal predicted by market research has been evident in the demand for posters and fliers of this 'national breast-feeding mother'.

Of greatest importance is the rainbow distribution of growth curves on the face of the card. Only the first three years are portrayed, as field experience showed that attendance of children above this age fell off considerably, that mothers are most concerned about children in the younger age group, and that children, once they reached 30–36 months, tended to grow consistently at whatever nutritional status they had by then obtained. Thus, the programme emphasis falls naturally to the child under three. The rainbow pattern is arrayed as a series of coloured channels based on the international (Harvard) standard of weight-for-age, with each channel width 5 per cent of the standard weight. No channel is considered to be normal or abnormal unless the child falls below 60 per cent of the Harvard standard. Each child is said to have his 'own colour and

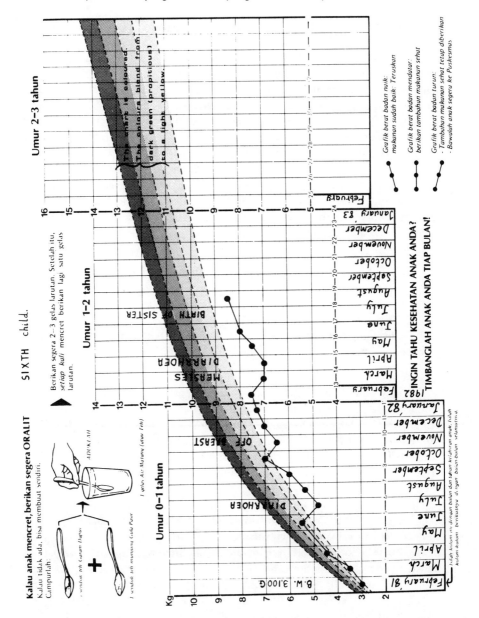

Fig. 16.2. Weight chart: only the first three years of the child's life are portrayed.

he should grow along that channel or above it'. Mothers felt that a deeper green colour represented greater health (a not surprising finding in this predominantly agricultural society), and so the colour arrangement moves from pale yellow to rich green from the lower colours to the upper ones.

However, while growth on higher channels is encouraged, there is no indication that regular growth along a lower channel is not good. Thus, children growing regularly at a weight considerably lower than the international standard continue to receive encouragement and positive feedback. Of even more importance, deviation from the normal trend of growth, even when the child is still above the arbitrary line considered as the 'border of malnutrition', is treated as an important sign of faltering growth and indicates the need for nutritional intervention by the mother to assure that the child regains his own growth pattern. Displayed prominently on the face of the card are three trend lines showing growth patterns in children:

1. A rising line accompanied by the statement that the child is healthy and growing well: 'Continue what you are doing in the month ahead'.
2. A flat trend showing no growth between two months stating: 'This is an important sign that the child is not receiving optimal food; give more food daily during the month ahead'.
3. A declining line stating: 'Mother should seek specific health advice and be certain the child is not ill, in addition to providing extra food and nutrition attention during the month ahead'.

The new weight chart was not only effective but also inexpensive. The cost of producing the card, when printed in millions of copies, is a mere US $0.05, compared with US $0.03 for the standard WHO card. Many international nutritionists who saw the card without knowing its cost stated that it must be too costly to justify its publication in full colour. This reaction is proof of the appeal of the card, and reflects in a small way the desire mothers have to own such a card and the care with which they keep the card in their homes.

The new weight chart proved to be an effective educational tool, modifying the concept of nutritional health toward one of *weight gain* rather than one of attained nutritional status.[2] With this card, the attention given to the monthly village 'score', expressed as proportion of children weighed who are gaining weight, made obvious sense. The monitoring of the programme by this single 'score' for each village became both possible and logical to mothers and the village leaders. In Godean, mothers had focused on the location of their children on a weight card (nutritional status), while the village evaluation was based on percentage gaining weight (growth). This new weight card made a consistent and uniform evaluation and monitoring system possible, stressing 'growth' of each child and 'growth' of the village.

The response to non-weight gain in many Banjarnegara villages was the establishment of a *taman gizi*, or neighbourhood nutrition club. This activity placed mother-to-mother communication in a culturally acceptable context. Using food available in their own homes, or produced in their own kitchen gardens, mothers gathered periodically to cook and serve a nutritious meal, discussing food choice among themselves and discovering methods of preparation that would make a well-rounded diet both affordable and acceptable to their children. This culturally appropriate forum based on action brought mothers together to share relevant experience without having the stigma of 'successful' and 'unsuccessful' mothers, or advisors and advisees. A *taman gizi* is a group actively based on local resources and local knowledge and it has become a popular social affair. The programme extended naturally in Banjarnegara as communities were increasingly seeking action programmes that they could carry out themselves. Women in each community became the prime motivators for neighbouring groups, and within five years weighing programmes were established in more than half the villages of the regency.

The Banjarnegara programme proved that community nutrition activities are inherently a part of a broader community development programme, and thus must adhere to community development principles of self-reliance and genuine, responsible participation. The very absence of material incentives for community nutrition workers and food supplementation, particularly with strange products from outside, proved to be a strength in this programme. The Banjarnegara approach showed what the existing government funds could do. The approach to the community and their true involvement in the evolution of this programme were not only its hallmark but also its key to success.

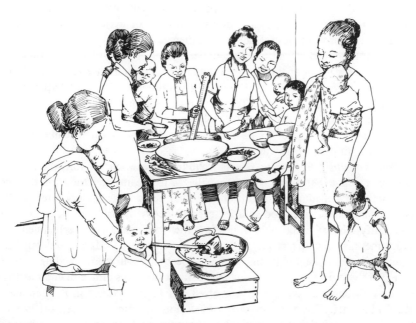

Fig. 16.3. *Taman gizi*: the neighbourhood nutrition club has become a popular social affair.

During the second Five Year Development Plan of 1974–79, the Ministry of Health adapted many of these principles in the revised Applied Nutrition Programme covering more than 800 villages in selected sites throughout the country. During a two-week field-training experience, provincial, regency and subdistrict nutritionists were exposed to the Godean and Banjarnegara communities, and they initiated the programme in one new community during the training course.[3] They then implemented, with Government budgetary and logistical support, similar activities in villages of their own provinces. The main components consisted of the following:

— monthly weighing of children under five;
— daily food supplements for four months to those 10 per cent of children in the community with the lowest weight-for-age;
— distribution of vitamin A and iron tablets;
— nutrition education; and
— oral rehydration for diarrhoea.

A review at a national workshop in 1978 demonstrated a number of common operational weaknesses. The programme had no clear objectives, which made evaluation difficult. Locations were extremely scattered and coverage was limited even within project villages; therefore, impact was difficult to see. No training network existed and there was no follow-up to the initial training of the leaders in the programme. Thus, implementation frequently deviated markedly from the planned activity. Communication support was weak, with a total absence of manuals for field staff and lack of useful media or even guidelines for clear feeding directions of practical value to mothers.

Attempts to include all children under five in a village led to considerable difficulty with the cooperation from the older children in that age group, whose mobility and general independence made the influence of maternal attention to their diet somewhat marginal. This detracted considerably from the attention that should have been given to the children in the six-month to three-year age range, when the choice of food, feeding patterns, hygiene, and the like can have the greatest impact on growth.

Supplementary feeding of selected children overwhelmed both the mothers and programme personnel. In many villages it became the focus of the programme, the weighing and nutrition messages being of secondary interest. The dependence on outside food sources, even if locally available, made programme continuity almost impossible following the four months of scheduled free supplementary feeding. Thus, rather than a sustained, village-based nutrition education effort, the programme tended to become a four month feeding activity.

From these field experiences, which involved hundreds of health and nutrition workers throughout the country, evolved the Family Nutrition Programme of REPELITA III. This national programme aims at community self-sufficiency, home food production, redistribution of existing food resources within the family setting, and greater emphasis on preventing malnutrition rather than on rehabitation of malnourished children. By focusing on the successive cohorts of nutritionally healthy children under three years old, the programme aims to achieve good nutrition in these children throughout, at least, their third year, thereby drastically reducing malnutrition among all children in the areas where the programme is operating. On this basis, guidelines for admission to the programme are to restrict eligibility to children under three years of age, and preferably those who are 6–18 months old. Six critical programme elements can be summarized:

Clear, simple, achievable, and objectively measurable programme objectives. These are (i) all children under three years of age should gain weight every month, and (ii) all children who reach the age of 36 months should have reached a weight of 11.5 kg. The development of clear programme goals, specific actions, and unequivocal objective monitoring indicators has led to a high degree of accountability by local administrators and assured their participation and involvement in reaching programme goals. The demystification of nutrition goals as exemplified in this programme has attracted the commitment of lay persons involved in programme implementation. This is a critical element in the success of making a transition to a truly community-based activity.

Emphasis is entirely on behavioural change leading to the goal 'every child should gain weight every month'. Mothers can easily understand, appreciate, and achieve this goal monthly. By contrast, improved nutritional status (or maintenance of 'normality') has less psychological attraction, is relatively static, and often leads to complacency or resignation on the part of mothers who see their children classified in a single, broad, nutritional category. Monthly growth is a self-motivating goal with recurring rewards.

A specific series of 12 messages tailored for each age grouping of several months provides a prescription for each mother to follow for any month in which her child does not gain weight. Each message specifies a feeding action, the amount of food, and the frequency with which it is to be given over the period of the next month in order to achieve the desired goal: 'weight gain'. Each message is printed on one page of a colourful flip chart, in a brief and carefully worded instruction. Thus, desired messages are uniformly transmitted, yet their local adaptation is assured by the directions to the kader to use local practices to illustrate the message.

Kaders are chosen from, among, and by, the participating village women. They are trained in a highly standardized series of five lessons teaching them: (i) how to weigh the children and fill out the weight card; (ii) how to interpret the resulting growth line; (iii) how to give nutritional advice using the weight chart; (iv) what to do for diarrhoea; and (v) what advice to give pregnant women. The nutrition kaders are encouraged to 'pair' with mothers of children who are faltering in growth and to visit them occasionally in their homes to share their own knowledge and experience in an informal setting.

A high degree of community participation and self-reliance is encouraged.

Programme goals embody the principle that all children under three years of age in the community should be weighed monthly. The monthly report form includes a statement of how many eligible children are in the community, how many have been issued weight cards, and how many came to the weighing that month. The provision of free food supplements has been avoided, and in its place communities are encouraged to use their own resources for occasional common meals, during which they discuss home food production, preparation, and feeding. Except for the initial investment in equipment: weight chart, manuals and flip chart; and recurring costs: supplies of high-dose vitamin A, iron tablets, and oral rehydration fluids, the programme will be managed and financed by the community.

Highly standardized procedures have been carefully detailed for the programme elements.[4] Use of the weight chart, the dacin scale, and the flip chart are described in a programmed text for self-learning. Organizational and management aspects of the programme in such elements as referral and monthly report forms are standardized in a manual used by the field worker advising the village. This manual is at the same time a trainer's manual for use by these field workers, containing one chapter detailing the specific objectives and methodology to be used in training community nutrition kaders. This 100-page manual forms the basis for training at all levels, from the provincial nutritionists and related administrative staff down to the field workers in the village. This 'vertical approach' to training was adopted in preference to the more usual approach whereby persons 'higher' in the system received a far more complex and detailed training, which was then abbreviated and simplified at each level as it reached down to the village level. Experience through the Ministry of Health showed that such broad-level training at the higher level resulted in considerable variation in programme implementation in the more peripheral sites, a problem that has been avoided by uniform training at provincial, Regency, and subdistrict as well as village level.

In the community, however, considerable latitude is encouraged in the choice of programme activities and implementation. The community is invited to choose its own nutrition kaders and to establish its own programme goals for coverage and targets over a given period of time. While the monthly weighing forms the backbone, they may choose to emphasize a variety of activities, such as *taman gizi*, home-garden food production, small-animal raising, treatment of minor illness and nutrition problems, such as vitamin A deficiency and anaemia, or improving their own access to the formal health care system through a programme of voluntary contribution toward health insurance schemes. Family planning clubs are often interested in a variety of welfare activities for their members, among which nutrition may be but one. Nutrition activities complement and enhance interest in village level programmes from other sectors and can be flexibly adapted to any village forum or organization.

The monitoring and reporting system is designed primarily as a stimulating and motivating tool and only secondarily as an information collection device.

REPORT FORM

Monthly report for ....
(month)

Weighing group (hamlet) .... Village .... District ....

Date of weighing .... Field Worker .... Number of kaders helping ....

Total hamlet population .... in .... families

1. Total children under 36 months old ....

2. Total children with weight charts ....

3. Total newly entered this month ....

4. Total with increased weight this month ....

5. Total with no increase in weight ....

6. Total weighed with last month weight unknown ....
   (therefore, do not know if weight increased)

7. Total weighed this month ....

Participation score   = # 2/1
Activity score   = # 7/2
Growth score   = #4/(7 − (3 + 6))
Overall score   = # 4/1

Use of supplies this month:
  Weight charts ....
  Oralyte packets ....
  Vitamin A high-dose capsules ....
  Iron folate tablets ....

Fig. 16.4. Monthly report form for village weighing post. The same form is used for summarizing results from all hamlets in each village, all villages in each subdistrict, and all subdistricts in each regency. Subdistrict and regency summaries are sent to the national capital, Jakarta, for data processing.

The coloured weight chart retained by the mother remains the basic information tool, and the monthly weight is recorded graphically on this chart. No effort is made to keep a master record of this weight, since such records were generally found not to be useful and, more importantly, to detract from the nutrition education work of the kaders.

The monthly report form is designed to encourage a clear view by the weighing group of their success toward their programme goals. The same form is used to summarize all the hamlets in the single village, all the villages in a single subdistrict, all the subdistricts in a single regency, and all the regencies in a province. The total target population, the number holding weight cards, and the number participating in monthly weighing are important participation indicators. Programme success is measured by the number of children gaining weight each month, and, for those passing 36 months of age, their attained weight at that one time. The other information on the form facilitates resupply of expendable items. The data from the monthly form are graphically displayed in each hamlet as a single vertical bar for each month, with lines at each level to indicate participation and weight gain. Programme goals as set by the community can be easily viewed from such a monthly record.

Thus, through repeated evolution of several field action projects, beginning in a single village and extending through a subdistrict and regency, and refined through experience of several years at the national level, a culturally acceptable and affordable programme has been designed. With this 'appropriate technology', including field manuals and communication tools, and the basic strategy now known, understood, and accepted by policy makers, the challenge was to find the organization and management approach that could expand the programme to reach a substantial proportion of the target population in Indonesia.

ORGANIZATION

While numerous successful nutrition *pilot projects* have been developed in Indonesia and elsewhere, the transition from small project to national programme has frequently resulted in failure. The charismatic leadership often associated with successful pilot projects tends to be lost in its transition to a nationwide programme. This is particularly true where the 'grass-roots social qualities' of the programme, such as community participation and self-reliance, appear to be key elements.

In the search for an organizational structure for broad-reaching community nutrition programmes, an analysis of the characteristics of the charismatic leader indicates some of the essential qualities of the charismatic organization necessary for mass implementation. Leadership must inspire, motivate, and engender enthusiasm and a sense of purpose for all involved. Leaders offer training, usually of a highly personal and action-orientated nature, that is geared to the level of trainees and that stimulates their responsible participation in an active learning process. Leaders provide on-going encouragement, technical supervision, and back-up in a flexible way, assuring evolution of the programme to meet local contingencies. Leaders give a sense of purpose and accomplishment, both through personal encouragement and recognition of success in all those participating. The leader leads by example, becoming a role model for those around him, who come to realize the importance of dedication to the task and respect for the role of others in programme success. While these are generally personal characteristics, they also describe the elements of a successful organization and management structure.

Indonesia's National Family Planning Coordinating Body (*BKKBN*), which, in 1980, was given overall responsibility for coordinating the National Family Nutrition Improvement Programme, embodies many of these characteristics.

Provided in 1972 with a mandate to coordinate and facilitate all involved sectors of the government in the National Family Planning effort, the BKKBN has evolved a highly successful management structure to meet these aims. BKKBN hired 7000 family planning field workers (FPFWs) to be the major communicators of the family planning message. Recruited from villages in which they would work, these FPFWs were given a short, uniform training course at 16 national training centres and have continued to receive periodic refresher courses as well as continuous education through monthly newsletters and technical bulletins. Their tast was highly target-orientated, with recruitment of new acceptors the clear goal. The terminology of family planning and its goals were supported by a mass communication effort involving simple slogans through posters, radio, newspapers, and other mass media.

By 1975 the number of current users of modern contraceptives became so high that FPFWs spent a majority of their time in resupply activities. They then established village resupply posts staffed by acceptor volunteers who received and distributed contraceptive supplies for their neighbours. From these posts developed acceptor clubs, which held monthly meetings, and they increasingly became a major factor in the extension of family planning goals and recruitment of new acceptors. These groups became highly articulate in their own communities, branching out into areas other than family planning and involving community members in other issues of common interest, such as health, nutrition, income production, village beautification, handicrafts, village art, and entertainment. Increasingly, FPFWs were called upon to address these groups about subjects beyond the boundaries of clinical family planning. By 1978, more than 40 000 acceptor clubs existed throughout Java and Bali, many of which had changed their name and primary focus to become family welfare clubs.

The Family Planning Programme in Indonesia has achieved remarkable success in the past decade. With 65 per cent of the total population of 150 million crowded onto the island of Java (representing only 7 per cent of the total land area), a crude birth rate of over 40 per 1000 threatened the future welfare of the population. Over the past decade, 14 million couples in fertile age groups have become new acceptors of family planning. The crude birth rate has declined by almost 20 per cent over a five-year period. In some large areas such as East Java, with a population of 25 million, over 50 per cent of eligible couples are currently practising family planning.

The organizational factors contributing to the BKKBN-led success in family planning are highly relevant for nutrition programming. The BKKBN has achieved:

- A high level of political commitment, starting from the President of the Republic, and extending to all civil leaders and bureaucrats in all sectors.
- A strong communication strategy, exemplified in the recruitment of village workers for face-to-face communication, use of mass media, and the formation of acceptor clubs.
- A young, flexible bureaucracy functioning as a coordinating unit among existing sectors. As a coordinating unit, the BKKBN must work with and

through other departments, providing concise goals and actions for co-operating sectors.
- A high degree of community and local leadership responsibility in programme planning, implementation, and evaluation.
- An effective programme information system working in both directions to hold the various levels together.

Appropriate as the BKKBN is, it could not implement the nutrition programme alone. Several important elements are missing. First, the credibility of any primary health care effort is closely linked to the availability of secondary back-up services for individual cases and situations that cannot be managed at the village level. Technical advice and particularly management of malnourished or continuously faltering children are necessary if FPPWs are to command the respect and support of the communities they serve. Second, programme focus on additional feeding assumes that such food is available, while in many households it clearly is not. Increased home food production thus becomes an action focus of the programme and specific family-oriented activities are needed. Third, in an Asian agricultural society, the acceptance of a family planning organization is limited, particularly among the more traditional elements of that society. In spite of the widely hailed success of the BKKBN, there still exists in many villages a substantial minority of people who are suspicious of the aims and messages of the Family Planning Programme.

An intersectoral programme was therefore designed where Health would provide the technical guidance and clinical backup. Agriculture extension workers would provide inputs for intensified home gardening, and Religion would actively seek social outreach through the mosques and churches of the country; meanwhile the BKKBN assimilated nutrition activities into its large organizational network. For months, the appropriate responsibility of each sector remained a point of contention. Factions within the BKKBN feared that a broadening of the mandate and task of the FPFWs could have a negative effect upon the family planning performance. On the other hand, many Health Department officials believed that nutrition matters should remain in the hands of health professionals, and that a detrimental diminution of programme effectiveness would result if FPFWs were given responsibility for village-level implementation. Programme supporters replied that a broader view of family welfare would strengthen family planning acceptance and continuation. Also, the current emphasis on primary health care and the present world emphasis on the 'demystification of medical technology' strongly supported the concept of turning over nutritional management to the people themselves in the village.

An important turning point in this stalemate came with a national seminar on the community nutrition programme that was conducted in a very remote rural setting in Central Java in January 1979. Top decision makers from BAPPE-NAS, the Ministries of Health and People's Welfare and the BKKBN met for several days in the field and visited numerous villages where FPFWs were effectively initiating and nurturing the village nutrition programme. Agricultural extention workers and religious leaders and other socially respected figures were actively involved. The health centre doctors provided the major motivation and guidance. Integration was de facto. This field exposure for top decision makers was one of the crucial steps in the acceptance of an inter-ministerial national programme in nutrition.

By early 1979 the Department of Health, assisted by university and private groups with extensive field and training experience, had defined the details of the programme described in a manual to be used by all workers. They designed a curriculum for a two-week field course for the purpose of retraining all BKKBN staff. Teachers from the 16 BKKBN training centres were the first to follow this course, which was run in Yogyakarta and the surrounding areas of Godean and Banjarnegara.

The Department of Agriculture developed new manuals on home food production and began retraining extension workers in the use of improved seed for vegetable, legume, and root crops. These new services would be made available through the FPFWs to the weighing groups. The Department of Religion has joined in to make the village nutrition programme one of its major social messages. Islamic scholars are preparing a booklet indicating passages from holy writings that support good nutrition and child care. Posters showing a breast-feeding mother, and using quotes from the Quran, are calling upon women to breast-feed for two whole years. The Department of Religion's backing of the national nutrition programme is leading to a much broader base of opinion-forming and respected support than had previously been thought possible for a nutrition activity.

Standardized retraining of 2000 FPFWs was carried out in the 16 regional training centres of the BKKBN from July to October 1979, using the national village nutrition workers' manual as the course guide and fieldwork manual. Supplies of *dacin* scales, weight charts, vitamin A and iron tablets, rehydration fluids, flip charts, and field manuals have flowed through the BKKBN's well-developed logistic system that effectively meets resupply needs for millions of contraceptive users. The monitoring and information system of BKKBN has been modified to receive and analyse information on monthly participation and on weight gain of children under three years of age, thus providing a sensitive index of nutritional status and growth from villages throughout Java and Bali. This rapid information collection system will become a key element of a national nutrition surveillance system, with the percentage of children gaining weight being a sensitive indicator of the need for health and nutrition inputs in food-short or epidemic-prone areas.

By mid-1982 all 7000 FPFWs were retrained and had begun weighing programmes in over 15 000 villages throughout Java and Bali. Some 2.5 million children under three years of age were enrolled and monthly reports of weight gain were being processed by the BKKBN computer in Jakarta. In addition, the Department of Health is continuing to expand its own efforts to reach into villages not yet served by the FPFWs. By 1984 this programme should reach into 40 000 villages, providing regular nutrition activities to more than half of the children under three years of age in the country. Only then will the transformation of village project to national programme truly be a reality.

CONCLUSIONS

The National Family Nutrition Improvement Programme in Indonesia was built on the development of a broad-based political commitment extending throughout many levels of government. Founded on representative national data, the importance of the nutrition situation was presented to professionals and policy makers in understandable terms and in a political context in keeping with the national objectives of development. This political commitment, reflected in the current five-year plan, is critical to the support necessary for mounting a national effort.

The specific intervention programme has adapted and refined a village-level nutrition technology that is at once culturally acceptable, understandable, and effective. Based on clear, simple, and measurable objectives, a communication strategy aimed at behavioural change to reach a national goal of every child gaining weight each month has brought a clear focus to the programme. Standardized procedures described in a simple lucid manual ensures appropriate programme actions, while a high degree of flexibility is encouraged at the field implementation level. Community participation and self-reliance are keynotes of the programme. The monitoring and information system is simple, sensitive, and oriented to both the need of the community for self-analysis and to the need to provide operational indicators for the success and extent of programme outreach.

The organizational responsibility for programme outreach has been accepted by the BKKBN, whose management structure is highly attuned to the needs of a national village-based effort. Their successful experience in training, supervision, information flow, and use of communication strategies in family planning has been adapted for use in the nutrition effort. The institutionalization of charismatic leadership in the form of a charismatic organization promises to extend the benefits of the field nutrition programme to a nationwide coverage.

These are the critical elements comprising the evolution of the national nutrition programme in Indonesia. They are an intricate and complex series of events and interactions among multiple sectors of government and private organizations, bound together by commonly accepted goals and technically appropriate activities, transmitted through a highly focused communication strategy aimed at behavioural change throughout the population. This approach should make the nutrition programme in Indonesia a truly national, self-reliant, and living example of the call by Alma Ata for 'Health for all by the year 2000'.

NOTES

1. See Rohde, J.E., Ismail, D., and Soetrisno, R., Mothers as weight watchers: the road to child health in the village. *Journal of Tropical Pediatrics and Environmental Child Health* **21**, 295–7 (1975).

2. See Haliman, A., Indonesia: community development through primary health care – the Banjarnegara experience. In *Community action – family nutrition programmes* (ed. D.B. and E.F.P. Jellife). UNICEF/Scaro, New Delhi (1977).

3. See Hendrata, L. and Rohde, J.E., Measuring weight gains. *Journal of Tropical Paediatrics and Environmental Child Health* **24** (1978).

4. Rohde, J.E., Ismail, D., Sadjimin, T., Suyadi, A., and Tugerin. Training course of village nutrition programmes. *Journal of Tropical Paediatrics and Environmental Child Health* **25** (1979).

REFERENCES

Presidential Instruction Number 14, Republic of Indonesia (1974).

Sayogyo, *ANP Evaluation Study, 1973*, Institute of Rural Social Research, Agricultural College, Bogor, Indonesia (1975).

17 A primary health care strategy for Ghana*

Richard H. Morrow examines how the Ministry of Health developed, promoted, and gained acceptance for a detailed primary health care strategy in Ghana.

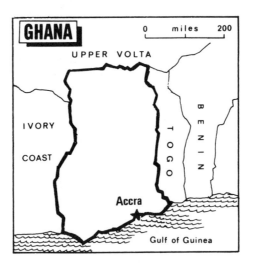

Richard H. Morrow, M.D., was Senior Health Planning Associate in the Ministry of Health, Ghana, from 1976-79. He is now Secretary of the Scientific Working Group on Epidemiology, Special Programme for Research and Training in Tropical Diseases, World Health Organization, Geneva.

This is the story of how a health planning unit (HPU) was started within the Ministry of Health (MOH), Ghana; how, as the HPU developed a rational approach to health planning, it reached conclusions that would require a radical restructuring of activities within and beyond the Ministry; and how this restructuring came to be accepted within the Ministry of Health and the Ministry of

*The work described in this article was a team effort involving colleagues from the Ministry of Health, the University of Ghana, the Kaiser Foundation International, and USAID, in particular Dr Mek Adibo, Mr A.R. Neill, Dr K.P. Nimo, Dr E.G. Beausoleil, Professor S. Ofosu-Amaah, Dr F.T. Sai, and Mr P.G. Smith amongst others. The project was supported by USAID Contract No. AIR/afr-C-1116, project No. 641–0068. Although the work was conducted by the entire team, this account is the author's own responsibility.

Economic Planning on a technical basis, and within the top decision-making levels on a political basis. A detailed strategy for primary health care (PHC) was developed, widely promoted and generally accepted.

The acceptance of the strategy was greatly aided by two special features in the approach to planning taken by the HPU. First, there was widespread involvement of individuals both within and outside the MOH in the analysis of problems and in the planning process itself. Second, a methodology was developed for quantifying the importance of the different diseases in Ghana and the impact that intervention programmes would have upon them. By quantifying the benefits that could be achieved by alternative programmes per cedi[1] expended, the methodology put health care decisions into a framework that could be appreciated by economists and decision-makers. The methodology involves estimating the cost and the amount of healthy life which may be saved by different health programmes. It clearly demonstrates that the introduction of a PHC strategy should provide a much greater improvement in the health of the Ghanaian people than an equivalent expenditure of resources put towards expansion of the conventional hospital-based system.

Although a good start towards implementation of the primary health care (PHC) system was made, this story also relates difficulties encountered and problems yet to be surmounted.

BACKGROUND TO GHANA AND ITS HEALTH ACTIVITIES

Of all the countries in Africa, Ghana should be among the most able to conduct an effective primary health care programme. Ghana has had the best education, the most developed infrastructure, the largest number per capita of well-trained health personnel, a relatively equitable distribution of resources, strong family and community traditions, and particularly able leaders in the health field.

Ghana, located on the Gulf of Guinea, in West Africa, has a population of nearly 11 million (1980) and extends about 450 miles from north to south and 250 miles from east to west. Geographically the country can be divided into three areas starting from the southern narrow coastal strip of savanna land, followed by a broad tropical rain forest extending 150–200 miles north which then merges into the northern savanna area. The Volta Lake, formed when the Akosombo Dam was constructed in the mid-1950s, is the largest manmade lake in the world and is an important geographical feature of the country.

Politically, Ghana is divided into nine regions, and the regions in turn are divided into an average of seven districts each (a total of 64 districts in 1979) with populations of about 150–180 thousand per district (see Fig. 17.1). Ghana's population has been increasing rapidly with an annual growth rate of over 3 per cent a year. The major cities have experienced very rapid growth: 30 per cent of the population now live in communities of over 5000.

In 1957 Ghana was the first of the many colonial countries in Africa to achieve independence, and it established a leadership position among the newly

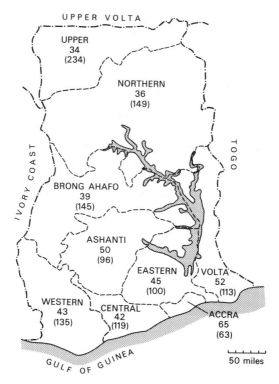

Fig. 17.1. Expectation of life and (infant mortality rates). Ghana 1976.

emerging African nations. Universal education has been an important goal for the country, and more than 50 per cent of the school-age children receive a primary school education, giving Ghana one of the highest literacy rates in Africa.

The most important export continues to be cocoa, by far the largest source of foreign exchange for the country, with timber being second. The largest industry is VALCO (Volta Aluminium Company) powered by the electricity generated at the Akosombo Dam. A modern industrial complex has been developed at the new port city of Tema near Accra. However, the major occupations continue to be those of traditional farming, fishing along the coast, and trading. For a combination of reasons, Ghana's economy has been undergoing a phenomenally destructive inflation rate in recent years, and the many, once flourishing small businesses have been dying out.

The pattern of health problems in Ghana is characteristic of most countries in Africa. The overall infant mortality rate is about 130 per 1000 live births but with a wide variation geographically. It ranges from a low of 63 per 1000 in the Greater Accra Region to a high of over 200 per 1000 in the Upper Region (see Fig. 17.1). Maternal mortality persists as a major problem ranging from an observed figure of 5 per 1000 under hospital conditions to an estimated 18 per 1000 in rural areas.

Communicable diseases such as malaria, measles, tuberculosis, onchocerciasis, and tetanus are major causes of morbidity and mortality. The disease problems of children — with malnutrition interacting with gastroenteritis, intestinal helminths, and other communicable diseases — are particularly severe. In addition, there are serious non-communicable disease problems, including sickle-cell disease, cirrhosis, hypertension, and stroke, which though very important, are not readily controllable.

Although there are a number of doctors and midwives in private practice in the large cities, most doctors are employed by and virtually all medical care is provided by the MOH. Mission hospitals, which account for about 30 per cent of the nation's hospital beds, are partially funded and staffed by the MOH and are closely coordinated with the Ministry. There are also paragovernmental military and mines hospitals and medical services which provide care to limited population groups. Figure 17.2 shows the sources of health inputs.

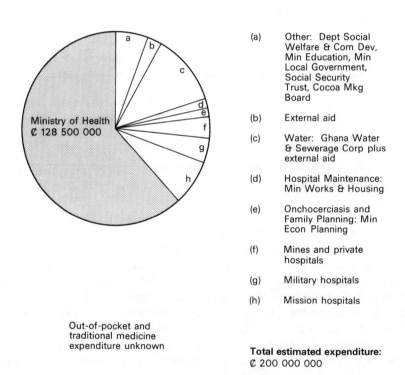

(a) Other: Dept Social Welfare & Com Dev, Min Education, Min Local Government, Social Security Trust, Cocoa Mkg Board

(b) External aid

(c) Water: Ghana Water & Sewerage Corp plus external aid

(d) Hospital Maintenance: Min Works & Housing

(e) Onchocerciasis and Family Planning: Min Econ Planning

(f) Mines and private hospitals

(g) Military hospitals

(h) Mission hospitals

Ministry of Health
¢ 128 500 000

Out-of-pocket and traditional medicine expenditure unknown

Total estimated expenditure: ¢ 200 000 000

Fig. 17.2. Sources of health inputs. The Ministry of Health controls about 65 per cent of total spending on formal health care and health-related activities. Source: 1976–77 Budget Estimates. External aid is for 1975 from the UNDP. Prepared by National Health Planning Unit. December, 1976. From Health Planning Data Book for Ghana (1977).

In the eighteen years since independence, there has been a great increase in the resources going into health – a threefold increase in the number of doctors, a fourfold increase in the number of nurses, and a more than twofold increase in the number of hospital beds (see Table 17.1). Furthermore, there has been a substantial increase in the complexity of services being provided. Ministry of Health expenditures rose fourfold in real terms, peaking in 1974–75 at Cedi 5^{80} (= US \$5.04) per capita (adjusted to consumer price index of 1963 and at the official exchange rate of US \$1.00 = Cedi 1^{15} in 1977).

Table 17.1. Manpower and facilities

Category	1960	1977	Percentage increase 15 years	Population per health professional/bed 1960	1977
Physicians	383	1100	187	17 564	9600
Dental surgeons	19	60	216	354 052	176 000
Nurses	1554	7840*	405	4329	1347
Midwives	130	1500	1054	51 746	7040
Hospital beds and cots	5787	13 500	133	1162	782

*4200 professional nurses and 3640 auxiliary nurses. In addition 860 nurses were also qualified as midwives.

Source: 1960 figures, *The health services in Ghana*, 1961, D. Brachott.
1977 figures, National Health Planning Unit. 1977 population estimate: 10 560 000.

In spite of this significant increase in health resources and complexity of health services, there has been little change in the administrative and managerial machinery to run the Ministry. For these reasons the MOH had a serious interest in strengthening the planning and management capacity within the Ministry. In the past, both before and since independence, a number of health plans were generated by the Ministry. These plans were put together either by a visiting consultant or, in some cases, by a specially selected committee. The Brachott Report of 1961 was perhaps the most comprehensive of these plans in scope and served as the basic plan of the Ministry for the next ten years. In addition, Ghana has a rich history of creative health schemes (e.g. the Medical Field Units, the Reindorf Yaws Campaign, etc.), several of which anticipated the underlying concepts of the present primary health strategy (Sai 1982). For some time, however, there has been an appreciation of the need for an on-going planning capability within the Ministry.

ESTABLISHMENT OF A NATIONAL HEALTH PLANNING UNIT (HPU) WITHIN THE MINISTRY OF HEALTH

The MOH in 1976, following a lengthy preparation period, established a health planning unit (HPU) assisted by the Kaiser Foundation International with funding from USAID. The objectives were: (i) to institutionalize an on-going planning process within the MOH and (ii) to establish a system of planning and delivery of low cost-effective health services for the entire country.

The responsibilities of the HPU were divided into five functional areas as follows:

1. Policy formulation.
2. Health assessment, programme evaluation, and health systems design.
3. Human resources.
4. Finance, budget, and control.
5. Logistics and delivery of health care services.

Although the first efforts were addressed to the MOH itself as an organization, it was recognized that the health of the people depended on many factors outside the direct control of the MOH. Therefore, the Planning Unit developed early relationships with other Ministries, particularly the Ministries of Economic Planning and of Finance. Later, with the development of the PHC strategy, there was more active cooperation and interchange with the Ministry of Local Government, the Department of Social Welfare and Community Development, the Ministry of Education, the Ministry of Agriculture, the Ghana Water and Sewerage Corporation and the Church Hospital Association of Ghana, and others. From the beginning the HPU worked closely with individuals from the University of Ghana and especially with the Department of Community Health.

During the first phase of building the base for the HPU, a series of workshops (referred to as 'Operation Dialogue' in keeping with the then military government) involving key decision-makers both within and outside the MOH was conducted to promote an understanding of the value of a Planning Unit within the Ministry of Health, to dispel possible suspicion and misunderstanding of what a Planning Unit might be doing, and to gain considered opinion on the problems and possible solutions that the MOH was facing.

The Planning Unit developed the following principles:

1. Planning should be linked with budgeting to ensure that plans can be translated into action.
2. Effective planning requires contributions from all levels in the system. From the top political and technical echelons must come policies, guidelines, overall priorities, and strategies, whereas from the district and community levels must come data evaluation and recommendations for operational activities based upon experience (Fig. 17.3).
3. Decentralization of the planning and budgeting should be carried out as far as possible so as to involve those responsible at the operational level directly in the planning of their activities.
4. Planning and coordination of activities should be carried out in cooperation with ministries and units both within and outside the MOH.

In order to carry out the work of planning, the Planning Unit developed two important mechanisms:

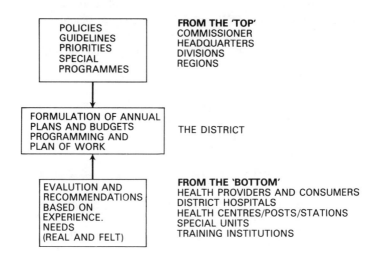

Fig. 17.3. 'Top-down/bottom-up' planning. (From: An Approach to Planning the Delivery of Health Care Services. Manual No. 1. National Health Planning Unit, Ministry of Health, Accra, Ghana (1979).)

1. The plan of work.
2. Project teams to carry out the work.

The plan of work was organized into five sections according to functional areas of responsibility as indicated above; specific tasks were defined in each area, starting and completion dates for each task were listed, and the estimated staff time required for each was worked out. Thus the 'what, when, and who' were detailed.

The project team approach was developed in order to carry out much of the work of the Planning Unit. Team members were drawn from senior staff of the Planning Unit and were supplemented by others from the MOH, the University, and other Ministries, thus adding expertise in specific subject areas, creating useful linkages with other groups and increasing the participation of many others in the planning process. Short-term consultants were sometimes used for specific subject areas, but they always worked with a project team in order to provide for coordination and continuity when the consultant departed.

PLANNING THE PRIMARY HEALTH CARE STRATEGY

In planning of any sort there are three major needs:

A. The need to know where we are ('here').
B. The need to know where we want to be ('there').
C. The need to know how to get from 'here' to 'there'.

A. For national health planning knowing 'where we are' involves:

- Assessment of the health status of the population, i.e., information about demography, vital statistics, morbidity, and mortality.
- Inventory of the health resources, i.e. the human resources, the facilities and equipment, and finances available.
- Evaluation of the current health-related programmes, i.e. the effectiveness, efficiency, and coverage achieved by the present use of the health resources.
- Appreciation of community perspectives about health.

B. The knowing 'where we want to be' involves:

- Formulation of explicit national health policies stated in operationally useful terms.
- Clearly defined goals stated in terms of specific objectives with time-limited targets to be achieved.

C. The knowing how to get from 'here' (A) to 'there' (B) involves:

- Deciding the right things to do, i.e. establishing health programme priorities.
- Doing the right things in the right way, i.e. proper management of the programmes established.

Health status assessment — the 'where we are?' need

The first project team was assigned to carry out a health status assessment by assembling the available data, largely from the Centre for Health Statistics, in order to establish the 'where we are?' need. However, assessment of the health status indicated that despite the remarkable increase in resources going into the health sector, the general health status of the population was still low (see Fig. 17.4). In the previous ten years there had been little or no improvement in the infant mortality rate, the maternal mortality rate, nor in communicable disease rates. Indeed, the incidence of yaws and cholera had increased dramatically.

Just at this time the Ministry of Health and the University of Ghana collaborated with the Institute of Development Studies at the University of Sussex, England (IDS 1978), to study the existing health-care system in two districts of the country. The 'where are we?' question was thus answered both by identifying the pattern of ill-health and by identifying the pattern of health-care resources and the shortcomings as well as strengths in the way they were being used (de Kadt and Segall 1978). A document prepared by the HPU entitled 'A primary health care strategy for Ghana' (HPU, MOH, 1978) gave the following analysis:

'The basic reason (for the lack of progress) is that the health services have been doing the wrong things because of misplaced priorities. The existing health services system funnels resources towards the minority of the population having access to hospital-based services which cater to specialized health problems.

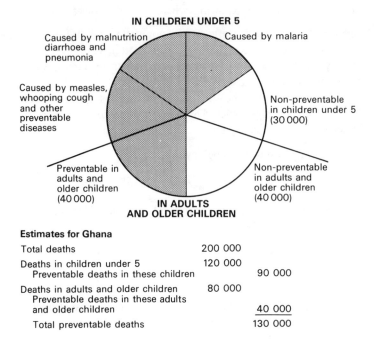

Fig. 17.4. Preventable deaths in Ghana per year. (From: A Primary Health Care Strategy for Ghana, April 1978, Ministry of Health, Accra, Ghana.)

The situation is strikingly illustrated in Fig. 17.5 referring to Ghana's 'health care dilemma'. It shows how the financial resources of the nation are being allocated in reverse proportion to the numbers of people in need!

Four conditions have been identified as the root cause of this situation in which Ghana, like many other countries, finds itself. These conditions are:

1. Emphasis on the construction of facilities rather than the provision of services.
2. Over-sophisticated training with emphasis on specialized hospital-based services for the few, rather than preventive and promotive services for everyone.
3. Poor and unequitable deployment of health staff.
4. A 'top-down' health care delivery system with a noticeable lack of co-ordination with other sectors (social welfare and community development, water and sewerage, agriculture, etc.) and little or no community involvement.

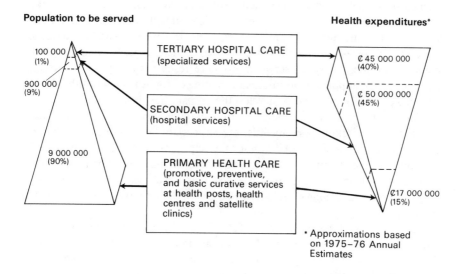

Fig. 17.5. The health care dilemma in Ghana. The distribution of funds and personnel for primary health care compared to costly hospital-based care is in inverse proportion to the numbers of people that need to be reached. The health care pyramid for Ghana is upside down! (From: A Primary Health Care Strategy for Ghana, April 1978, Ministry of Health, Accra, Ghana.)

The present health care system of Ghana can be likened to a pyramid with the Korle Bu Teaching Hospital (in Accra) at the top and a network of health posts and dressing stations at the bottom.

This is a system based on service delivery points (i.e. facilities). It focusses attention on bricks and mortar rather than on health services for the people.

This emphasis on facilities creates false 'needs' among the people for more facilities. Good health becomes synonymous with the provision of a doctor and a hospital rather than the enjoyment of a disease-free environment.

Under these conditions, each community without a health post believes it should have one; each community with a health post wants to expand it to a health centre; and each community with a health centre sees a 'need' to add a surgical theatre and ward and bring a surgeon to town. The pressure continues upward to regional levels with attendant burgeoning demands for financial and manpower resources.

This upward pressure absorbs all available resources and leaves an ever-increasing vacuum at the bottom of the pyramid where the real health needs of the nation continue to multiply.

A health care system whose priority is to directly address the diseases suffered by the majority of people will lead to a direct decline in the need for costly secondary and tertiary hospital services. Hospital-based curative services have received the greatest amount of attention in Ghana. But they require highly

trained personnel and expensive equipment, and have consumed the bulk of resources set aside for health care by the Government. Because of inadequate
public health and primary care services, patients with preventable conditions
continue to over-load the hospital services which in itself leads to greater
demand for more hospital services. As more resources are put into the construction and equipping of hospitals and training of sophisticated health workers,
even fewer resources are left to develop the primary health care system.

For most preventable conditions (moderately advanced leprosy, schistosomiasis, kwashiorkor, poliomyelitis, etc.) the elaborate hospital care required
after the damage is discovered is not only expensive, but is also only partially
effective, thus compounding the consequences of this inappropriate allocation
of resources. It is an unfortunate paradox that the *demand* for services occurs
only after illness becomes evident; while the *need* for services is before illness
occurs.

The people, their elders, leaders and chiefs, and therefore the political decision-
makers perceive the basic issues of health care in terms of hospitals and doctors.
This view is reinforced by doctors themselves who have been trained in the
sophisticated, intellectually intriguing disciplines of diagnosis and therapy of
individually ill people. Their attention is focused on the *sick who seek their
help*. But the need is to maintain the health of *those who are not yet ill*.

National health policy — 'the 'where we want to be'

From the beginning of the Planning Unit's establishment, it was appreciated that
explicit formulation of the policies of the Ministry would be necessary to carry
out effective planning. During 'Operation Dialogue' this need for clear policy
guidelines was emphasized time and again by the participants as a prerequisite
to planning. As with most nations, Ghana's policies were unwritten and somewhat vague. The generally understood policy of 'the best health care possible
for everyone' was subject to a great variety of interpretations and could not
serve as a firm basis for planning an overall health-care system.

The role of the Planning Unit in policy formulation was to serve as a secretariat to the Directorate of the Ministry, to circulate drafts of the policy for
broad review, and to conduct workshops for discussion of the draft policy
statement in preparation for final acceptance.

Following a series of meetings in 1977, the Director of Medical Services (DMS)
prepared a draft statement for the Planning Unit to develop. Because of its
importance and its sensitivity, the policy draft was widely circulated, discussed
at workshops, and revised several times until a consensus within the Ministry
was reached.

The policy explicitly stated that the goals of the Ministry of Health were the
following:

— 'To maximize the total amount of healthy life of the Ghanian people', and

— To assure that 'Every Ghanian shall have ready access to basic and primary health care' . . . and that there will be 'mechanisms for prompt referral' of those requiring higher levels of care.

The primary health care concept paper of 1977 went on to specify two objectives to be met by 1980:

— To achieve basic and primary health care for 80 per cent of the population of Ghana, and
— to attack effectively the disease problems that contribute 80 per cent of the unnecessary death and disability afflicting Ghanaians.

More specific sections of the policy statement dealt with the strengthening of the management of health services, health manpower development, and the organization of comprehensive health services. The primary health care strategy for Ghana, discussed below, fully incorporates the principles and guidelines of these new health policies.

The development of a primary health care strategy — 'The 'how to get from here to there'

Establishing health programme priorities — 'deciding on the right things to do'

The HPU developed a method for assessing the health status of the population in order to compare the relative importance of the different disease problems in Ghana. Since the health policy stated that the goal of the MOH was to maximize the total amount of healthy life of the Ghanaian people, an approach was developed to measure loss of healthy life due to the various diseases.

The three most important effects that a disease may have in a community are as causes of illness, disability, and death. With some exceptions, other social and economic effects of a disease are directly related to its severity as measured by these three factors. Each of these factors was quantified in terms of the number of days of healthy life lost due to a disease; the total number of days lost in the community was used as a measure of the health impact of the disease.

The major information needed included the following:

— The annual incidence of the disease.
— The disability caused by the disease.
— The case fatality rate of the disease.

These data are not routinely available, but the project team was able to make best estimates obtaining data from a variety of sources including: the National Census; age-, sex-, and region-specific death rate estimates from a special sample of the census (Gaisie 1976); cause of death from death certificates (available on about 12 per cent of all deaths in Ghana — mostly deaths in hospitals and therefore a biased, but useful sample); in-patient and out-patient statistics, special surveys and published studies; and interviews with experienced clinicians.

Table 17.2. Disease problems of Ghana — ranked in order of
healthy life lost*

Rank order	Disease	Days of healthy life lost per 1000 persons per year	Percentage of total
1	Malaria	32 600	10.2
2	Measles	23 400	7.3
3	Pneumonia (child)	18 600	5.8
4	Sickle-cell disease	17 500	5.5
5	Malnutrition (severe)	17 500	5.5
6	Prematurity	16 800	5.2
7	Birth injury	16 400	5.2
8	Accidents	14 900	4.7
9	Gastroenteritis	14 500	4.5
10	Tuberculosis	11 000	3.5
11	Cerebrovascular disease	10 400	3.3
12	Pneumonia (adult)	9100	2.9
13	Tetanus (neonatal)	6900	2.2
14	Cirrhosis	6600	2.1
15	Congenital malformations	6000	1.9
16	Complications of pregnancy	5900	1.8
17	Hypertension	5100	1.6
18	Intestinal obstruction	4900	1.6
19	Typhoid	4800	1.5
20	Meningitis	4600	1.5
21	Hepatitis	4600	1.5
22	Pertussis	4600	1.5
23	Other birth diseases	4600	1.5
24	Tetanus (adult)	4500	1.4
25	Schistosomiasis	4400	1.4
Total of first 25 diseases		270 200	84.9

*Modified from Ghana Health Assessment Project Team (1981).

By the use of these estimates, it was possible to approximate the amount of healthy life lost through illness, disability, and death as a consequence of each disease. Table 17.2 ranks the first 25 diseases in order of their importance, measured in terms of the days of healthy life lost per 1000 population attributed to onset of the disease in one year (Ghana Health Assessment Team 1981).

Developing a measure for the relative importance of disease problems is only the first step towards establishing health programme priorities. The second step is to estimate the effects of different health interventions on the incidence (such as immunization, vector control, treatment of infectious cases, etc.), case fatality and disability (by treatment, early case finding, etc.) due to the diseases and work out the benefits of each intervention as measured by the number of healthy days of life saved. The third step is to determine the costs of each intervention procedure or programme and calculate the benefit to cost ratios (healthy days of life saved per cedi expended).

Several levels of priorities were considered. First, all procedures that might affect each of the disease problems were considered. Then programme alternatives consisting of different combinations of procedures or methods of administering them were examined; and finally, different systems incorporating programme alternatives were studied. By comparing the amount of healthy life saved per cedi expended, health programme priorities could be established on a technical basis. This approach makes every assumption and each step explicit so that if there are disagreements with conclusions, the underlying assumptions and data can be re-examined.

The primary health care strategy itself

The analysis of the impact of the major disease problems in Ghana was summarized above in Table 17.2. Examination of the effects of possible health-directed activities towards these problems and the costs that would be required for their implementation reinforced the importance for community and family involvement if these activities were to be effectively carried out. Further, the analysis pinpointed very clearly a limited number of highly specific, but relatively simple activities that would be most cost-effective.

The general framework of the primary health care system – anticipating the recommendations put forth at the Alma Alta Conference in 1978 – was based upon a three-tier system as follows (see Table 17.3).

At the community level, labelled level (A), there are community health workers selected and compensated by the community itself, but trained by the Ministry of Health in primary preventive and promotive procedures for simple, first-level curative measures, with emphasis on pregnancy management, child health promotion, environmental protection, and mobilization for health-related community projects. There are at least two types of level (A) workers: the traditional birth attendant (TBA) who usually is illiterate and middle-aged; and community health workers (CHW) who generally have a primary school level education. A third function, organizing for community development, may involve a village development worker (VDW) or, more commonly, this function is the responsibility of a village development committee.

At the second level, level (B), there are community health nurse-midwives (CHN/MW) who have additional minimal training in therapeutic procedures, and community environmental development officers who are assistant health sanitarians with additional training in therapeutic procedures as well. These are people with middle-school leaving certificates, though some have a secondary school education, who have completed two years of Ministry of Health training. Their principal responsibilities include the technical supervision of the village health workers, all routine immunizations and care of patients referred from level (A). They are employees of the Ministry of Health.

The district level, or level (C), with a population of 150–200 000, is the key

Table 17.3. The number of personnel needed for the primary health care system. Approximations

Level	Name of team	Catchment area Radius (km)	Area (km²)	Population per team	Health workers	Usual number per team	Number per district (range)	Number for country
A	Local community	2	12	500	1. Community health workers (CHW)	1-3	500	30 000
					2. Traditional birth attendants (TBA)	1-5	3-500	20 000
					3. Village development worker (VDW) or community committee	1	300	18 000
B	Health station	8	200	5000	1. Community health nurse/midwife (CHN/MW)	2-3	40-60	3000
					2. Community environment development office (CEDO)	1-2	20-40	1500
C	District	40	5000	200 000	District Health Management Team			
					District medical officer	1	—	65
					District public health nurses	2-4	—	130-260
					District community health specialists (district health inspectors)	1-2	—	65-130
					District health administrator	1	—	65
					Senior medical officer (hospital)	1	—	65

level for management of the entire system. A district health management team, consisting of a district medical officer who has special postgraduate training along with a district public health nurse, a district health administrator, and a district health inspector, works in direct relation with the district chief executive to facilitate an integrated approach to total community development. Each district will also have a small team of medical field unit personnel trained for communicable disease surveillance, although in many regions not all districts would have such a group and regional medical field unit teams would have to divide their time amongst a number of districts. Figure 17.6 shows how this is integrated with the health system.

The implementation of the strategy over the next ten years will be the principal instrument for carrying out the major objectives of the Ministry as stated in the health policy. To be emphasized, however, is that the PHC system supplements and extends the present largely hospital-based health services, rather than supplanting them; it should enable the hospital-based services to concentrate on rendering the specialized referral care for which hospitals are designed.

IMPLEMENTATION OF THE PRIMARY HEALTH CARE SYSTEM

The HPU in conjunction with others from the MOH including the regional medical officers and the Department of Community Health conducted a five week intensive training programme for the first nine (one from each Region) District Health Management Teams before they began their new responsibilities in early 1979.

In addition, the HPU identified and initiated project teams to develop a number of key aspects of the PHC system. These included the following:

- An analysis of the health manpower situation and an outline of the major training and retraining programmes required for the PHCS. The most important changes involved the enhanced role and increased responsibilities of nurses.
- A model district health action plan.
- The basic drug and medication requirements for the PHC system for a district and for the whole country when full implementation was achieved.
- The development of a health data system for the PHC system.

Analysis of the health manpower situation

An important task carried out by the HPU that had direct bearing on the planning for the PHC strategy was an analysis of the health manpower and training situation. As indicated earlier, health manpower for Ghana has increased greatly over the past 10 years. The training programmes developed over this time were geared to continually increase the numbers of trained health personnel for most major categories of health workers. The total number of newly trained health workers for 1977 was nearly 1500, an increase of 15 per cent over the 1976 total of 9500 personnel employed. This increase was much greater than the population growth and greatly exceeded the economic growth rate.

The overwhelming number of health workers has been trained for and

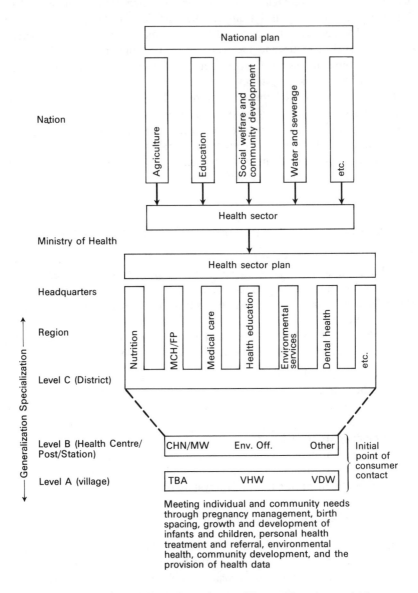

Fig. 17.6. The integration of health services. (From: Planning and Management of Health Services at the District Level. Manual No. 2. National Health Planning Unit, Ministry of Health, Accra, Ghana (1979).)

deployed to hospital positions. Those trained for environmental services, epidemiological services, public health and community health nursing, and nutrition extension work, together constituted less than a quarter of all trained health workers. With the re-examination of health service priorities and the development of the PHC strategy, major new training and retraining programmes were clearly required. By retraining presently available health personnel and by converting some of the present training programmes, particularly those for enrolled nurses and community health nurses, it seemed possible to meet the requirements of the PHC system with little increase in personnel costs over the current projections.

Nurses are by far the largest group of trained health personnel, and the most important issues raised by the health manpower analysis concerned the training programmes for nurses (see Table 17.4). The state registered nurse training programme had commendably high quality and broad coverage, but with so many graduates scheduled for specialized areas there was virtually no increase projected for SRNs for the general services. For example, psychiatric nursing was the single largest specialized area and as projected, would claim one-third of all SRN graduates over the next ten years, primarily for institutionalized psychiatric care.

The Health Centre Superintendent Programme had been designed to train senior nurses to provide PHC at the Health Centre and Health Post level, but it had evolved to emphasize curative care provided to out-patients. If midwifery were to be added and emphasis restored to community health practice, then the Health Centre Superintendent would be an ideal choice to serve as a Level B community health nurse midwife. However, the numbers being turned out are far too few for this purpose, and the number of SRNs being trained would have had to be more than double to meet the needs. Nevertheless, expansion of this sort of training would come close to meeting some important needs of the PHC system.

The projected increase in trained midwives was enormous, but this was largely because of the policy adopted to train all nurses in midwifery. Nevertheless, properly deployed, the 6000+ midwives projected for 1990 would be sufficient to deliver the 720 000 births anticipated that year at the rate of 10 births per month per midwife. This potential should be borne in mind in relation to plans for the extensive retraining of traditional birth attendants.

The very large projected increase in enrolled nurses was much greater than could be absorbed by the health system and constituted a very serious problem. The quality of training for these nurses was highly variable and all required considerable supervision on the job by qualified professional nurses who would continue to be in short supply. Analysis of the training programmes for other categories of health workers revealed similar problems.

Although health personnel needs should be established on the basis of the health needs of the people, the major constraining factor for further growth in health manpower is the economic capacity of the country to pay for the services. This is particularly true for the most highly trained: the doctors, the professional nurses, and the technologists. These groups have alternatives to the MOH for employment, and increasing numbers are departing from the service. If the present output of trained health personnel is continued, Ghana will soon be using its very costly training programmes, especially those for doctors and nurses, largely for the benefit of other countries.

A health data system for PHC

A most important tool for management and evaluation is a satisfactory record system. The system in use by the MOH had major defects which to a large extent reflected the deficiencies of the health system itself. Many forms were overly complicated and were intended for use at the central level rather than for use at the point of collection. Little use was made of the large amount of information gathered – the principal purpose seemed to be that of satisfying the requests of WHO for information!

On the other hand, there was no information available about who should be receiving the various services such as ante-natal care, immunization, tuberculosis therapy, etc. Thus, there was no way of establishing targets to be achieved or work to be conducted.

With the introduction of the PHC system, in which promotive and preventive care were emphasized and for which there was a clear need to know the denominator targets to be reached, a complete revision of the data system was required. A first approximation to the data system needed was worked out. Although it had not yet been tested, the principles upon which it was based are important. Simplified records for each level of personnel were devised. Emphasis throughout was on the collection of the minimum amount of data necessary in the simplest possible fashion. In every case, the fundamental purpose in collecting information was for the management and evaluation of the activity being carried out at that level. Data collected by level A personnel was to provide the basis for the planning of that person's work, to evaluate his/her accomplishments, and to form the basis for supervision and evaluation by the level B workers when they visited level A.

Output of the data system at each level was to assist in the establishment of the target group for each of the programmes and to provide some data for evaluation of the programme. However, to evaluate the health status of the population while the PHC system was being implemented, an approach based upon a periodic health examination of a sample of the population was devised. The examination, of a random sample to include about 2000 persons every two or three years in a district, was to consist of questions concerning the use of health services, the present state of health, pregnancy history from women, anthropometric measures on children, physical examination, and blood, urine, and stool examinations for a limited number of indicator conditions (adapted from Belcher *et al*. 1976). Thus the major instrument for evaluation was a separate assessment of the system's output determined by objective measures in the change of health status

Table 17.4. Health personnel titles and description in Ghana

Title	Description	Approx. annual median salary
Enrolled nurse	A two-year course following Middle School Leaving Certificate or some secondary school. Hospital oriented	₵1044
Community health	A two-year course after Middle School Leaving Certificate or some secondary school. Public health oriented	₵1380
Qualified registered nurse (QRN)	Three-year course after Middle School Leaving Certificate. Recently discontinued	₵1500
State registered nurse (SRN)	Three-year course after secondary school	₵1620
Midwife	Two-and-half year course after Middle School Leaving Certificate or some secondary school	₵1620
Enrolled nurse/ midwife	Two years midwifery training after Enrolled Nurse	₵1380
SRN/midwife QRN/midwife	One to one-and-half years of midwifery training after nursing course	₵1620–1800
Ward sister	SRN/midwife or QRN/midwife	₵1800–2100
Public health nurse	SRN/midwife plus one year course	₵2172
Health centre superintendent	Male QRN or SRN or female QRN/ midwife or SRN/midwife plus at least five years working experience plus one-year course with emphasis on primary clinical care	₵2556

Notes: Qualifying examinations are required for admission to all training schools.
These professional health personnel are each entitled to subsidized housing and other benefits.
Source: Health Planning Data Book for Ghana, National Health Planning Unit, Ministry of Health, Accra, Ghana (1977).

of the population.

A third feature of the data system was that individual patient records would be retained by the patient (or mother in the case of children). Studies in Ghana indicated that patient-retained records were lost less frequently than those kept by the teams of out-patient clerks in the health facilities; they speeded up registration at out-patient centres; and with the high mobility of the Ghanaian population, the records remained with the patient (Danfa Project 1979).

LESSONS LEARNED AND PUZZLES REMAINING

By 1980 genuine progress had been made in getting a functioning primary health care system started in Ghana. An effective health planning unit had been established within the MOH. An overall strategy for PHC had been worked out which, following widespread discussions with personnel at all levels and in all regions both from the MOH and with key individuals from the University, other Ministries, and other agencies, was accepted and adopted as the principal means to fulfill the goals as stated in the health policy statement of the Government of Ghana. Implementation of the programme had begun with the identification, training, and installation of District Health Management Teams in the first nine districts, one district in each Region. Much had been accomplished; yet much more remained to be done.

The following paragraphs outline important issues and problems identified by the HPU that would require careful consideration in the future. In some cases, crucial decisions could only be made at the local and district levels, especially those concerning community activities. Considerable effort in the micro-planning for the logistical support and the training and retraining programmes for the District and Regional level would be required. For some issues, new approaches would have to be tried. Finally, there were some problems encountered that were beyond the control of the MOH.

Issues concerning community health workers

From the experience gained from the Brong Ahafo Regional Integrated Development Project (BARIDEP) (World Health Organization 1979) and in the Danfa Comprehensive Rural Health and Family Planning Project (Danfa Project 1979), it seemed that in Ghana, community health workers could be chosen by the community and adequately compensated for their activities provided that the MOH undertook the training, technical supervision, and provision of the necessary supplies. In some communities these community health workers, who usually were relatively young people with secondary school-leaving certificates, worked nearly full-time for the community, but in other communities they worked part-time or even on a voluntary basis.

There are large differences in the capacity of communities to provide compensation for community health workers (CHWs). In the Brong Ahafo Region, where there was a relatively healthy agricultural economy, the communities generally found little difficulty in compensating the community health workers to mutual satisfaction. Compensation was provided during the training period largely by cash; thereafter CHWs were paid either in cash or in kind or both. Some village development committees also helped the CHW with his/her farm work (Kintampo Workshop 1979). Experiences in other districts, however, were not all satisfactory. Most communities were quite happy to work out a once-and-for-all, one-shot payment for any particular project, but many communities had difficulty in obtaining revenues on a regular basis for local expenditures. Some community health workers quit their activities when they no longer received regular compensation. Nevertheless, this was the minority experience. District Health Management Teams were looking into possible alternatives, there being considerable variation in the way that local taxes were collected and dispersements made from the local, district, and regional levels. Possibilities included rebates from regional sources for those communities embarking on the PHCS. These are issues that can only be settled at the local and district level.

The local selection and compensation of community health workers by the communities themselves was in marked contrast to the course being followed in Nigeria where all workers in the health system were to have a career position within the Ministry or Government services. But in Ghana, particularly as a result of the experiences in **BARIDEP** and Danfa, the consensus was that the success of community health workers would depend upon their being members of the community, having intimate knowledge of their community and having the community's full trust. Further, since their role was clearly limited and often part-time, it was felt that such individuals would be more likely to continue in their positions without moving away, thus providing stability of service.

This principle of local responsibility, however, is in conflict with the principle of equity. It was often pointed out that those living in urban areas had access to free medical care; yet under this scheme for community health worker compensation, the rural communities would pay for their own health workers, albeit that drugs and supplies would be provided by the MOH. This inequity seemed particularly unfair since in Ghana the principal exports and sources of wealth for the country were from the rural areas. In practice, however, this conflict did not seem to be of great importance to the communities; most communities in which the programme was started were quite satisfied with the arrangements.

Problems with community health workers included a few instances in which they overplayed their role, charging for drugs, etc., but the responsibility for discipline and control of supplies was that of the community, and generally this seemed to work well. A much more serious problem was the maintaining of supplies for the community health workers and community health nurses/midwives. There were insufficient supplies going from regional stores to the District Health Management Team; this, in turn, was related to a general, national shortage of drugs and supplies.

There were also serious shortcomings with transport. All District Health Management Teams were to be provided with a vehicle and level B personnel with bicycles or motorbikes. Vehicles and their maintenance were budgeted and allocated but there were delays in the delivery of the vehicles. Again this was a reflection of the national situation, but it caused disruption in the continuity of both supervision and supplies. This sort of disruption is probably the single greatest threat to the system. In general, communities met their commitments in terms of the selection and remuneration of community health workers, but all too frequently, the District Health Management Teams were unable to keep their commitments due to deficiencies beyond their control in transport and supplies.

An important lesson is that there must be a guarantee to provide the necessary transport and supplies for the District Health Management Team and for the community health nurse-midwives at level B to ensure continuing supervision and support for the community health workers. Promises to communities that are not kept will doom future efforts. Programmes must not be expanded or, indeed, even started until there is reasonable assurance that the supervision and supplies can be maintained.

The retraining of traditional birth attendants was well received and caused few problems, but they required frequent revisits and review of the new delivery procedures. Compensation was continued in the traditional manner. However, the assignment of ante-natal care activities, which was not part of their tradition, has not met with great success in several communities. In these communities ante-natal care might need to be included in the responsibilities of community health workers, leaving only the actual delivery to the TBAs.

Issues of decentralization

Because of the heterogeneity in the nature of communities and districts throughout Ghana, the principle of decentralization with basic responsibility for implementation to lie with the District Health Management Team was built into the strategy for PHC. The success of the programme was considered to depend very much upon the capability and dedication of the DHMT and their ability to adapt the general principles of the total programme to their specific situations. However, decentralization with considerable flexibility for local decision-making requires highly skilled and responsible personnel. The selection of the first nine District Health Management Teams was quite difficult and in some regions stretched the availability for personnel within the region. Extension of the system requiring such able personnel to the remaining 55 districts constitutes a formidable problem even when spread over the planned 10 year phase-in period.

Retraining and redeployment

The issues of retraining and redeployment of community health nurses and the training of sufficient numbers of them over the next 10 years remain a major challenge. In a very important sense the level B community health nurse, with training in midwifery and simple curative procedures as well as additional training for the teaching and supervision of community health workers, is the key to the actual operation of PHC. The community health nurse midwife is the one truly new category of health worker required for the PHC system as it was designed. The two major pilot projects, the BARIDEP and the Danfa programmes, generally used more highly trained nurses such as SRNs and Health Centre Superintendents in their community health worker programmes and so, too, did the first DHMTs. The use of community health nurses who have two years' post-primary school training with the additional training in midwifery, selected curative measures, and management-teaching skills have not yet been adequately tested. If the timetable for extension of the PHC system to cover the country by 1990 is to be met, then there is no hope of meeting the numbers required (see Table 17.3) by using more highly trained nurses according to the health manpower analysis noted above. Further, the posting of CHN/MWs to level B health post facilities means posting them to generally small and rather remote villages lacking the amenities and companionship that could be found in most of the level C district level towns. The system as designed is expecting miraculous results from personnel with limited education and outlook. Nevertheless, the early experience of the District Health Management Team in recruiting nurses for this level was encouraging and seemed to be reasonably satisfactory in the case of the first few. Recruiting, training, and maintaining the personnel needed for level B, however, will require continuing efforts and probably new approaches.

The role of nurses

Although nurses were involved in all workshops concerning the PHCS and con-tinuing contact was maintained with the top echelons of the nursing establish-ment, there seemed to be little dissemination of information among the nursing force. The early efforts to develop retraining programmes for CHN/MWs and the new curricula that would be required for training new CHN/MWs were met with fairly widespread resistance. The need to expand the nurses' roles and their responsibilities — indeed, even the idea that nurses should work on their own in making patient-care decisions and in supervising the activities of com-munity health workers — was contrary to deeply ingrained nursing principles. Certainly in Ghana and probably in most countries, nursing education does not prepare nurses for the often independent leadership roles required for PHC responsibilities.

Perhaps one of the HPU's greatest shortcomings in the early planning of the PHC system was its failure to recognize some of the constraints on nurses and to make more concerted efforts to gain their understanding and support. Later in the project, when nurses were more widely involved and had a fuller understanding of PHC concepts with a concomitant appreciation of the need for changed roles and responsibilities, they became staunch supporters and major contributors to the PHC system. In Ghana and any other country introducing a PHC system of similar nature, women, and the nursing profession in particular, will have the central role to play. It is crucial therefore, that they be fully involved at all levels in the planning and policy making process.

Transport and logistics

Strong logistical back-up for transport required for supervision and for distri-bution of supplies is a prerequisite for a PHCS. Inadequate attention to the management of the support functions of transport and communication leads to serious problems affecting efficiency and effectiveness of the system which in turn causes a deterioration in the morale of the personnel. If the needed drugs and vaccines cannot be obtained by the community health workers and CHN/MW, the system will break down. While attempts were made as part of the PHC programme to strengthen the transport support function of the MOH, little progress, in fact, was made. This was largely due to the inertia of a highly bureaucratic civil service in which there was little appreciation of the high-level skills required for managing the maintenance and control of the large fleet of vehicles. It seemed impossible to obtain the approval from the Establishment Secretariat to upgrade the needed positions to a level to attract and keep those with the necessary managerial skills to run the transport and maintenance systems. An additional serious problem quite beyond the control of the MOH was the increasing scarcity of spare parts. This was directly related to the deteriorating economic condition of the country.

The procurement and distribution of drugs and supplies requires major high level managerial and logistical support and, as with the management of transport, it seemed impossible to obtain the needed upgrading of civil service posts to reflect their high degree of responsibility. Another problem that went unrecognized in the early efforts of the HPU was that drug procurement was largely outside the authority of the MOH. The true authority lay with those making decisions about import licenses. As the economic situation worsened it became increasingly difficult to obtain any items requiring import.

The economic situation

The deteriorating economic situation in Ghana may have helped our early efforts in the Planning Unit in the development of the PHC system. It became evident by 1977 that more hospital construction was not possible and that it was essential for the MOH, as for the country as a whole, to become cost-conscious and develop alternative low-cost approaches to health care. Thus the fact that the PHC system required relatively little capital construction was welcomed, particularly by the Ministries of Economic Planning and Finance.

A point that required continued reiteration, however, was that the PHCS was not a low-cost, cheap or inferior substitute for hospitalization. Over and over it was necessary to make clear to the health professionals as well as the public that the specific health improvement procedures being introduced by the PHC system were those that would have the greatest impact on the health of the people – and that hospitals and doctors, in fact, had little direct relevance to the effective delivery of these particular procedures.

By the time of the installation of the first District Health Management Teams in 1979, the economic situation had become so bad that the morale of the teams was difficult to maintain. Transport and supply deficiencies rendered their work virtually impossible. Almost certainly, the economic and political turmoil since

1980 has contributed to the lack of progress in further extending the primary health care programme.

The time factor

An important lesson that we seemed to have to learn over and over was that if plans were to be implemented, then everyone concerned must be involved in the thinking and planning. There must be widespread understanding of the objectives, of the proposed plans and of the required activities at all levels. To achieve this understanding requires time, effort, and considerable repetition. Intellectual planning may be relatively straightforward, but active involvement of those who will be carrying out the plans is a long-term process. New ideas should not be, and indeed cannot be, rushed. Otherwise there will be serious delays through misunderstanding and even active obstruction in the future. In nearly every case that the Planning Unit or Project Teams developed aspects of plans ahead of the rest of the Ministry, much time was required to bring everyone else up-to-date. Attempts to hurry things through were generally counter-productive.

Capacity to absorb change

The capacity to absorb change in an organization such as the Ministry of Health is highly limited. The installation of a strengthened, but not really new, budget estimate system within the Ministry took three years of intensive effort on the part of the Planning Unit. The recommended changes in the out-patient and in-patient forms will require a similar prolonged effort, with workshops to be held in every region and every district, probably for several years. For such procedural changes to occur throughout the system, it will require a minimum of two to three years of persistent exertion. The establishment of an effective planning unit really took five years. Even with the best of intentions and generally enthusiastic support, a three to five year time horizon should be allowed for similar projects elsewhere.

CONCLUSIONS

In the final chapter of *Health by the people* (1975), Newell categorized the examples from the nine countries in the book into three overlapping groups: those examples that represent profound national changes (China, Cuba, Tanzania), those that represented extensions of the existing system (Iran, Niger, Venezuela), and those of local community development (Guatemala, India, Indonesia). In Ghana, the Planning Unit clearly started from within the establishment, looking at its problems and possible solutions through the eyes of the MOH. The original objective was to extend the existing system of hospitals, health centres and health posts in order to increase coverage of the professionally provided outpatient services available. However, the HPU became convinced that the only way to make a major impact on the health of the Ghanaian people was through the implementation of very specific intervention procedures. These could be carried out only by the direct involvement of the family and community in their homes and neighbourhoods, backed by an effective primary health care system.

Experiences in Ghana from the several local community development programmes indicated that mobilization for community involvement in health-related programmes could be successfully carried out; the challenge was to extend the lessons learned to the entire nation working through an established bureaucracy using available personnel imbued with a civil service mentality. For the implementation of the primary health care strategy there had to be a profound change in the approach and organization of the health service programmes, which in turn required major political commitment. In order to obtain the understanding and commitment at the highest political levels, it was necessary to put the argument for PHC in terms that the economists and decision-makers could clearly understand. The HPU developed a methodology that demonstrated in a quantitative manner that the introduction of a primary health care strategy should provide a much greater improvement in the healthy life of the Ghanaian people than an equivalent expenditure on the extension of the conventional hospital-based system. By making a sound technical case in economic terms, the HPU was able to obtain the backing of, first, the Ministry of Economic Planning, and then the political policy makers at the cabinet level. With approval from the top and with widespread acceptance within the health establishment for the primary health care strategy, implementation was begun with the training and installation of the first nine District Health Management Teams, one in each Region.

This story provides an account of the steps leading from the establishment of a Health Planning Unit within the MOH, Ghana to the planning, development, acceptance, and initial implementation of a national primary health care strategy. Although there remain crucial issues to be resolved and much detailed planning at the district and local levels to be carried out, a good start towards a functional PHC system has been made.

REFERENCES

Belcher, D.W., *et al.*, A comparison of morbidity interviews with a health examination survey in rural Africa. *American Journal of Tropical Medicine and Hygiene* **25**, 751–8 (1976).
Brachott, D., *The health services in Ghana*, Ministry of Health, Accra, Ghana (1961).
World Health Organization, *Community involvement in primary health care.* Report of a Workshop, Kintampo. PHC/79.2. WHO, Geneva (1979).

The Danfa Comprehensive Rural Health and Family Planning Project, Ghana. Final Report. University of Ghana Medical School, Accra, Ghana (1979).

Gaisie, S.K., *Estimating Ghanian fertility, mortality and age structure.* Population Dynamics Programme, University of Ghana, Legon, Accra (1976).

Ghana Health Assessment Project Team. A quantitative method of assessing the health impact of different diseases in less developed countries. *International Journal of Epidemiology* **10** (No. 1), 73–80. (1981).

Health planning data book for Ghana. Ministry of Health, National Health Planning Unit, Accra, Ghana (1977).

IDS Research Reports. *Health needs and health services in rural Ghana,* Vols. 1 and 2. Institute of Development Studies, University of Sussex, Brighton, England (1978).

de Kadt, E., and Segall, M., Health needs and health services in rural Ghana. *Social Science and Medicine* **15A** (Special Number), pp. 397–513 (1981).

Manual No. 1. *An approach to planning the delivery of health care services.* National Health Planning Unit, Ministry of Health, Accra, Ghana (1979).

Manual No. 2. *Planning and management of health services at the district level.* National Health Planning Unit, Ministry of Health, Accra, Ghana (1979).

Newell, K.W. (ed.), *Health by the people,* World Health Organization, Geneva (1975).

Primary health care strategy for Ghana, National Health Planning Unit, Ministry of Health, Accra, Ghana. (1979).

Sai, F.T., *History of the health services in Ghana.* Draft (1982).

18 Primary health care in Democratic Yemen: evolution of policy and political commitment

Malcolm Segall and **Glen Williams** analyse the interactions of socialist development policies, community initiatives, external influences, and planning processes — and conclude that 'Health for All by the Year 2000' is not an impossible goal for Democratic Yemen.

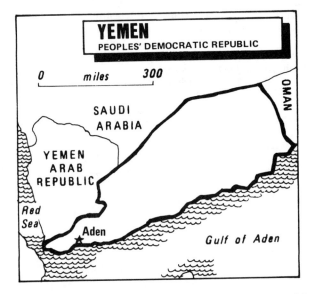

Malcolm Segall, a paediatrician, is now a Fellow of the Institute of Development Studies, Sussex, England, and specializes in health policy and planning. He has worked in Tanzania, Mozambique, Zimbabwe, and Ethiopia, and is a WHO consultant in primary health care.

Glen Williams is a writer on Third World development issues, based in Oxford.

*This chapter is based on a report written in 1980 by the Ministry of Public Health of Democratic Yemen with the support of Malcolm Segall. The report was the country's contribution to a comparative study sponsored by the Joint Committee on Health Policy of WHO and UNICEF on the subject of political decision-making processes for primary health care. The full report from Democratic Yemen may be requested from the Strengthening of Health Services Division of WHO, Geneva. The complete study has been published under the title *National decision-making for primary health care*. WHO, Geneva (1981).

Despite official declarations in support of primary health care (PHC) and 'Health for All by the Year 2000', practical progress and concrete results are hard to find in many countries. A recent joint UNICEF-WHO study noted that the term 'primary health care' is often being applied to approaches that are really a continuation of the conventional 'basic health services' strategy, sometimes extended further by the use of cheaper village health workers. Thus the scope and depth of community involvement are often very doubtful, and as the study report continues: 'The coordination of health and development planning is often poor and intersectoral health-related activities are frequently rudimentary. Vertical single disease programmes are often not yet integrated with PHC in practice' (UNICEF/WHO 1981, p.27).

Such problems are in fact not too surprising as PHC is, so to speak, quite 'strong medicine'. It demands a reordering of priorities at all levels of the health-care system and in other sectors related to health. It requires political commitment to equitable socioeconomic development at the national level, the decentralization of decision-making processes, an integrated development effort by many sectors, a high degree of community involvement in deciding priorities and implementing programmes, and a preferential allocation of resources to promoting the health of the least healthy – usually the poor majority of the population living mainly in rural areas. It is not surprising that many governments prefer to take their 'dose' of PHC well diluted.

One country which appears now to be making encouraging progress is the People's Democratic Republic of Yemen.[1] It did not reach this situation from one day to the next, but only in stages over several years, and this article attempts to relate and analyse the historical process leading towards PHC in this country.

BACKGROUND

Situated in the south-western corner of the Arabian Peninsula, Democratic Yemen has a population of about two million, of whom just over a half live in rural areas, a third are urban dwellers, and a tenth are nomads. The rugged terrain and harsh, dry climate are unfavourable for agriculture, on which most of the population depend for their livelihood. GNP per capita was estimated at US $480 in 1979 – among the lowest in the region. Aden, the capital city, was a British colony from 1839 until 1967. The rest of the country was divided administratively into 32 Sultanates, Emirites, and Sheikdoms, which enjoyed 'independent' status under British Protection. Used originally as a coaling station for the steam ships of the East India Company, Aden became an important British military base after the Second World War.

All decision-making power during the colonial period was invested in the British administration; there were no organizations to represent the people's interests. Divided tribally and ruled in a feudal manner by Sultans and Sheiks, the vast majority of the people lived under social, economic, and political oppression. Most arable land was the property of a few landlords and was tilled by share croppers and labourers. Educational and health facilities were virtually confined to Aden and other places where they could be enjoyed by the ruling elite, both local and foreign. Some 90 per cent of the population was illiterate. There was no legislation protecting the rights of women, who could not participate in political, economic, or community affairs. Women were regarded as the husband's property, to be bought and sold like a commodity. A woman had no choice of husband or any say in divorce. The limited educational opportunities available were open only to men.

Nurses and health assistants were the only categories of health personnel produced at the two local training hospitals, and these only in small numbers. At the time of independence in 1967, there were only eight national physicians and very few paramedical personnel in the entire country.

The National Liberation Front (NLF), formed in 1963, led the independence struggle which triumphed on 30 November 1967. The people in the countryside supported the NLF guerillas by providing them with food, shelter and medicines, carrying their arms, and building their barricades. This active participation proved to be an invaluable experience upon which popular mobilization has been built for the post-independence struggle against underdevelopment − in health as in other fields.

The new state inherited a huge legacy of political, socioeconomic, and administrative problems. The economy was characterized by low per capita income, chronic budgetary deficits, a negative balance of payments, underdeveloped natural resources, and low agricultural production and productivity. These problems were exacerbated by the high rate of illiteracy, the rigid social class stratification, and the mass exodus of trained personnel who identified their interests with those of the colonial power. But while people demanded reforms, employment opportunities and better living standards, the NLF was unable to take decisive action during the first two years of independence, because of internal differences between its progressive and more right-wing factions.

The turning point came on 22 June 1969, when the progressive wing gained control of the Front's 'Political Organization', expelled the right-wing elements, and announced new social policies known as the 'Corrective Measures'. The main features of the new policies were:

− the establishment of the public sector as the dominant force in the national economy;
− the spread of agricultural and fishery cooperatives on a broader scale;
− the development of the national economy on a planned, programmed, and coordinated basis.

One of the most far-reaching economic reforms made after the Corrective Measures was the Agrarian Reform Law No. 27 of 1970, which confiscated without compensation the land and property of the Sultans, Emirs, and Sheiks, and of their vassals, collaborators, and associated trusts. All land officially became the property of the state, which distributed it to the farmers. Limits were set to individual landholdings and the formation of cooperatives was encouraged. A vast network of schools was established, particularly in the rural areas. Education of women and girls was encouraged, and technical education was developed to meet the growing needs of the country. Adult literacy campaigns cut the illiteracy rate from about 90 to 40 per cent over a decade. The State also took actions guaranteeing equal rights for men and women in all aspects of political, economic and social life. The Family Law of 1974 aimed to support the institution of marriage as a cornerstone of socialist society. It provided for complete freedom of choice of a marriage partner and prohibited divorce by one partner unilaterally. The Basic Labour Law of 1978 guaranteed equal pay for women and provided pregnant workers with maternity leave and other benefits.

Present political, social, and economic structures

Political authority is vested in the Yemeni Socialist Party. The Supreme People's Assembly, whose members are elected by universal suffrage, is responsible for legislation. Executive authority resides with the Council of Ministers, headed by the Prime Minister. In each of the six Governorates there is a Local People's Council, elected by universal suffrage, and represented by an Executive Office between meetings.

'People's Organizations' play an important role in economic, social, legislative and cultural affairs. The General Federation of Workers' Unions, for example, looks after the welfare of workers and contributes to the formulation of legislation relating to work, social welfare, health insurance, the penal code, and family matters; it also has economic and political functions. Each People's Organization has a role in a particular field of health policy and practice, as for example:

— the Workers' Union in occupational health;
— the Women's Federation in mother-and-child health and family planning (MCH/FP);
— the Youth Federation in school health;
— the People's Defence Committees in the development of public health activities and health education.

Economic development aims to achieve more equitable and rising levels of income. Key sectors of the economy such as banking, insurance, foreign trade, and shipping are now publicly owned. Some private enterprises continue to exist, however, notably in local trade, handicraft, and manufacture. Foreign enterprises are encouraged to take part in oil exploration. Arable land amounts to less than 1 per cent of the country's land surface, and much of it has been turned into cooperative or state farms. The main food crops are wheat, millet, and sorghum, though productivity remains low. The country's main exports are fish, cotton, and salt. Aden is the region's best natural harbour. Many men work in neighbouring oil-exporting countries and send remittances back to their families.

One of the revolution's most fundamental achievements is the radically changed social structure and income distribution. The process of change began as large tracts of the country were liberated just before independence, forcing the Sultans and Sheiks, with their families, to quit the country. The major economic measures of the early 1970s — nationalization of the 'commanding heights' of the economy, agrarian reform, the cooperative movement, and the establishment of central planning of the country's development — removed the economic bases of the classes and groups hostile to social change. Though many small-scale tradesmen, retailers, artisans, and manufacturers have remained in the country, they generally work in cooperation with the revolution, often in mixed enterprises in which the State owns a majority of the shares.

Considerable progress has been made in meeting the basic needs of the population. Essential food supplies are available in sufficient quantity in the urban areas, where the people can afford them due to the policies of minimum wages and selective food subsidies. A programme to create adequate food supplies in the countryside has also made some progress, though rural food consumption is probably still inadequate. Yet despite encouraging achievements to date, the thorny problem of urban/rural disparities still remains to be solved: incomes in agricultural and fishing communities may be only about one-third of those of urban workers.

Major health problems

The pattern of health problems in Democratic Yemen is similar to that of other countries recently emerged from a long colonial history of underdevelopment: poor nutritional status, high incidences of communicable diseases (especially among children), and problems related to pregnancy, childbirth, and the new-born period. The fundamental cause of this disease profile is poverty, with its associated poor diet, housing, and environmental conditions, and low educational levels.

Despite progress since independence, basic health-care facilities and personnel are still insufficient in quantity and quality, and promotive and preventive activities need to be greatly increased. Supervisory, logistic, and administrative support from the higher levels of the health service for mass work at the base is still deficient.

This combination of factors results in high levels of morbidity and mortality, the most vulnerable groups being the very young and women of child-bearing age: the national infant mortality rate is estimated to be 152 per 1000 live births (see Table 18.1).

The greatest health problems include the following:

- *protein-energy malnutrition* (*PEM*): at least half of all pre-school children have a body weight of less than 75 per cent of the Havard international standard, and thus fall into grades two or three of 'weight for age'. Apart from being a killer in its own right, PEM is a common accomplice of diarrhoea and other infections in children.

— *common infectious diseases of childhood*: diarrhoea is a serious and common problem in pre-school children, and conditions such as pneumonia, measles, whooping cough, tuberculosis, poliomyelitis, and tetanus of the newborn also have high incidence rates.

— *malaria*: one in every three to five people carry malaria parasites in their blood; about 5000 children die yearly from this disease.

— *active pulmonary tuberculosis*: reliable statistics are not available but data from the main tuberculosis centre in Aden and from WHO reports (1974–79) suggest a prevalence rate of about 2.6 per cent.

Table 18.1. Estimated vital statistics of People's Democratic Republic of the Yemen, 1980

Crude birth rate	45 per 1000 population
Crude death rate	19 per 1000 population
Annual natural increase	2.6 per cent
Infant mortality rate	152 per 1000 live births
Life expectancy at birth	45 years of age

Other major health problems include acute respiratory infections, communicable eye diseases, schistosomiasis, anaemia, and perinatal disorders.

Most of these conditions are preventable through improved nutrition, housing and environmental sanitation, an adequate supply of safe water, higher levels of literacy and education, and the provision of basic health care.

Health care facilities and personnel

In 1980 there were 28 hospitals at regional and governorate levels with a total capacity of less than 3000 beds – a ratio of about one hospital bed per 700 persons. Nearly 40 per cent of health facility beds were in Aden, which contains nearly 20 per cent of the population. There were 18 health centres, a further 60 special-purpose clinics such as those for MCH/FP, and 17 tuberculosis centres; again these smaller units were concentrated in urban and semi-urban areas. Limited care was provided outside these areas through 252 rural health units. It was estimated that only 16 per cent of the rural population had reasonable access to these units, most of which were curative in orientation and were not yet adequately staffed or equipped.

Fully-trained health professionals included 250 physicians and 200 nurses, equivalent to about one physician for every 8000 population and one nurse for every 10 000; however, almost half of these personnel were located in Aden.

In rural areas, advice and assistance in pregnancy and childbirth still usually come from female relatives, and deliveries are mostly conducted at home. Only a minority of women enjoy the services of even a traditional birth attendant (TBA).

The Institute of Health Manpower Development, however, has trained over 100 TBAs, and more are attending courses.

EVOLUTION OF PRIMARY HEALTH CARE SINCE INDEPENDENCE

The leaders of the Political Organization, who had led the armed struggle for independence, came from the rural labouring class. They had lived with the huge problems affecting the people in the rural areas, and they were acutely aware of the great disparity in the level of development between the towns and the countryside. After independence the people, for their part, felt for the first time that their country was one nation, rather than fragmented into tiny states. They expected some dramatic changes to be made in their favour, and in particular expected rapid economic and social transformation of the rural areas.

Only after the Corrective Measures of 1969, however, was the Political Organization able to formulate a clear policy of developing the rural areas and raising the living standards there. In the new political situation the rural people became increasingly aware of three facts of life that would come to influence their role later: first, that resources were scarce; second, that despite this, the Political Organization was determined to give the highest priority to developing the countryside; and third, related to the previous two, that the people must depend in large measure on their own creative initiatives. The people's readiness to accept the guidance of the Political Organization was a valuable inheritance from the national liberation struggle, and reflected the high prestige of the Organization among them.

The Plan replaces 'development by spontaneity'

There was no national development plan for the first three years of independence. Rural development activities were carried out by spontaneous community effort. Community actions were not conceived in sectoral terms but were developed according to priority needs as perceived by the local population. Where they felt the need for a school, they built one. Where they needed drinking water, they sank a well. Projects received the agreement and guidance of local members of the Political Organization, and were given technical and material support by the government sector concerned.

Many communities constructed rural health units and health centres, and this generated a demand for trained health personnel. In 1970 four United Nations agencies combined to support the establishment of the Institute of Health Manpower Development which was to train auxiliary health workers, particularly those for service in the rural areas. In the same year, the College of Higher Education and the High Institute of Agriculture were established to train teachers and agriculturalists respectively.

'Development by spontaneity', however, could not continue indefinitely. To meet community needs more effectively and to accelerate the pace of development, the state decided to plan the economy more systematically and to match community action with public resources. The first three-year National Development Plan was issued on 1 April 1971.

The plan included a literacy campaign but little else that would now be regarded as relating specifically to the PHC concept. The small, vertical malaria and tuberculosis programmes already in existence were not included in the plan. The health sector was in fact still strongly oriented towards curative care, concentrating on the expansion of hospitals, health centres and rural health units. There were two main reasons for this. First, curative services were certainly needed urgently all over the country; and second, many of the health facilities which had been constructed by community effort during 1969 and 1970 still needed equipment and trained personnel.

An evaluation of the plan three years later found that a total of 11 health centres and 42 health units had been established in the rural areas. In addition, a total of five hospitals, with 220 beds, had been constructed or upgraded.

Beginnings of primary health care and the abolition of private medicine

The Ministry of Public Health convened its first National Health Conference in 1972 to discuss how best to develop the health services to meet the growing demands of the people. Participants came from all sectors of the economy, the People's Organizations and the Political Organization. For the first time, recommendations were made which contained elements of PHC, such as the expansion of MCH services, occupational health care, environmental sanitation, safe village water supplies, and other preventive actions, as well as the elimination of illiteracy. Active community participation was to be a notable feature in all promotional activities. Yet at the time participants in the conference were not even aware of the term primary health care, let alone of the concepts of the approach.

Of the conference's many resolutions, only one was implemented immediately: the creation of a High Drug Council, and the establishment of the National Drug Company to manage the importation and distribution of drugs and children's food. Although private pharmacies were still permitted to operate, they had to comply with the directives and guidelines of the Drug Council.

The recommendations and resolutions of the conference were the subject of much political debate over the following year, leading to some important government decisions. First, it was decided to expand the vertical programmes of tuberculosis and malaria control. Second, a dialogue was established between the Ministry of Public Health and other health-related bodies, such as the Ministry of Agriculture and Agrarian Reform, the Ministry of Education, and the Water Corporation. Third, it was decided that the necessary integration of preventive and curative care would be greatly facilitated by the nationalization of the health services. As a result, Law No. 17 was issued in September 1973, abolishing private medical practice and private clinics, and introducing People's Clinics in their place. This law had the following immediate effects:

— health services became non-profit making;
— health care was made free of charge for all citizens;
— the State shared the responsibility for health services with the population through the People's Organizations.

1974–78 National Health Plan

Nevertheless the 1974–78 Health Plan was still mainly curative in emphasis. It provided for the addition of 980 general beds to hospitals and health centres — an increase in bed capacity of 45 per cent — in addition to a central children's hospital of 300 beds (which included a maternity unit). The Plan also called for the construction and/or expansion of 20 rural health units.

Some shifts, however, were made towards preventive activities: the malaria and tuberculosis control programmes were expanded and some more MCH services were provided. This was a direct result of the Health Conference held in 1972. Yet it was too late to influence the five-year National Development Plan for 1974–78. Although the Development Plan embodied some water supply projects, the malaria and tuberculosis programmes were still not included. The Ministry of Public Health, however, was given the go-ahead to seek external assistance for these programmes, and to promote community participation in all its preventive activities.

Cuba visits and intenational support

In 1974 two delegations went from Democratic Yemen to Cuba, and each visit in a different way had an important influence on health policy. The first was by a health delegation and this resulted in the decision to establish a Faculty of Medicine in Aden, building on Cuba's experience of training medical personnel, as well as on the success of the local Institute of Health Manpower Development started four years earlier. The Faculty of Medicine took in its first medical students in October 1975. The second delegation was from the Political Organization and this visit was one of the turning points in the development of PHC concepts in Democratic Yemen. This delegation was impressed by Cuba's system of Committees for the Defence of the Revolution and it recommended a similar system for Democratic Yemen. As a result, the decision to establish Civil Defence Committees was made in 1975. These Committees have a number of secretaries each responsible for a particular sector, and the Secretary for Health is becoming a key cadre in the interface of the PHC system and the community.

The trend towards promotive and preventive activities continued during 1975 and 1976. Approaches were made to multilateral and bilateral sources for assistance to the preventive programmes. In 1975 a schistosomiasis control programme was started with WHO assistance, and in the same year a MCH/FP programme was established with UNFPA help. In 1977 the Arab League granted help through WHO for the malaria control programme. Study tours on preventive

medicine were made to socialist countries, some of which provided vaccines for
the immunization programme.

Intersectoral coordination at local level

In 1976 the Local Government Administration Law was enacted and the following year the Local People's Councils were elected in all six Governorates, creating
the political foundation for intersectoral coordination at the local level. The
Local People's Councils each have an Executive Office comprised of representatives of important sectors of the economy: agriculture, fisheries, education,
health, finance, supplies, and social affairs. This office coordinates and integrates
all local development activities.

The Local Government Administration Law marked the beginning of decentralization of authority to the Governorates. In 1977 further devolution in
the health service took place when the Ministry of Public Health established in
each Governorate a Directorate of Health Services with administrative and
financial authority. The Directorate is responsible for all health activities in the
Governorate, thus ending the previous separation between the preventive vertical
programmes and the curative health facilities. The Director is a member of the
Executive Office of the Local People's Council.

The National Health Programme — preventive but vertical

In 1978, the last year of the National Development Plan, preparations gathered
greater momentum for the next five year plan. In close collaboration with WHO,
the Ministry of Public Health undertook a National Health Programme (NHP)
exercise. The Ministry grasped this opportunity to plan for the integration of the
preventive and curative health services, with a greater emphasis on the former, as
recommended by the Health Conference of 1972. The NHP exercise listed the
priority health programmes as follows:

- Expanded Programme of Immunization;
- malaria control;
- PHC, with components for malnutrition, diarrhoeal diseases, acute respiratory diseases, anaemias, and perinatal disorders;
- tuberculosis control;
- communicable eye diseases control;
- schistosomiasis control;
- strengthening of MCH/FP services;
- urban polyclinics;
- health service administration;
- health manpower development;
- environmental health;
- occupational health.

The dominant trend of the NHP exercise was thus the perpetuation of vertical programmes. Most of the components of PHC, as understood today, were presented as vertical programmes *outside* the 'PHC' package. In fact 'PHC' itself emerged as a vertical – and separate – programme!

Influence of the Alma Ata Conference

At this point the WHO–UNICEF International Conference on Primary Health Care held at Alma Ata in September 1978 played a crucial role. A high level delegation, headed by the Minister of Public Health, attended the conference. The delegation became convinced of the need to restructure 'PHC' as then understood, and in particular to integrate at least most of the vertical programmes to create a comprehensive PHC 'package'.

While the Alma Ata Conference was taking place, however, the earlier NHP document was already being discussed with the Ministry of Planning and as a result the vertical programmes became incorporated into the 1979–83 National Development Plan. As had happened five years earlier, shifts in Ministry of Public Health thinking came just too late to influence the official government plan. They were also not in time to be fully represented in the National Health Plan of 1979–83.

Nevertheless, the Health Ministry moved rapidly to formulate its PHC policy. First, a Primary Health Care Office was established and a Director appointed on 1 January 1979. Second, the Ministry organized a high-level five-week seminar on Health Administration and Planning, to work out fresh approaches to PHC planning problems. In November 1979 the MCH/FP programme was integrated with PHC and the Programme Director became Deputy–Director of PHC.

The Ministry's Department of Planning and Statistics and the newly-formed PHC Office began evaluating the National Health Programme and the health-related parts of the National Development Plan in the light of the insights gained from the Alma Ata Conference. WHO and UNICEF helped to improve the conceptualization of PHC by facilitating exchanges of information with other countries. For example, the Director of the PHC Office attended PHC seminars organized by WHO in Thailand and Yugoslavia in 1979. UNICEF assigned a team to Democratic Yemen to assess the need for training PHC workers and to design curricula. In early 1980 UNICEF arranged the visit of three PHC programme officers to Ethiopia to observe the achievements in PHC there. This visit reinforced the importance to be assigned in Democratic Yemen to the Health Secretaries of the Civil Defence Committees: since 1980 these Secretaries have been among the cadres being trained in basic health care to function as part-time health workers at the community level. The participation of Democratic Yemen in a study organized by the Joint Committee on Health Policy of WHO and UNICEF on 'National Decision-Making for Primary Health Care' was another factor promoting the development of ideas in the country. The study was conducted by the Ministry of Public Health but involved wide-ranging consultations with other sectors, which as a result became increasingly aware of the health-related nature of their work.

All these events led during 1979–80 to a growing awareness at top government level that the target of 'Health for All by the Year 2000' (HFA/2000), to be achieved through PHC, was much more than a simple medical question: it required high-level political commitment and intersectoral coordination. Thus the Council of Ministers' Order No. 35 of 1979 established official committees to pursue specific tasks in this area including: the formulation of a policy, strategy, and plan of action to achieve HFA/2000; the review and revision of health legislation to support PHC; the convening of a second health conference; the convening of a donors' meeting; and the establishment of a Primary Health Care Council. The latter came into operation in April 1980 with the task of coordinating the activities of some of the vertical programmes (to begin with those for immunization and malaria control) as a first step to their full integration with PHC.

These were technical operations set in motion by political sanction, but on 17 June 1980 the Council of Ministers passed a resolution of more thorough-going political significance. It established a Health Promotion Council with high-level participation from the economic and social sectors involved in HFA/2000, and chaired by the Minister of Planning. This influential body is charged with the responsibility to develop a coordinated, intersectoral attack on the health problems of the country, and is an indicator of the government's commitment to PHC in the broad 'health/development' sense of the term.

Thus, over the past decade, the concepts of PHC in Democratic Yemen have progressively matured by a process of evolution, so reaching the policies of the present day.

The PHC approach today

Primary health care in Democratic Yemen is no longer confined to medical actions but has been broadened to encompass many health-related activities, like the provision of safe water and the production and consumption of nutritious foods. As a result, PHC is not the exclusive responsibility of health personnel. Responsibilities at the local level are shared among a broad range of people and social institutions, including agricultural and fisheries cooperatives, local government authorities, the Political Organization, the People's Organizations, and technical staff of various sectors. Financial responsibilities are also shared: the People's Organizations, communities and production cooperatives lighten the financial burden on the Ministry of Public Health by making contributions in labour, cash, or kind to particular projects and programmes. Supervision of PHC personnel is shared between the health service and the community: while health professionals at the secondary and tertiary levels are responsible for technical supervision, the community – supported by the People's Organizations and local Party members – controls the manner in which the PHC workers discharge their functions.

The integrated PHC 'package' in Democratic Yemen today includes the following elements:

— MCH care, including ante-natal, delivery, and postnatal care, a family planning service, immunizations, nutritional surveillance, health and nutrition education, oral rehydration for diarrhoea, and inservice training and supervision of TBAs;
— environmental hygiene and provision of safe water;
— control of major specific communicable diseases;
— health education (including information on personal hygiene);
— management of common diseases and injuries, and referral of more complex problems;
— reporting on vital statistics and epidemics, and other basic items of health information.

A major feature of the approach is the importance given to popular participation in all stages of the PHC process, from planning through implementation to evaluation.

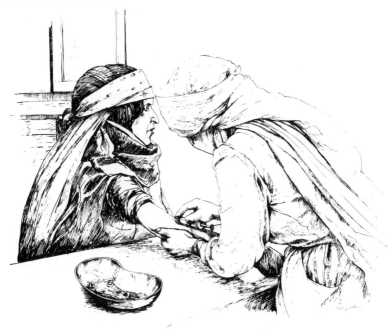

Fig. 18.1. Maternal care is part of primary health care in Democratic Yemen.

Frontline health workers

Originally the Ministry of Public Health envisaged that full-time PHC workers, paid by the Ministry, would perform all health-care activities on the periphery of the system. After the health delegation's study tour in Ethiopia, however, this concept came under critical review. The insights gained from studying Ethiopia's health system enabled the Ministry's planners to pinpoint some serious weaknesses in the original concept. First, it would be a heavy financial burden on the Ministry and would not tap local resources. Second, it would not be substantially different from the old Basic Health Services concept, with its one-sided emphasis on health service units and cadres. Thus, it would not involve the community and local People's Organizations in the planning and implementation of health activities, and it would not provide a framework for a collaboration between TBAs and PHC workers.

For these reasons the frontline health care structure was completely redesigned. The new model still included a well-located PHC unit, run by one or more salaried workers, who would be mainly retrained health or medical assistants or community nurse-midwives. But the unit would now be supported by at least four part-time community health workers, as well as the local TBAs, living in the villages served by the unit and responsible to local social structures.

The activities of the community health worker should be primarily promotive and preventive, aiming especially to achieve a reasonable level of environmental hygiene and safety in water supply. He or she will also treat the most common diseases, give first aid for minor injuries, and make referrals of more complex problems to the local PHC unit.

The village TBA, after attending a training course, should identify all pregnancies and refer those women with a high risk of complications to the PHC unit. She should advise pregnant women on nutrition and the need for tetanus immunization, and generally promote family planning, breast-feeding, and infant care. In performing normal deliveries she is trained to use the principles of asepsis, and she should report all births, and maternal and neonatal diseases and mortalities to the PHC unit.

Frontline PHC workers are to be supported by a supervisory team attached to the nearest health centre or district hospital. Apart from providing on-going guidance and training, the team should ensure an adequate supply of essential drugs and vaccines to PHC units, handle clinical referrals, and analyse the data reported from their area.

Selection and training of frontline health workers

Frontline health workers are selected by the community from men or women who are active in the People's Organization or a cooperative, are literate, and are permanently resident in the community. The selection is likely to include the Health Secretaries of the Civil Defence Committees, and TBAs are also eligible. So far about 90 per cent of community health workers have been men – a legacy from the past which is only gradually changing. Training is for three periods of 10 days, spread out over three months.

Rather than begin with an untried programme all over the country, the

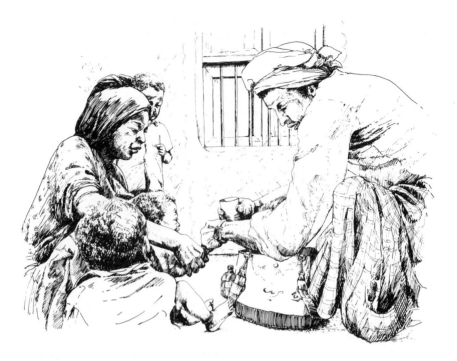

Fig. 18.2. Nine out of every ten community health workers so far are men — a legacy from the past, which is gradually changing.

Ministry of Public Health decided to initiate the new PHC approach with a pilot experience in one area. One of the first tasks was obviously the training of personnel and, rather than approach this on an *a priori* basis it was decided to build up curricula on the basis of practical experience. Thus a training team was established of health workers from the Ministry, the Governorate Directorate of Health Services, and the local supervising health centre. This team went to serve in the pilot area as PHC workers, to learn about the local conditions and the present capabilities of the future frontline cadres. With this experience the team determined what tasks the local workers could realistically be expected to perform, and it then devised pilot training (or retraining) programmes for the community health workers, TBAs and PHC unit cadres.

This first pilot experience in PHC and training was begun in the village of Musemir in August 1980. A group of about 50 community health workers was trained and have returned to their villages to work. Initial results have been generally encouraging and the project is being closely monitored to provide guidelines for an expanded, countrywide programme.

CONCLUSION

The evolution of PHC in Democratic Yemen and of the Government's commitment to it have resulted from the operation of four main factors which have interacted with each other to move the process forward.

The first has been the socialist orientation of the country. This political perspective of the Party and Government did not arise as a random phenomenon, but as a specific response to a long period of feudal and colonial oppression of the people. These historical conditions both created the popular basis for social transformation and threw up the political leadership to bring it about. The struggles first for independence and then against underdevelopment have created a situation in which problems of health — as of other areas — are thought through in a radical manner, and the institutional changes necessary to resolve such problems are made. The nationalization of the health sector and the prohibition of private medical practice in 1973 was in many respects a turning point in the history of health development in Democratic Yemen. For the first time it became possible to mobilize and plan all the country's scarce health resources to meet the urgent needs of the people. This legislative action was taken more from the general perspective of equity than from specific notions of PHC, which were still embryonic at that time.

While the political context has laid the basis for the evolution of PHC, it has not been a unique determinant. Another important factor has been community initiative. This began as popular support for the national liberation struggle and was then carried over in the post-independence period in the struggle for development. The maintenance of community activity has been provided for by specific new social structures, such as the People's Organizations, the Civil Defence Committees and the Local People's Councils. The combination of political will and community action led initially to a strong curative emphasis in health care. The people constructed rural health units and the Government responded by providing curative personnel and supplies. In terms of technical content this may seem a far cry from PHC, but in one important respect it did mark the beginning of this approach. There was an urgent need and demand for curative care in the countryside, and the allocation of government resources to the rural areas in response to local demand and action was a positive — if spontaneous and limited — move in the right direction. There were also other popular initiatives, however, in the fields of water supplies, environmental hygiene and rural development. These were in fact PHC activities, although they were not at first recognized as such.

A third factor then came into operation which introduced some key ideas into the situation of committed spontaneity. This factor was conceptual influence from abroad, so that Democratic Yemen did not have, so to speak, to rediscover the PHC wheel, but could benefit from the experience of other countries. This external influence has been of two main types. The first was the experience of other socialist countries, especially developing socialist countries; of these the two most influential have been (at different times and in different ways) Cuba and Ethiopia. The other type of external influence was that of the United Nations agencies, especially WHO. The thinking of that organization was itself undergoing a transformation during the 1970s, and it was particularly towards the end of that decade that WHO's more systematized conceptualizations of PHC began to have a major impact.

At each stage of the evolution of PHC, however, it was necessary to synthesize the current state of thinking, translate it into national policies, put those policies into practice, and evaluate the outcomes. This function of centralizing and distilling experience, and drawing practical conclusions, has been realized through the planning activities of the Ministry of Public Health, operating within the broader framework of government development planning. This technical health planning and programming work constitutes the fourth factor in the evolution of PHC in Democratic Yemen. Beginning after independence with a curative orientation, health-sector policy shifted gradually towards prevention, especially after the first National Health Conference in 1972. The preventive activities were seen first in terms of vertical programmes, but in the last few years these have given way to the concept of an integrated PHC approach, with a strong component of organized community responsibility in the context of socioeconomic development.

During the 15 years since Democratic Yemen achieved independence, ideas about health have thus evolved as a result of the interactions of political processes, community initiatives, external influences, and health-sector planning and practice. The Ministry of Public Health has only recently formulated its comprehensive PHC policy, and indeed new ideas are still coming off the drawing board. Yet, though only a few steps have been taken along the long road of implementation, the gap between rhetoric and reality seems smaller than in many developing countries. For the people of Democratic Yemen, 'Health for all by the Year 2000' may not be an impossible goal.

NOTES

1. Also known as 'South Yemen'.

REFERENCES

Ministry of Public Health, *Country decision-making for the achievement of the objectives of primary health care: report to WHO/UNICEF by the People's Democratic Republic of Yemen,* Aden (1980).
UNICEF/WHO, *National decision-making for primary health care: a study by the Joint Committee on Health Policy,* WHO, Geneva (1981).

Part IV

Conclusions

19 Practising health for all

'Health for All by the Year 2000' sounds much too optimistic. What does it really mean? It cannot possibly mean that everyone on earth will be healthy by the end of the century. There are no valid reasons to expect humanity to achieve such Utopian conditions within such a short space of time. Is 'Health for All' just an idle slogan, the latest fad in international development jargon? Halfdan Mahler, Director General of the World Health Organization, thinks not. According to Mahler, 'Health for All' means

'. . . that people will use much better approaches than they do now for preventing disease and alleviating unavoidable illness and disability, and that there will be better ways of growing up, growing old and dying gracefully. And it means that health begins at home and at the work place, because it is there, where people live and work, that health is made or broken. And it means that essential health care will be accessible to *all* individuals and families in an acceptable and afford-able way, and with their full participation' (1982).

This sounds like something rather less than Utopia, but it is still a very optimistic prediction. Optimism, of course, has much to recommend it. As Charles Medawar has observed, 'Optimism is the hope of progress, an essential part of both wanting to and being able to face a future' (1983). In overdose it can be dangerous, but a certain amount of optimism is a prerequisite to success in any field.

But what counts as 'success' in primary health care, the route to 'Health for All' recommended by WHO? How is it assessed or evaluated? Obviously, any programme must be evaluated in terms of its stated goals. The goals of PHC, as Newell noted in *Health by the People*, 'are much wider than conventional ones and range from that of health as a political and social right to that of health as an expression, or spin-off, of a quietly functioning informed community' (1975, p. 192). Yet no matter how broadly the goals of PHC are defined, two valid criteria of a particular programme's success are its *medical effectiveness* and *social impact*.

MEDICAL EFFECTIVENESS

This information is expressed through quantitative indicators such as rates of morbidity and mortality, nutritional status, and life expectancy. It is important for several reasons. First, it can encourage and stimulate a community by providing feedback on the results of their efforts to improve their health status. The Serabu Hospital in Sierra Leone; for example, has developed a method known as 'community assessment' using indicators such as infant mortality and nutrinonal status as a motivational tool. In Indonesia, the government health service in Banjarnegara regency on the island of Java has promoted the use of simple indicators such as the number of under-five children weighed each month to help village communities monitor the results of their health programme.

Second, health professionals need reliable information to check the effectiveness of their own work. The staff of the Comprehensive Community Development Project at Pachod in India, for example, have devised an accurate statistical method based on monthly reports from village health workers, enabling them to monitor changes in health status within the villages covered by the programme.

Third, health information expressed in simple, quantitative form can be highly useful to health professionals when communicating with political decision-makers. Since all health programmes depend on decisions made at various levels of the political hierarchy, health professionals must be able to communicate in terms which clarify, rather than obscure, the main issues at stake. In Ghana, for example, the Health Planning Unit of the Ministry of Health has developed a methodology which demonstrates quantitatively that a PHC strategy can provide a much greater improvement in the healthy life of the Ghanaian people than an equivalent expenditure on a conventional, hospital-based system. This methodology can also be used to monitor and evaluate the medical effectiveness of the programme. Similarly in Indonesia, the National Family Nutrition Improvement Programme has developed an excellent system for collecting and analysing information on monthly participation and the weight gain of children — thus providing a sensitive index of nutritional status and growth from villages throughout Java and Bali.

Programmes with a reliable system of monitoring and evaluating medical effectiveness are rare. Yet such a system is almost as important for a programme's effectiveness as vaccines, syringes, and oral rehydration salts. Few health professionals — let alone volunteer community health workers — have been adequately trained to collect, analyse, and interpret health data relevant to medical effectiveness. That so few PHC programmes are able to monitor and evaluate their own medical effectiveness is, however, more disappointing than surprising, given the lack of international agreement in this field. Long overdue is a set of quantifiable indicators of community health status, internationally accepted and promoted, and adaptable for use in the semi-literate communities where the struggle for 'Health for All' is taking place.

SOCIAL IMPACT

A second useful criterion of the success or failure of PHC programmes is *social impact*. At least as important as medical effectiveness, social impact is even more difficult to quantify. Interpretations of the concept itself vary considerably.

Muller, in his perceptive study of PHC programmes in four communities in Peru, suggests that 'social impact . . . is indicated by the community's increased awareness of health problems and capacity to organize itself to solve these problems'. It is manifested in the development of the knowledge, skills, and attitudes of community members in relation to health, nutrition, and fertility. In assessing social impact it is especially important to observe the changes in the health, social status, and responsibilities of women in society. Women constitute a major 'at risk' group while of child-bearing age, and play important roles in treating illness and promoting good health — either in the home or as traditional midwives or folk healers. But they are rarely given any training, formal responsibility, or status for carrying out these roles. Yet in PHC programmes where women are actively involved and treated as capable, responsible, and concerned individuals, they play an enormously effective and important part, not just in improving health but in winning more social justice within their own communities. In the south-west corner of the Dominican Republic, for example, rural women have developed the skills and confidence to run successful nutrition and literacy programmes. They have built up a strong women's movement aiming at social and political changes. Even in the most rigid, caste-ridden communities of rural India, deeply rooted prejudices and practices of social discrimination are being broken down by womens' organizations taking community health as their starting point.

Yet although there is widespread agreement on the importance of social impact in PHC, there is still no general consensus on how to measure and assess this phenomenon. Evaluation in this field is therefore bound to involve much subjectivity and to result in widely differing viewpoints.

INTEGRATING THEMES

Two integrating themes run through the chapters of this book: the importance of political commitment to equitable socioeconomic development, and the need for community participation in planning, implementing, and evaluating PHC.

An essential precondition to successful PHC is a supportive political climate in which health is viewed as part of total human development and the right of every individual. Political support for high coverage health services and the integration of health with other sectors of development thus provide the best possible starting point for a PHC programme.

Community participation, as envisaged by WHO and UNICEF, is 'the process by which individuals and families assume responsibility for their own health and welfare and for those of the community, and develop the capacity to contribute to their and the community's development' (1978, p. 20). Participation implies not just the mobilization of the community's resources, but a process through which people gain greater *control* over the social, political, economic, and environmental factors affecting their health.

David Werner, author of two widely used PHC manuals, has frequently observed that, as people look more deeply into the reasons for their ill-health, they recognize that sickness, disease, and malnutrition are merely symptoms of a deeper malady stemming from social inequality, economic exploitation, and political oppression. PHC in the true sense threatens inequitable socioeconomic or political structures. It implies a redistribution of responsibility and power of a much more radical kind than is generally realized or accepted. It means shifts in power from top to lower levels of government administration; from the government itself to people's organizations; from military to civilian administrators; from doctors to paradedics; from health professionals to ordinary people; from the village elite to landless and marginal farmers; and from men to women.

This book examines several widely different examples of the complex relationship between community participation and political commitment to equitable development.

In socialist countries with strong political commitment to 'Health for All' – such as China and Cuba – the one-Party state system is highly successful in mobilizing community resources for health and educating people about the socioeconomic causes of hunger and disease. But there is also a political 'cost' involved: conformity to the one-Party state. To some outside observers, this 'cost' seems dauntingly high. David Werner, in assessing Cuba's health system, asks whether 'benevolent coercion and authoritarian enforcement of conformity are necessary to get people sharing and working to help each other, rather than greedily hoarding and taking unkind advantage of one another'. Werner also questions Cuba's reliance on a doctor-centred health system which seems at variance with the PHC principle of the community taking maximum responsibility for its own health care. Yet Cuba's achievements cannot be denied – universal health coverage of the population and levels of life-expectancy, morbidity, and mortality comparable with those of many industrialized countries, all in the short space of two decades. If health has a political 'cost', it seems acceptable to most Cubans.

China's approach to 'Health for All' differs from Cuba's by avoiding heavy reliance on highly trained doctors. Instead, China has trained a huge cadre of paramedical workers who are accountable to the community rather than to the medical hierarchy. Greater stress is also laid on the responsibility of the individual and of the community as a whole for taking charge of their own health care, both curative and preventive. Health is the right, and the duty, of every citizen. Recent trends towards modernization and professionalization in health care, however, may carry China away from the very principle of full community involvement which has made China's health system a model for other developing countries.

Yet even with strong political commitment to equity and broadly based people's participation, a country may still need several years to develop an appropriate PHC programme. In the People's Democratic Republic of the Yemen, for example, a whole decade elapsed before a complex process of interaction between health planners, people's organizations, political bodies, and international agencies produced a PHC programme worthy of the name.

The appearance of political commitment to equity and community partici- pation in health should not be mistaken for the reality. India, for example, led the Third World in health policy when the Bhore Report — which anticipated the basic principles of PHC by 30 years — was published in 1946. Yet efforts by the Indian government to establish a viable PHC programme on a nationwide basis are still beset with seemingly intractable political problems at every level from the village to the central government. Likewise in Tanzania, where equitable development and health for all has long been official policy, insufficient political commitment at all levels results in high expenditure on hospital-based care for the urban minority and few resources going to the rural majority.

These examples are typical of many countries in the Third World.[1] Since the Alma Ata conference, which stressed the need for 'full community participation in the planning, organization, and management of primary health care', many — probably most — PHC programmes throughout the Third World have laid claim to high levels of community involvement, or participation. On closer examina- tion, however, such 'participation' usually amounts to the government coercing the people to mobilize their own resources to subsidise a government-planned and -operated programme in which the people have little or no say. This approach repeats itself again and again, invariably resulting in failure as the people become the victims of a condescending, bungled outreach effort inspired by the current vogue in international health policies. Lower level health workers, far from feeling responsible to the community, look up to the higher echelons of the government hierarchy for rewards and support, constantly complaining, taking little pride in their work and considering themselves the most neglected corner of the massive, impersonal government bureaucracy.

Emanuel de Kadt, writing about Latin America, concludes that community participation will prosper 'only under governments with a substantial measure of genuine commitment to overcoming poverty and social inequality'. Since such governments are the exception rather than the rule throughout the world, is the PHC approach therefore bound to meet with failure? Not necessarily. 'Within any large state bureaucracy', de Kadt writes, 'there are always nooks and crannies where an orientation can cooperate which is more progressive — or conservative! — than the dominant government line'. Indeed, in many coun- tries PHC programmes based on genuine community participation have been relatively successful — though on a limited scale — despite an unfavourable political climate at national level.

For example in India, where the central government has experienced great difficulty in promoting PHC on a national basis, the State of Kerala has had remarkable success because it has created a political climate favourable to equitable development and widespread community participation. Though one of the poorest States in the country, Kerala has the highest levels of life- expectancy, literacy, and utilization of health services, as well as the lowest levels of the infant and child mortality. Kerala demonstrates that equitable socioeconomic and health policies are not necessarily incompatible with democratic government and that a high Gross Domestic Product is not essential for health: fair shares for the many are better than large shares for the few.

In Indonesia, where the political conditions created by the military-led government are hardly ideal for equity-orientated development, progressive voluntary agencies and sections of the government have succeeded in promoting PHC in parts of the country during the past decade. Newell's *Health by the people* contained the story of a community-based PHC project started in the late 1960s by a Christian agency in the city of Solo. Newell was not optimistic, however, about the chances of this programme spreading to other areas or influencing government policy. Yet Mary Johnston presents an account of how this community-based approach to PHC was extended by the local municipal government, how it was adapted and developed in the rural regency of Banjarnegara, and how the progressive National Family Planning Coordinating Board adopted one aspect – nutritional surveillance of under-five children by mothers' clubs – as a national programme. The example of Sukodono village, however, introduces a more cautious note. Here a group of young men and women, inspired by the example of health care in Banjarnegara, tried to start a PHC project but were thwarted by the rigidly centralized village power structure.

Other chapters in this book illustrate various aspects of community participation in relation to political commitment to equity in countries as diverse as the Dominican Republic, the Philippines, Peru, and Sierra Leone. Two clear lessons emerge. First, the *mobilization* of the community's human, financial, and material resources for PHC activities is highly desirable – not just to ease government resource constraints but to help the community achieve a sense of responsibility. Second, this sense of responsibility will develop only if the community is involved in *every* stage of the project – the initial assessment and definition of problems, planning, implementation, and evaluation. In these ways the members of the community gain more *control* over the social, political, economic, and environmental factors affecting their health.

POLITICS AND THE HEALTH PROFESSIONAL

The political dimensions of PHC place health professionals in a dilemma with which they are generally poorly equipped to deal. Tan gives a vivid account of how he, a young doctor in the Philippines, has tried to cope with the unforeseen stresses of working in rural communities charged with political tensions. 'My work with the peasants has led me to a rude awakening that the health problems of our country are inter-related with problems of economics, politics, and culture. How should a Filipino doctor answer this challenge? It is not enough to attend to health needs. If being a Filipino is foremost, then it certainly means going beyond medicine and health.' Most health professionals – whether in the North or the South – still resist Tan's conclusion that it is necessary to 'go beyond medicine and health'. Most succumb rapidly to the temptation to ignore or trivialize sociopolitical issues. They concentrate instead on purely technical problems. Why not just get on with implementing the effective and affordable health technologies already available, and leave the political and socioeconomic problems to others?

Some health professionals move in the opposite direction, arguing that there is no point trying to start PHC work under governments only superficially committed to equitable development.

Both these approaches are understandable, but misguided. There are simply no purely technical solutions to community health problems. The political process intrudes everywhere — whether at national or community level. To ignore or underestimate it is equivalent to discounting malnutrition as a prime contributing factor in the diseases of infants and children in the Third World. To retreat into a world of purely technical 'solutions' is an abdication of social responsibility.

But health professionals who despair of ever achieving anything worthwhile under governments insufficiently committed to equity and genuine community participation should also reconsider their position. The processes of human and community development set in motion by a sensitive, well-designed PHC programme can make a substantial contribution to social and political change at the local level. We have read of how, for example, traditional midwives in India and village women in the Dominican Republic are winning new dignity and social justice within their own communities. Neither of these programmes would be possible without the contribution of health professionals prepared to work towards what is possible *at the moment*, while not ignoring the deeper issues which must be resolved if health is to become the right of everyone. The 'seeds of change', as de Kadt observes, may *need* to be sown in unfavourable circumstances. The results may sometimes surprise even the most sceptical observer.

SUMMARY

The basic principles of success in primary health care can be summarized as follows:

1. *Political commitment to social equity*: A supportive political climate, in which health is viewed as part of human development and the right of each individual, is an essential starting point for a successful PHC programme. Although this commitment is rare on a national basis, it is often found to some extent within a community or at an intermediate level of the government hierarchy. Neither high income levels nor technically sophisticated medical services can ensure health for all. What really counts is political commitment to ensuring universal coverage by health services and the integration of health with other sectors of development.

2. *Community participation*: Community participation should not aim simply to mobilize the people's human, financial, and material resources. Abo

all else, participation should help the people gain greater *control* over the factors affecting their health – by making their own decisions, organizing their own activities, and taking greater responsibilities. This will require considerable de-centralization in decision-making within the health system and society. All members of the community should be involved in some aspect of the health programme. The role of women is crucial to the success of PHC. As health professionals, volunteer community organizers, traditional midwives, folk healers, and mothers, women are in the frontline of primary health care.

3. *Technical fit*: Although not analysed in detail in this book, the techno-logical appropriateness of PHC interventions is critical to success, whether measured by medical or social criteria. Thus, an initial epidemiological analysis of health problems can help the community to focus on the most prevalent and important conditions for which affordable solutions exist. Involvement of the community in this planning stage does not obviate the need for sound epidemiological principles. Appropriate technology also extends to training and management strategies, and to monitoring and evaluation using precise indicators by which a community can gauge its progress in solving health problems. These technical factors alone will not guarantee a successful PHC programme, but they are essential and tend to be overlooked by those for whom social goals are paramount in PHC.

CONCLUSION

By the end of the 1980s the governments of many countries will have to admit that, with their existing policies, 'Health for All' will still be a distant dream by the year 2000. The strategy of primary health care will not be at fault: in many countries it will not have been even tried, except in some superficial, token form. Health is a function of the political process. We all take part in that pro-cess, either through political parties, trade unions, churches, community organ-izations, voluntary agencies, the armed forces, government bureaucracies, or health services. And we all share the responsibility for either maintaining existing inequalities or for building a new social order based on greater equity and human dignity, in which 'Health for All' will be no mere dream but a fact of life.

NOTES

1. For an excellent study of the lessons learned about community partici-pation from many UNICEF-supported programmes in health, education, nutri-tion, water supply, and sanitation, see *Assignment Children*, 59/60 (1982).

REFERENCES

Mahler, Halfdan, 'Essential drugs for all'. Address given by the Director General of the World Health Organization to the Eleventh Assembly of the Inter-national Federation of Pharmaceutical Manufacturers' Associations, Washing-ton, DC, 8 June 1982.

Medawar, Charles, 'Hoping for health for all'. In *Rapport fran SIDA*, Stockholm, Spring 1983.

Newell, Kenneth (ed.), *Health by the people*, WHO, Geneva (1975).

UNICEF, *Assignment children*, 59/60. Geneva (1982).

Werner, David, *Helping health workers learn*. Hesperian Foundation, Palo Alto (1982).

Werner, David, *Where there is no doctor*. Hesperian Foundation, Palo Alto (1977).

WHO–UNICEF, *Primary health care*. WHO, Geneva (1978).

Index

Alibag district (India), Foundation for Research in Community Health project 135
Alma Ata Conference (1978) vi, 310–11, 323

Banjarnegara Regency (Java) 176–82
  community participation 257–66
  crude birth rate 182
  Family Nutrition Programme 262–6
  growth curve chart 258–60
  infant mortality rate 181
  kaders 177–8, 257, 258, 263
  kring 180
  maternal mortality rate 181
  neighbourhood nutrition club (*Taman Gizi*) 260–1
  nutritional status, under-fives 182
  nutrition programme 262–6
  primary health care programme 176–82
  weighing of children 258, 263–4
    report form 265
  weight chart 258–9
  see also Indonesia
Bhore Report (1946) 39, 323
Brazil, health policy 239

Castro, F. 18, 22
Chile 234
  health policy 238, 240
China
  Barefoot doctors 3, 6, 7–9
  doctors 7
  health services
    access 15
    accountability 10
    community participation 14
    decentralization 10–11
    developments 12–13, 13–14
    monitoring and evaluation 11
    politics 13
  health workers and community 15
  primary health care system 10–15
  public health 3, 5–16
  rural areas 7

  self-reliance 14
  traditional medicine 11, 15
Colombia:
  Escuela Nacional de Salud Publica 245n
  statutory participation bodies 234
community participation for health:
  decision-making 234–6
  implementation 231–4
  opposing views 190–1
conscientisadores 230
CUAVES (Urban Community of Self-Sufficiency, Villa el Salvador) 200, 203
Cuba 3, 17–37, 234
  birth rate 21–2, 37n
  childbirth 29
  Democratic Yemen, relations with 308–9
  diarrhoea, child with 267
  doctors:
    centre of health service 322
    exodus 22–3
    hierarchy 26–7
    supply 24–5
  family planning 21–2
  health education, anti-educational 28–9
  health policy 240
  hospital services 23
  infant mortality 19
  life expectancy 19
  limited access to non-approved information 30–2
  Ministry of Public Health 23–4
  mortality from infectious and contagious diseases 19 (fig)
  newborn baby–mother separation 29–30, 31 (fig)
  new man (*hombre neuvo*) 18
  organizations 234
  people's power (*poder popular*) 37n
  polio vaccination 23
  politics of health 34–7
  polyclinic 24
  public health system 22–33
    community health workers' minimal responsibility 27–8
    cost-effectiveness 32–3